Emotions in Social Life

The development of a sociology of emotions is crucial to our understanding of social life. Emotions are 'social things', they are controlled and managed in our everyday lives and transcend the divides between mind and body, nature and culture, structure and action. In this way, they hold the key to our understanding of social process and can push forward the boundaries of sociological investigation.

Throughout western social thought emotions are seen to be the very antithesis of the detached scientific mind and its quest for 'objectivity'. However, as the course of human history has testified, crucial implications stem from the separation of reason and feeling. Accordingly, emotions have a fundamental import for all pertinent sociological themes and issues, in particular, social action and social identity, gender, sexuality and intimacy, the embodiment of emotions across the life-course (from childhood to old age), health and illness, and the social organization of emotions in the workplace.

Unique and timely, *Emotions in Social Life* acts to consolidate the sociology of emotions as a legitimate and viable field of inquiry. It provides a comprehensive 'state of the art' assessment of the sociology of emotions, drawing upon work from scholars of international stature, as well as newer writers in the field. It presents new empirical research in conjunction with innovative and challenging theoretical material, and will be essential reading for students of sociology, health psychology, anthropology and gender studies.

Gillian Bendelow is a Lecturer and **Simon J. Williams** is a Research Fellow, both at the University of Warwick, Coventry.

Emotions in Social Life
Critical Themes and Contemporary Issues

Edited by Gillian Bendelow and
Simon J. Williams

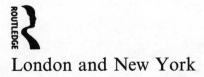

London and New York

First published 1998 by Routledge
11 New Fetter Lane, London EC4P 4EE

Simultaneously published in the USA and Canada
by Routledge
29 West 35th Street, New York, NY 10001

Typeset in Times by BC Typesetting, Bristol
Printed and bound in Great Britain by
TJ International Ltd, Padstow, Cornwall

British Library Cataloguing in Publication Data
A catalogue record for this book is available from the British Library

Library of Congress Cataloging in Publication Data
Emotions in social life: critical themes and contemporary issues/
    edited by Gillian Bendelow and Simon J. Williams
        p.   cm.
    Includes bibliographical references and index.
    1. Emotions—Sociological aspects. 2. Social psychology.
3. Social medicine. 4. Sex—Philosophy. I. Bendelow, Gillian,
1956– . II. Williams, Simon J. (Simon Johnson), 1961– .
HM291.E59 1998
302–dc21   97–11499
                                                         CIP

ISBN 0–415–13798–5 (hbk)
ISBN 0–415–13799–3 (pbk)

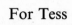
For Tess

Contents

Notes on contributors

Gillian Bendelow is a lecturer in Applied Social Studies at the University of Warwick. She worked in community psychiatry in East London before completing her doctoral thesis on the role of gender in beliefs about pain at the Social Science Research Unit. She is the convenor of the BSA study group for the Sociology of the Emotions, and current book projects include, with Simon J. Williams, *Embodying Sociology: Critical Perspectives on the Dualist Legacies* (Cambridge: Polity Press) and *Pain and Gender: A Sociocultural Analysis* (Harlow, Essex: Addison Wesley Longman).

Debora Bone is a doctoral candidate in sociology in the Department of Social and Behavioral Sciences, School of Nursing, University of California, San Francisco. She is currently finishing her dissertation on nurses' emotional labour in rationalizing health care contexts. A graduate of Ecoles des Infirmières, Le Bon Secours, Geneva, she is interested in women's health, gender and the body, qualitative methods and international health issues.

Nick Crossley lectures on the sociology and philosophy of psychiatry at the Centre for Psychotherapeutic Studies, University of Sheffield. He is the author of *The Politics of Subjectivity: Between Foucault and Merleau-Ponty* (Aldershot, Hants: Avebury, 1994) and *Intersubjectivity: The Fabric of Social Becoming* (London: Sage, 1996) and numerous papers on the sociology and philosophy of the body. He is currently working on a study of mental health movements and their activities in the public sphere.

Norman K. Denzin is Research Professor of Communications at the University of Illinois, Urbana-Champaign, and the author of *On Understanding Emotion* (San Francisco, CA: 1984). He is the editor of the *Sociological Quarterly* and co-author of *The Handbook of Qualitative Research* (London: 1994). His most recent book is *Interpretive Ethnography: Ethnographic Practices for the 21st Century* (London: 1997).

Jean Duncombe is Senior Research Officer at Essex University on an ESRC-funded project, 'The role of ideologies of love in the social construction of coupledom', and has co-authored (with Dennis Marsden) a number of published papers on love, intimacy and sex in couple relationships, and also a discussion of the methodology and ethics of researching the private sphere. She has previously been involved in research on extra-marital relationships, Alexandra Kollontai, women's work, Household Allocative Systems in couples and families, and YTS.

Simon Forrest is a Research Officer at the Centre for Health Education and Research, Canterbury Christ Church College. He has undertaken developmental research on sex relationships leading to the production of resources for young people and investigations of sexual behaviour and attitudes among youth.

Peter E. S. Freund is Professor of Sociology at Montclair University, NJ. His current interests are in theory, sociology of the body, sociology of health and illness, environmental sociology and the sociology of transportation. He is author of *The Civilized Body: Social Domination, Control and Health* (Philadelphia, PA: 1982) and, with M. McGuire, *Health, Illness and the Social Body* (New Jersey and London: 1991, 1995).

Mike Hepworth is Reader in Sociology at the University of Aberdeen. Originally a criminologist, he became interested in sociological approaches to the ageing process during the late 1970s when he began, in collaboration with Mike Featherstone, to study changing images of middle age. As a result of this work, he became increasingly interested in the social categorization of old age and the construction of distinctions between 'normal' and 'deviant' ageing. He is a member of the Association of Educational Gerontology and the British Society of Gerontology.

Arlie Russell Hochschild is Professor of Sociology at the University of California, Berkeley, and the author of the acclaimed work on emotion, *The Managed Heart: The Commercialization of Human Feeling* (Berkeley, CA: 1983). Other books include *The Second Shift* (London: 1989) and *The Time Bind* (New York: 1997).

Margot L. Lyon is an anthropologist in the Department of Archaeology and Anthropology at the Australian National University, Canberra. Her recent work has been focused primarily in the areas of critical medical anthropology and emotion. Her publications include 'Emotion as mediator of somatic and social processes: the example of respiration' in *Social Perspectives on Emotion*, Vol. II (New York: 1994), 'C. Wright Mills meets Prozac: the relevance of social emotion' in *Sociology of Health and Illness Monograph on Emotions* (Cambridge: 1996) and, with J. Barbalet, 'Society's body: emotion and the "somatization" of social theory' in *Embodiment and Experience: The Existential Ground of Culture and Self* (Cambridge: 1994).

Dennis Marsden is Professor of Sociology at the University of Essex. In addition to works co-authored with Jean Duncombe, he has published *Mothers Alone* (London: 1969), *Workless* (London: 1975) and, with David Lee, *Scheming for Youth* (Milton Keynes, Bucks: 1990). Other research areas include family violence, the social costs of community care, and step-families.

Berry Mayall is Assistant Director of the Social Science Research Unit, Institute of Education, University of London, and has carried out many research studies of children's daily lives. With Alan Prout, she has co-ordinated the ESRC seminar series on the Sociology of Childhood and her publications include *Children, Health and the Social Order* (Buckingham, Bucks: 1996), *Negotiating Health: Children at Home and at Primary School* (London: 1994) and an edited volume, *Children's Childhoods: Observed and Experienced* (London: 1994).

Liz Meerabeau has recently become Head of the School of Health at the University of Greenwich, having spent four years as a research manager at the Department of Health, and twelve years in various posts in nursing education. Her doctoral research was on the experience of fertility treatment. Apart from the sociology of emotions, her other main area of interest is professional knowledge and practice.

Tim Newton is a Senior Lecturer in Organization Studies at the University of Edinburgh. He is presently engaged in research related to debates surrounding subjectivity and the self; postmodernism; the management of knowledge; organizations and the natural environment. Recent publications include a book, with Jocelyn Handy and Stephen Fineman, examining Foucauldian, Eliasian and labour process perspectives on the psychological stress discourse: *'Managing' Stress: Emotion and Power at Work* (London: Sage, 1995).

Virginia Olesen is Professor Emerita of Sociology in the Department of Social and Behavioral Sciences, School of Nursing, University of California, San Francisco. Her publications include, with Sheryl Ruzek and Adele Clarke, *Women's Health: Complexities and Differences* (Ohio: Ohio State University Press, 1997) and her research interests include scepticism in analysis, and the place of evocative transformations in health care contexts.

Susie Page is a Senior Lecturer in Research Studies at Thames Valley University. After qualifying as a nurse, she gained considerable experience caring for high-dependency patients both in the UK and overseas. She is particularly interested in the sociology of 'high drama, high technology' scenarios, and plans to research the management of sudden death for her doctorate.

Shirley Prendergast is Senior Research Fellow in the Department of Sociology at Anglia Polytechnic University, Cambridge. She has researched and written in the area of young people, gender and schooling and is currently developing work on gender groups in the classroom.

Victor Jeleniewski Seidler is Professor of Social Theory in the Department of Sociology, Goldsmiths' College, University of London. His recent work includes *The Moral Limits of Modernity: Love, Inequality and Oppression* (London: Macmillan, 1991), *Unreasonable Men: Masculinity and Social Theory* (London: Routledge, 1994) and *Recovering the Self: Morality and Social Theory* (London: Routledge, 1995).

Keith Tester is Professor of Social Theory at the University of Portsmouth. He is the author of a number of books, including *Civil Society* (London: Routledge, 1993) and *The Inhuman Condition* (London: Routledge, 1995). He has also edited a volume on *The Flâneur* (London: Routledge, 1994).

Simon J. Williams is a Warwick Research Fellow in the Department of Sociology, and co-director of the Centre for Research in Health, Medicine and Society, University of Warwick. He has published extensively in the field of medical sociology and, more recently, on the problem of embodiment in social theory, particularly pain and emotions. Current book projects include, with Gillian Bendelow, 'Embodying sociology: critical perspectives on the dualist legacies' (Cambridge: Polity Press), a single-authored text 'Emotions and social theory' (London: Sage) and a co-edited volume 'Theorising medicine, health and society' (London: Sage).

Cas Wouters is a researcher at the Faculty of Social Sciences, Utrecht University, and is involved in research on informalization and the civilizing of emotions in the Netherlands, Germany, the UK and the USA. As well as numerous articles in Dutch, English and German, on dominant codes of behaviour regulating the relationships between the dying and those who live on, he has published *Van Minnen en Sterven* (On Loving and Dying) (Amsterdam: 1990, 1995) and, with Bram von Stolk, *Vrouwen in Tweesrtijd* (Women Torn Two Ways)/*Frauen im Zwiespalt* (Amsterdam: 1983, 1985, 1987).

Acknowledgements

This book is an important 'stepping stone' in the establishment of emotions as a viable area of sociological study, building as it does on the legacies of the BSA study group for the Sociology of the Emotions, established by Veronica James in 1989, and convened by me since 1992. It also reflects the diverse international links and growing network of researchers whose common aim has been to put emotions 'on the map', especially my colleagues at the Social Science Research Unit and the organizers of the Theory, Culture and Society conferences. However, certain individuals deserve particular recognition for their encouragement and support, namely Ann Oakley, Arlie Hochschild, Berry Mayall, Priscilla Alderson and Colin Samson. Last, but not least, I would like to thank my co-editor, Simon J. Williams, for his support and determination to see this project through and his unwavering dedication to the theoretical and sociological development of emotions in this book, and beyond.

Gillian Bendelow

Introduction: emotions in social life
Mapping the sociological terrain

Simon J. Williams and Gillian Bendelow

Despite their obvious importance to a range of issues within the social sciences, emotions, like the body to which they are so closely tied, have tended to enjoy a rather 'ethereal' existence within sociology, lurking in the shadows or banished to the margins of sociological thought and practice. Certainly, it is possible to point towards implicit if not explicit emotional themes in classical sociological writing. Marx's emotions, for example, were grounded in the social, historical and material conditions of existence; conditions which led to feelings of alienation and estrangement, from our species being under the capitalist mode of production. Durkheim, in contrast, in keeping with his claim that social facts are 'things in themselves', chose to emphasize the collective, moral nature of human feelings and sentiments, solidified into rituals, both sacred and profane. To this we may also add Weber's deliberations on processes of western rationalization, asceticism and the emotional significance of the charismatic leader, together with Simmel's analysis of the senses and the sociological significance of embodied gesture. None the less, in conjunction with the recent upsurge of interest in the body and society (Turner 1996; Grosz 1994), it is really only within the last decade or so that a distinct 'corpus' of work, mostly American in origin, has begun to emerge in the sociology of emotions.[1]

The roots of this neglect lie deeply buried in western thought: a tradition which has sought to divorce body from mind, nature from culture, reason from emotion, and public from private. As such, emotions have tended to be dismissed as private, 'irrational', inner sensations, which have been tied, historically, to women's 'dangerous desires' and 'hysterical bodies'. Here, the dominant view, dating as far back as Plato, seems to have been that emotions need to be 'tamed', 'harnessed' or 'driven out' by the steady (male) hand of reason. Seen in these terms male rationality becomes wholly 'unreasonable' (Seidler 1994 and this volume; Rose 1994; Bordo and Jaggar 1989). Historically, we should have learnt the important lessons which stem from the 'irrational passion for dispassionate rationality' (Rieff 1979): an ideology devoid of feeling, empathy and compassion for the plight of one's fellow human beings (Bauman 1989; Lynch 1985).

Even to the present day, emotions are seen to be the very antithesis of the detached scientific mind and its quest for 'objectivity', 'truth' and 'wisdom'. Reason rather than emotions is regarded as the 'indispensable faculty' for the acquisition of human knowledge. Such a view neglects the fact that rational methods of scientific inquiry, even at their most positivistic, involve the incorporation of values and emotions. Rather than repressing emotions in western epistemology, therefore, it is necessary fundamentally to rethink the relation between knowledge and emotion and to construct conceptual models that 'demonstrate the mutually constitutive rather than oppositional relation between reason and emotion' (Jaggar 1989: 157). This critical attack on the Cartesian rationalist project, in turn, keys into recent postmodernist/poststructuralist perspectives that have sought to (re)open debates on the relationship between desire and reason, and to celebrate the corporeal intimacies and affective dimensions of social life.

As this suggests, emotions lie at the juncture of a number of fundamental dualisms in western thought such as mind/body, nature/culture, public/private. A major strength of the study of emotions lies, therefore, in its ability to transcend many of these former dichotomous ways of thinking, which serve to limit social thought and scientific investigation in unnecessary, self-perpetuating ways. All the contributors to Kemper's (1990a) volume, for instance, can be seen as actively engaging with or contesting divisions within sociology such as micro versus macro, quantitative versus qualitative, positivism versus naturalism, managing versus accounting for emotions, prediction versus description and, of course, the biological versus the social.

Whilst debates continue to rage as to *what*, precisely, emotions are and *how* they should be studied (Craib 1995; Williams and Bendelow 1996a) – a situation in which the sociology of emotions, with its proliferation of perspectives and research agendas, becomes a 'victim' of its own success (Wouters 1992: 248) – a potentially fruitful way out of these dilemmas is to view emotions as existentially *embodied* modes of being which involve an *active* engagement with the world and an intimate connection with both culture and self (Csordas 1994; Denzin 1984). From this viewpoint – one which is not merely *about* bodies but *from* bodies – embodiment is reducible neither to representations of the body, to the body as an objectification of power, to the body as physiological entity, nor to the body as the inalienable centre of human consciousness (Csordas 1994). Rather, as an 'uncontainable' term in any one domain or discourse (Grosz 1994), embodiment instead lies ambiguously across the nature/culture dualism, providing the existential basis of identity, culture and social life (Csordas 1994).

The interactive, relational character of emotional experience – what Wentworth and Ryan (1990) refer to as the 'deep sociality' of emotions – in turn offers us a way of moving beyond microanalytic, subjective, individualistic levels of analysis, towards more 'open-ended' forms of social inquiry in which embodied agency can be understood not merely as 'meaning-making', but also as 'institution-making' (Csordas 1994; Lyon and Barbalet 1994). In short, the emphasis here is on the active, emotionally expressive body, as the basis of self, sociality, meaning and order, located within the broader sociocultural realms of everyday life and the ritualized forms of interaction and exchange they involve. Seen in these terms, emotions provide the 'missing link' between 'personal troubles' and broader 'public issues' of social structure; itself the defining hallmark of the 'sociological imagination' (Mills 1959). Indeed, from this perspective, social structure, to paraphrase Giddens (1984), may profitably be seen as both the medium and the outcome of the *emotionally embodied practices* and *body techniques* it recursively organizes.[2]

It is within this exciting and challenging context, one in which previously ossified conceptual forms are seen as increasingly problematic, that the rationale for the present book emerges, the central aim of which is to present, within the scope of a single volume, a 'state of the art' assessment of current theoretical and empirical work from leading scholars within the sociology of emotions. This overarching aim, in turn, involves:

1 an epistemological challenge to the dominance of western rationality and an ontological commitment to alternative ways of being and knowing;
2 a critical exploration of the link that emotions provide between a number of traditional divisions and debates within the social sciences such as the biological versus the social, micro versus macro, public versus private, quantitative versus qualitative: divisions which have dogged sociology since its inception;
3 a substantive commitment to demonstrating the centrality of emotions to a range of key developments in contemporary social life, including the 'somatization' of society, the salience of health, the advent of cyberspace, the transformation of intimacy, together with changing styles of work and social organization in late twentieth-century capitalist society.

It is with these particular aims in mind that the organizing themes for the volume as a whole have been chosen; spanning as they do, a broad range of current theory and practice, both abstract and empirical, within the sociology of emotions.

1 CRITICAL PERSPECTIVES ON EMOTIONS

In the first part, readers are introduced to a number of differing theoretical perspectives on emotions in social life. Central issues here concern the relationship between biological and social explanations, and the importance of emotions for a more embodied approach to social agency and social (inter)-action. Certainly the role of the biological in social explanation has been an important topic of debate in the sociology of emotions. In this respect,

whilst few sociologists would deny the biological underpinnings of emotions, the key question concerns just *how* important this is (Kemper 1990a).

Taking a broadly 'interactionist' approach, one that sits in the analytical
space between 'organismic' (i.e. biological) and 'social constructionist' (i.e.
cultural) accounts,[3] Arlie Hochschild, in Chapter 1, argues that whilst a
sociological approach to emotions involves 'going beyond' the biological
to the social, cultural and ideological realms, this does not mean ignoring
or leaving out the physiological substrate altogether. In taking this position,
Hochschild revisits her earlier work on 'emotion management', using love as
an example. In doing so, she returns to central concepts such as 'feeling
rules', 'status shields', 'deep' and 'surface' acting; issues which have profoundly influenced the nature and development of the sociology of emotions
over the last two decades. It is on this basis that Hochschild is able to
fashion her sociological approach to emotions as a new 'way of seeing'
the world and our gendered modes of emotionally embodied being within it.

The relationship between emotions and social agency is also addressed in
the next chapter, by Nick Crossley, on the relevance of emotions for a
reconstructed Habermasian project of communicative action. As Crossley
argues, although Habermas has been influential in the current move
towards intersubjective approaches to social action, he can none the less
be criticized for failing to give adequate attention to the affective dimensions of communicative rational action. In this respect, drawing upon
existentialist-phenomenological approaches (i.e. Sartre and Merleau-
Ponty) to emotions as embodied, purposive, meaningful responses to situations, Crossley argues that Habermas's approach can usefully absorb and be
strengthened by an account of emotional life. Emotional life, in other words,
as an existentially embodied mode of being-in-the-world, can and should be
seen as interwoven with the fabric of communicative rational action and the
constitution of the social world.

The embodied nature of emotions as the active basis of social agency
and social life is also taken up and explicitly addressed by Margot Lyon in
Chapter 3 in her critique of the 'limits' of cultural constructionism. As she
argues, an expanded relational understanding of emotion and its social
and biological ontology is required in order to move beyond the limitations
of cultural constructionism. What is subject to social relations is not simply,
as cultural constructionists claim, the cognitive faculties, but living human
bodies. Society, in other words, ultimately consists of bodies in social
relations of motion and rest, animation and action. We must therefore,
as Lyon suggests, overcome our fear of biology, and seek to re-embody
sociology.

In the final chapter in this part, Tim Newton takes up these emotional
issues across the long historical curve of the civilizing process. As we have
argued elsewhere (Williams and Bendelow 1996a, 1996b), a particular
strength of Elias's approach to emotions and the 'civilized body' lies in
the manner in which, in considering the emotions, he is able to interlock

biological and social in a dynamic sociological way; one in which, through an evolutionary process of 'symbol emancipation', the balance has tilted ever more heavily in favour of learned versus unlearned forms of human behaviour and emotional expression. In taking these issues forward, Newton not only provides us with a detailed historical analysis of changes in emotion codes from the seventeenth- to nineteenth-century bourgeois society, he also critically re-examines, in the light of this Eliasian analysis, Hochschild's work on emotional labour. These insights, in turn, have implications for our understanding of twentieth-century social life; in particular, the theorization of gender, the public/private division and the development of emotion codes in the workplace.[4]

Taken together, these four chapters, in their differing ways, illustrate the lively nature of theoretical debate within the sociology of emotions, and the relevance of these issues for more general debates within mainstream sociological theory. The time for emotions, in short, has arrived.

2 THE 'MEDIATION' OF EMOTIONAL EXPERIENCE

Moving to our second major theme, a striking feature of contemporary western society concerns the exponential growth of information systems and communications technology. From radio, newspapers, television and film, to computer technology and the recent advent of so-called 'cyberspace', we live in an increasingly 'mediated' age; one which carries potentially important implications for traditional notions of (gendered) embodiment and self-identity (Featherstone and Burrows 1995; Stone 1991; Springer 1991). This, in turn, gives rise to a number of important questions regarding the 'fate' of human emotions at the turn of the century. Will this, for instance, lead to an intensification or a diminution of emotional experience, are new modes of emotional trust, intimacy and sharing beginning to open up in the (erotic ontology) of cyberspace (Heim 1991), and if so, what light does all this shed on existing categories and concepts within the sociology of emotions?

Clearly, definitive answers to these questions are well beyond the scope of a single volume such as this; for many, only time will tell. The three chapters contained in this second section of the book do, none the less, provide some provisional clues and tentative answers to these questions.

In Chapter 5, Keith Tester develops a general account of the emotional responses of television consumers to the images of war and violence they see daily on their screens. We are, Tester argues, the children of a tradition of the television, and that tradition is one which articulates the blasé and reserved attitudes emphasized by Simmel. These attitudes, he suggests, are defining of the emotional responses of individuals to all that we can know and see thanks to television.

If Tester comes down on the side of a blunting or diminution of emotional response in a digitally 'mediated' age, then Norman Denzin, in the next chapter, offers a very different view of the role of information technology (IT) through an exploration of the gendered, emotional talk and 'narratives of self' that are posted in an on-line Internet newsgroup called 'alt. recovery.codependency'. As Denzin argues, the advent of cyberspace has created a site for the production of new emotional self-stories, stories that might not be told elsewhere. These narratives, he suggests, are grounded in the everyday lives and experiences of the women who write them, yet they circulate in the anonymous, privatized territories of cyberspace. The gendered talk that occurs in this newsgroup does not connect to an oral tradition of group story-telling; there are no canonical texts that are referenced. Rather, their talk is personal and emotional, filled with evocative symbols connected to mothers, families, holidays and children. They are talking about things the men in their lives will not listen to, using this information technology to create new identities and lives for themselves whilst men still debate the rules of discourse. In this sense, the implications of cyberspace are truly revolutionary in their consequences for emotional democracy. Yet as Denzin also warns, these virtual reality (VR) relationships frequently tilt in the direction of men telling women what to do and how to feel. In this way, virtual reality reproduces the real world (RW) as gendered modes of being are upheld rather than unravelled.

These issues are further explored in Chapter 7 by Simon Williams, who offers a timely critical appraisal of the constraints as well as opportunities that cyberspace affords for contemporary forms of emotionally embodied experience. As he argues, the tensions between representation and reality, emotional involvement and detachment, together with the associated problems of high-tech dualism in cyberspace, suggest a number of dilemmas for the (post)modern individual: issues which defy easy answers or simple solutions. Moreover, the advent of cyberspace may also necessitate a fundamental rethinking of existing concepts within the sociology of emotions, including the 'self', the 'expressive' body, 'emotion work', 'feeling rules', 'deep' and 'surface' acting. In raising these issues, Williams's intention is not to play down or neglect the emotional opportunities which the advent of cyberspace affords, but to challenge some of the over-inflated claims and disembodied visions which it spawns. Only on the basis of our carnal bonds in the real world, he suggests, can a truly human ethics of trust, emotional intimacy and responsibility emerge; one grounded in a shared sense of bodily contingency, limitation and constraint.

3 EMOTIONS AND THE BODY THROUGH THE LIFE-COURSE

Building on some of these earlier themes, Part III seeks to extend and develop sociological approaches to emotions across the biographically embodied life-course. A central issue here concerns whether or not emotions, like the body, undergo some form of distinctive transformation over time, and if so, to what should we attribute these changes: biology, culture or both? The study of emotional continuity and change over the life-course, in other words, serves as an important 'test case' for a purely 'constructionist' approach; one which is forced to confront the physical as well as cognitive aspects of growing up and ageing, and the feelings associated with these distinct bodily states and physiological changes. More generally, it also enables us to question, again, dominant notions of western rationality; modes of thought which have sought to exclude children and the elderly, like women past and present, from the public world of (male) reason.

In Chapter 8, Berry Mayall makes a preliminary exploration of these issues through a focus on the neglected topic of children's bodies and emotional lives. In doing so, she highlights some crucial ways of incorporating children and childhood into sociological discussions on the importance of emotions in social life. As Mayall shows, children take their embodied selves daily across the private/public divide and in so doing encounter a range of adult-determined social structures. Key issues here include the 'civilizing', 'regulation' and 'construction' of children's bodies and minds, both at home and at school, together with the tensions between children's time and adults' time. Rather than being the passive recipients of these processes, children are in fact active participants in the construction of their bodies and minds. The quality of children's emotional and embodied living therefore depends, Mayall argues, on how far adults accept and value their personhood and contributions to the social order; a message as applicable to existing adult-centred approaches and perspectives within sociology as it is to society in general.

These issues are further explored in the next chapter, by Shirley Prendergast and Simon Forrest. Drawing upon empirical research carried out in secondary schools, they examine 'emotion work' in adolescent boys. Compared with girls, boys speak 'hard', act 'hard' and ultimately, perhaps to their detriment, learn to be 'hard'. In this respect, as Prendergast and Forrest suggest, definitions of (male) dominance and hierarchy based on embodied attitudes can be seen to play a significant role in the gendered construction of emotions. In particular, embodied metaphors of size, height and 'hardness', themselves indicative of male superiority, together with the enacted rituals of peer group behaviours and transitions, create a paradigm of 'proper' masculine selfhood that sharply proscribes emotional expression. Seen in these terms, hegemonic forms of masculinity are not only ritually embodied in adulthood, but enacted at an early stage in the life-course through stereotypical forms of gendered emotional behaviour.

Moving to the opposite end of the life-course, Mike Hepworth, in Chapter 10, takes up the controversial issue of ageing and emotion through a moving and sensitive analysis of the social construction of emotions in old age, set against the backdrop of historically changing conceptions of the life-course in western culture. For several centuries 'growing old' has been framed within a model of the 'ages', and more recently 'stages' of life, of (wo)man, which, in addition to defining age- and gender-related dress, comportment and conduct, is also emotionally prescriptive. Each 'age' or 'stage' of life incorporates definitions of desirable or 'normal' states of feeling. Yet, as Hepworth shows, beneath the surface of these public images and vocabularies of the life-course, there is evidence of a complex cultural and subjective imagery indicating a considerable degree of struggle, contest and conflict. In taking this position, Hepworth pays particular attention to the role of gender in the tension between public emotional prescriptions and private emotional expressions of later life, and their broader implications for the sociology of emotions.

Taken together, these chapters point to the culturally pre/proscriptive nature of western emotional styles over the biographically embodied life-course and the gendered forms of transition, struggle and resistance they involve across the public/private divide.

4 SEXUALITY, INTIMACY AND PERSONAL RELATIONSHIPS

An implicit, if not explicit, theme in many of the chapters considered so far has, of course, been the issue of gender. Certainly, exploration of the relationship between gender, emotions and the body opens up a vast array of important issues, spanning everything from feminist critiques of western being and knowing (mentioned above) and the newly emerging field of men and masculinities (Connell 1995; Hearn and Morgan 1990; Morgan 1992, 1993; Jeffords 1989, 1994; Kimmel 1987), to the gender division of emotional labour (Hochschild 1989b), domestic violence (Hearn and Morgan 1990), prostitution (Scambler and Scambler 1997), homosexuality (Plummer 1992) and the recent emergence of 'queer' theory (Burston and Richardson 1995).

The critique of (male) rationality is explicitly addressed by Seidler in Chapter 11. As he argues, masculinity and femininity are inevitably emotionally opposed in western society by the structuring of social theory into reason and nature. The Cartesian legacy renders sexuality 'animal', needing taming, regulation and control. Subsequently, dominant masculinist thought encourages the notion that nature is inherently flawed, intimacy becomes unworkable and men regard themselves as unlovable, whereas women, who are unable to be dissociated from those processes, become subject to male control. In exploring these issues, Seidler claims that a major influence in this development has been the impact of Weber's Protestant work ethic, with the subsequent moral culture of the rejection of the body and emotional life, and that other cultures (although still open to accusations of patriarchy) may offer different perspectives on carnality and sexuality. Inevitably, he argues, what is needed is a more unified 'feminine' concept of reason which accepts emotions and sexuality as having an important role in the acquisition of knowledge. In this respect he echoes the views of certain poststructuralist feminist thinkers such as Cixous and Irigaray who have sought to 'rewrite' western (masculine) thought through a more pluralized metaphysics of female desire, fluidity and flow.

Another important theme in current writing around gender, sexuality and the emotions concerns the issue of love and the transformation of intimacy in late modernity. Jackson (1993), for example, has recently focused on the cultural meanings of love as a neglected issue within sociological discourse, arguing for an approach to the emotion itself as just as much cultural as the conventions which surround it. Certainly it is clear, as a variety of commentators have suggested, that a profound transformation in the spheres of sexuality and interpersonal intimacy is currently taking place in late twentieth-century western society (Cancian 1987). Today, for the first time, women claim equality with men in a reflexive age where sexuality – freed from the rule of the phallus and the constraints of reproduction – becomes 'plastic' and 'pluralized' (Giddens 1992) and love becomes a 'blank' which couples must 'fill in' themselves (Beck and Beck-Gernsheim 1995). Increasingly, individuals who wish to live together are becoming the 'legislators of their own way of life', the 'judges of their own transgressions', the 'priests who absolve their own sins' and the 'therapists who loosen the bonds of their own past' (Beck and Beck-Gernsheim 1995: 5).

As critics have pointed out, the problem with this type of analysis is that, although suggestive, it tends to paint these transformations in broad brushstrokes with little attention to empirical detail. In this respect, not only is Giddens's 'pure relationship' best seen as an 'ideological ideal' of late modernity (Craib 1995), but recognition of the impact of differential power on actual relationships seriously undermines many of its 'core' features (Hey *et al.* 1993–4).

These issues are explicitly addressed in Chapter 12 by Jean Duncombe and Dennis Marsden. As they argue, the exploration of socially regulated or 'managed' gender divisions in intimate emotional behaviour entails two interrelated, yet distinct, questions: are men and women equally 'susceptible' to emotions or discourse of love and intimacy; and, do they handle such emotions in similar ways in the context of these close personal relationships? Using evidence from a variety of recent research, they begin by trying to find empirical examples of the kinds of emotion work that women and men do in heterosexual couple relationships. This evidence indeed *appears* to conform to gender stereotypes of 'Stepford wives' and 'hollow men'. However, as Duncombe and Marsden argue, this is partly a product of the conceptual and methodological problems involved in researching men's and women's performance of emotion work. In raising these issues, they then proceed to use recent theories of gender pluralism and 'doing gender' in order to discuss Hochschild's work and psychodynamic theory, which suggests that doing emotion work may lead to a loss of 'authenticity'. Finally, drawing upon their own research on couples, they show how attempts by individual men and women to preserve their sense of authenticity may vary, depending on what the authors term their 'core identities'. In doing so, they attempt to clarify some of the 'conceptual confusion' that surrounds the term 'emotion work'; a concept, they suggest, which has been adopted, adapted or criticized to such an extent that it is in danger of becoming a 'catch-all cliché'.

Finally, in an Eliasian vein, the 'emancipation of sexuality' and the transformation of intimacy are considered by Cas Wouters in Chapter 13. Focusing on the period from the 'sexual revolution' of the 1960s onwards, Wouters approaches these issues from the perspective of the 'lust balance', a concept inspired by Elias, which explores the tension that may arise between the longing for love and enduring intimacy, and the longing for sex. Using empirical evidence from the Netherlands, the chapter argues that since the sexual revolution, more and more men and women have been experimenting with the 'balance' in between the extremes of desexualized love (i.e. a relationship in which most or even all sexual longing has been subordinated to the continuation of the relationship), and depersonalized sexual contact (i.e. the idea of sex for the sake of sex). As the notion of erotic and sexual awareness increases both through increased (pleasurable) sexual contact, or through a more equal balance of power between the sexes and by mutual consent, both types of longings, Wouters suggests, intensify and feelings become tense and ambivalent.

In their different ways, each of the chapters in this part of the book underscores the point raised earlier about the extent to which notions of the pure relationship and emotional democracy remain ideological ideals in an era where traditional masculinist concepts of (un)reason, stereotypical gender divisions of emotional labour and tensions in the 'lust balance' between love and sex are still very much alive and kicking.

5 EMOTIONS AND HEALTH

Finally, in the last section of the volume we return to many previous themes and issues within the volume through an explicit focus on health. As we have argued elsewhere (Williams and Bendelow 1996b), the sociology of health and illness is a particularly fertile terrain upon which to explore the role of emotions, raising as it does deep ontological questions concerning the nature of embodiment as both nature and culture and the symbolic transformation of suffering into meaningful human experience (Scheper-Hughes and Lock 1987; Kleinman 1988).

These issues are clearly illustrated in Chapter 14 through a sociological focus on pain, emotions and gender. Drawing upon our own research in this area, we show how people's experiences of pain, far from being 'unscientific', are complex, subtle and sophisticated, incorporating not only physical and sensory components, but also feelings and vulnerabilities of an existential, moral or religious kind. Despite the widespread endorsement of emotional pain, significant gender differences were none the less evident in terms of the importance attached to emotions and in social expectations of men's and women's ability to 'cope' with pain. Here, as we show, the attribution by both sexes of women's superior capacity to cope with pain was not only linked in our respondents' minds to their biological and reproductive functioning, but also underpinned by a constellation of cultural assumptions about gendered roles and patterns of socialization, particularly in relation to 'emotion work'. Using a sociological perspective on emotions in this way, we suggest, helps transcend false mind/body dualism, thus facilitating an understanding of pain as an everyday emotional, as well as a 'medicalized', phenomenon, which, in turn, is crucially linked to gender, culture and embodiment.

Taking these arguments further, Peter Freund, in the next chapter, examines the interrelationship between social status, control, emotion work and bodily states, including those that may contribute to illness. In doing so, Freund advances what he refers to as a 'geography' of emotions and emotional relationships across social-physical and psycho-somatic space. The concept of 'dramaturgical stress' provides a tool, he suggests, for analysing the intermingling of bodies, emotions and social interaction, whilst emotional labour may be regarded as a 'stressor'. In particular, there are two main features of the sociocultural situation in which such dramaturgical stress takes place, namely the form of social control that prevails and the relative social positions of the actors involved. It therefore follows that those in subordinate positions (e.g. women and minority groups, workers in lower-class service occupations, etc.) are likely to be particularly vulnerable. Under such conditions, neuromuscular, hormonal and respiratory activity produced in response to dramaturgical stress may have an impact on health. Altered physiological reactivity may also influence moods and emotional states. Hence social performances and their 'discontents', and the capacity to cope with these, can, Freund suggests, contribute to illness.

Taking this critical exploration of the micro–macro divide further, the last two chapters in this volume build on previous studies of emotions in the workplace (Fineman 1993; James 1992, 1989; Smith 1992; Lawler 1991) through a focus on gender and the changing institutional dynamics of health care. The dramatic nature of such emotion work is perfectly illustrated in Chapter 16 by Susie Page and Liz Meerabeau in their analysis of nurses' (*post-facto*) accounts of cardiopulmonary resuscitation (CPR). As they show, preparation of nursing and medical personnel for such an event is fraught with difficulty, not least because the reality of the event frequently bears little resemblance to how it is presented in a training situation. In doing so, Page and Meerabeau insightfully link issues of emotion management to the medicalization of death and its subsequent amenability to human manipulation. As they argue, this manipulation is also true of the emotions engendered for those involved in 'body work', with its 'clean' and 'dirty' associations mediated by ritual. From this perspective, CPR is perhaps best seen as a symbolic event which often involves a loss of dignity for both parties, and an outcome which is all too frequently dichotomized into good/bad, desirable/undesirable or success/failure.

Finally, the last chapter by Virginia Olesen and Debora Bone moves the sociological analysis and understanding of emotions to considerations of processual and structural issues, located in the context of a discussion of US health care settings and organizations. These, they argue, represent prime cases of substantial ongoing change, especially increasing rationalization, in contexts where emotions are significantly embedded in the work, thus generating a theoretically intriguing tension between demands for affective neutrality and desires for particularity. Transitions in these health care systems bring forth new structures where expectations, deeply ingrained in professional care-givers and related to important emotional and social issues, are no longer appropriate and new emotional responses have not yet been sufficiently developed or are fragmented. In opening up these questions of emotions in cultural, social and economic change, a topic thus far little explored in the growing literature on emotions, Olesen and Bone therefore move the analysis of emotions from 'point in time' issues to a more dynamic view. In doing so, they draw on previously developed concepts and positions such as emotional labour, feeling rules, the sentimental order, and the relationship of structure to emotions and evocative transformations, concluding with an agenda for future research utilizing comparisons of other settings such as business and industry.

All in all, the chapters contained in this volume suggest an exciting future for the sociology of emotions, keying as it does into a number of important issues and debates within mainstream sociology, including the recent upsurge of interest in the body and society, and the critique of western rationality. In particular, as we have argued, one of the most important features of this newly emerging field of inquiry lies in the manner in which it is able to transcend many of the sterile divides and dualistic legacies of the past through a truly embodied form of sociology. Despite this promising start, much still remains to be done, particularly if we are to move from the current proliferation of competing perspectives and alternative research agendas, towards a more integrated phase of sociological theorizing on emotions in social life. Whilst this suggests constraints as well as opportunities, it none the less points to the fact that a sociology of emotions, alongside the body, could potentially become the 'leading edge' of contemporary social theory. Whatever the outcome, one thing remains clear: emotions, at the dawn of the twenty-first century, have truly come of age.

NOTES

1 Kemper, for example, traces the beginnings of American sociological interest in emotions back to the 'watershed year' of 1975, arguing that, by the brink of the 1980s, the sociology of emotions was truly 'poised for developmental take-off' (1990b: 4). Landmark texts here include Hochschild's *The Managed Heart* (1983) and, more recently, *The Second Shift* (1989b); Denzin's (1984) *On Understanding Emotion*; together with a variety of edited collections including Franks and McCarthy's (1989) *The Sociology of Emotions*, Kemper's (1990) *Research*

Agendas in the Sociology of Emotions, and two recent British texts, Fineman's (1993) *Emotions in Organisations* and James and Gabe's (1996) *Health and the Sociology of Emotions*. To this, we may also add other, populist texts, such as Goleman's (1996) recent number one best-seller: *Emotional Intelligence: How It Can Matter More Than IQ*.

2 For critical explorations of the role of emotions in micro–macro linkages see Collins (1981, 1990), Kemper (1990a), Gordon (1990).

3 Classic examples of 'organismic' approaches can be found in the work of Darwin (1955 [1873]), Freud (1923), James and Lange (1922) and Ekman (1982, 1984). In contrast, social constructionists, as the name implies, view emotions as capable of considerable historical and cultural variation: see, for example, Harré (1986, 1991), Stearns (1994), Stearns and Stearns (1988), Lutz (1989) and Rosaldo (1984).

4 For another lively and interesting debate, from an Eliasian perspective, on the historical merits of Hochschild's emotion management approach, see Wouters (1989a, 1989b) and Hochschild (1989a).

BIBLIOGRAPHY

Bauman, Z. (1989) *Modernity and the Holocaust*. Cambridge: Polity Press.

Beck, U. and Beck-Gernsheim, E. (1995) *The Normal Chaos of Love*. Cambridge: Polity Press.

Bordo, S. (1986) 'The masculinisation of Cartesian thought', *Signs* 11(3): 433–57.

Bordo, S. and Jaggar, A. (eds) (1989) *Gender/Body/Knowledge: Feminist Reconstructions of Being and Knowing*. New Brunswick, NJ, and London: Rutgers University Press.

Burston, P. and Richardson, C. (eds) (1995) *A Queer Romance: Lesbians, Gay Men and Popular Culture*. London: Routledge.

Cancian, F. (1987) *Love in America: Gender and Self-Development*. Cambridge: Cambridge University Press.

Collins, R. (1981) 'On the micro-foundations of macro-sociology', *American Journal of Sociology* 86: 984–1014.

Collins, R. (1990) 'Stratification, emotional energy, and the transient emotions', in T. D. Kemper (ed.) *Research Agendas in the Sociology of Emotions*. New York: State University of New York Press.

Connell, R. (1995) *Masculinities*. Cambridge: Polity Press.

Craib, I. (1995) 'Some comments on the sociology of the emotions', *Sociology* 29: 151–8.

Csordas, T. J. (ed.) (1994) *Embodiment and Experience: The Existential Ground of Culture and Self*. Cambridge: Cambridge University Press.

Darwin, C. (1955 [1873]) *The Expression of the Emotions in Man and Animals*. New York: Philosophical Library.

Denzin, N. K. (1984) *On Understanding Emotion*. San Francisco: Jossey-Bass.

Ekman, P. (ed.) (1982) *Emotion in the Human Face*. Cambridge and New York: Cambridge University Press.

Ekman, P. (1984) *Approaches to Emotion*. Hillsdale, NJ: Lawrence Erlbaum.

Elias, N. (1991a) 'On human beings and their emotions: a process-sociological essay', in M. Featherstone, M. Hepworth and B. Turner (eds) *The Body: Social Process and Cultural Theory*. London: Sage.

Elias, N. (1991b) *Symbol Theory*. London: Sage.

Featherstone, M. and Burrows, R. (eds) (1995) *Cyberspace/Cyberbodies/Cyberpunk*. London: Sage.

Fineman, S. (ed.) (1993) *Emotions in Organisations*. London: Sage.

Franks, D. and Doyle McCarthy, E. (eds) (1989) *The Sociology of Emotions: Original Essays and Research Papers*. Greenwich, CT: JAI Press.

Freud, S. (1923) *The Ego and the Id*. London: Hogarth Press and the Institute of Psycho-Analysis.

Gerth, H. and Mills, C. Wright (1964) *Character and Social Structure: The Psychology of Social Institutions*. New York: Harcourt, Brace & World.

Giddens, A. (1984) *The Constitution of Society*. Cambridge: Polity Press.

Giddens, A. (1992) *The Transformation of Intimacy*. Cambridge: Polity Press.

Goleman, D. (1996) *Emotional Intelligence: How It Can Matter More Than IQ*. London: Bloomsbury.

Gordon, S. (1990) 'Social structural effects on emotions', in T. D. Kemper (ed.) *Research Agendas in the Sociology of Emotions*. New York: State University of New York Press.

Grosz, E. (1994) *Volatile Bodies*. Bloomington and Indianapolis, IN: Indiana University Press.

Harré, R. (ed.) (1986) *The Social Construction of Emotions*. New York: Blackwell.

Harré, R. (1991) *Physical Being: A Theory of Corporeal Psychology*. Oxford: Blackwell.

Hearn, J. and Morgan, D. H. J. (eds) (1990) *Men, Masculinity and Social Theory*. London: Unwin Hyman.

Heim, M. (1991) 'The erotic ontology of cyberspace', in M. Benedikt (ed.) *Cyberspace: The First Steps*. Cambridge, MA: MIT Press.

Hey, C., O'Brien, M. and Penna, S. (1993–4) 'Giddens, modernity and self-identity', *Arena* 2: 45–76.

Hochschild, A. (1979) 'Emotion work, feeling rules and social structure', *American Journal of Sociology* 85: 551–75.

Hochschild, A. (1983) *The Managed Heart: The Commercialization of Human Feeling*, Berkeley, CA: University of California Press.

Hochschild, A. (1989a) 'Reply to Cas Wouter's review essay on the "Managed Heart"', *Theory, Culture and Society* 6(3): 439–45.

Hochschild, A. (1989b) *The Second Shift: Working Parents and the Revolution at Home*. London: Piatkus.

Jackson, S. (1993) 'Even sociologists fall in love: an exploration of the sociology of emotions', *Sociology* 27(2): 201–20.

Jaggar, A. (1989) 'Love and knowledge: emotion in feminist epistemology', in S. Bordo and A. Jaggar (eds) *Gender/Body/Knowledge: Feminist Reconstructions of Being and Knowing*. New Brunswick, NJ, and London: Rutgers University Press.

James, N. (1989) 'Emotional labour: skill and work in the social regulation of feelings', *Sociological Review* 37(1): 15–42.

James, N. (1992) 'Care = organisation + physical labour + emotional labour', *Sociology of Health and Illness* 14(4): 488–509.

James, V. and Gabe, J. (eds) (1996) *Health and the Sociology of Emotions*. Oxford: Blackwell.

James, W. and Lange, C. (1922) *The Emotions*. Baltimore, MD: Williams & Wilkins.

Jeffords, S. (1989) *The Remasculinisation of America*. Bloomington, IN: Indiana University Press.

Jeffords, S. (1994) *Hard Bodies: Hollywood Masculinity in the Reagan Era*. New Brunswick, NJ: Rutgers University Press.

Kemper, T. D. (ed.) (1990a) *Research Agendas in the Sociology of Emotions*. New York: State University of New York Press.

Kemper, T. D. (1990b) 'Social relations and emotions: a structural approach', in T. D. Kemper (ed.) *Research Agendas in the Sociology of Emotions*. New York: State University of New York Press.

Kimmel, M. S. (ed.) (1987) *Changing Men*. London: Sage.

Kirkup, G. and Keller, L. Smith (eds) (1992) *Inventing Women: Science, Technology and Gender*. Cambridge: Polity Press.

Kleinman, A. (1988) *The Illness Narratives*. New York: Basic Books.

Lawler, J. (1991) *Behind the Screens: Nursing, Somology and the Problem of the Body*. Melbourne and Edinburgh: Churchill Livingstone.

Lutz, C. (1989) *Unnatural Emotions*. Chicago: University of Chicago Press.

Lynch, J. (1985) *The Language of the Heart: The Human Body in Dialogue*. New York: Basic Books.

Lyon, M. and Barbalet, J. (1994) 'Society's body: emotion and the "somatization" of social theory', in T. J. Csordas (ed.) *Embodiment and Experience: The Existential Ground of Culture and Self*. Cambridge: Cambridge University Press.

Mills, C. Wright (1959) *The Sociological Imagination*. New York: Oxford University Press.

Morgan, D. H. J. (1992) *Discovering Men*. London: Routledge.

Morgan, D. H. J. (1993) 'You too can have a body like mine', in S. Scott and D. H. J. Morgan (eds) *Body Matters*. London: Falmer Press.

Plato (1961) *The Collected Dialogues*, ed. E. Hamilton and C. Huntington. Princeton, NJ: Princeton University Press.

Plato (1993) *Phaedo*. Oxford: Oxford University Press.

Plummer, K. (ed.) (1992) *Modern Homosexualities: Fragments of Lesbian and Gay Experiences*. London: Routledge.

Rieff, P. (1979) *Freud: The Mind of a Moralist*. London: Chatto & Windus.

Rosaldo, M. (1984) 'Towards an anthropology of self and feeling', in R. A. Shweder and R. A. Levine (eds) *Culture Theory*. Cambridge: Cambridge University Press.

Rose, H. (1994) *Love, Power and Knowledge: Towards a Feminist Transformation of Science*. Cambridge: Polity Press.

Sartre, J. P. (1962 [1939]) *Sketch for a Theory of the Emotions*. London: Methuen.

Scambler, G. and Scambler, A. (eds) (1997) *Rethinking Prostitution: Purchasing Sex in the 1990s*. London: Routledge.

Scheff, T. J. (1990) 'Socialization of emotions: pride and shame as causal agents', in T. D. Kemper (ed.) *Research Agendas in the Sociology of Emotions*. New York: State University of New York Press.

Scheper-Hughes, N. and Lock, M. (1987) 'The mindful body: a prolegomenon to future work in medical anthropology', *Medical Anthropology Quarterly* 1(1): 6–41.

Seidler, V. (1994) *Unreasonable Men: Masculinity and Social Theory*. London: Routledge.

Smith, P. (1992) *The Emotional Division of Labour in Nursing*. Basingstoke: Macmillan Educational Books.

Springer, C. (1991) 'The pleasure of the interface', *Screen* 32(3): 303–23.

Stearns, C. Z. and Stearns, P. (1988) *Emotions and Social Change*. New York: Holmes & Meier.

Stearns, P. (1994) *American Cool: Constructing a Twentieth Century American Style*. New York: New York University Press.

Stone, A. R. (1992) 'Will the real body please stand up?', in M. Benedikt (ed.) *Cyberspace: The First Steps*. Cambridge, MA: MIT Press.

Turner, B. S. (1996) *Body and Society*, 2nd edition. London: Sage.

Wentworth, W. and Ryan, J. (1990) 'Balancing body, mind and culture: the place of emotion in social life', in D. Franks (ed.) *Social Perspectives on Emotions*. Greenwich, CT: JAI Press.

Wiley, J. (1995) 'Nobody is "doing it": cybersexuality as a postmodern narrative', *Body and Society* 1(1:) 145–62.

Williams, S. J. and Bendelow, G. (1996a) 'Emotions and "sociological imperialism":
a rejoinder to Craib', *Sociology* 30(1): 145–54.

Williams, S. J. and Bendelow, G. (1996b) 'Emotions and health: the "missing link" in
medical sociology?', in V. James and J. Gabe (eds) *Health and the Sociology of
Emotions*. Oxford: Blackwell.

Wouters, C. (1989a) 'The sociology of emotions and flight attendants: Hochschild's
"Managed Heart"', *Theory, Culture and Society* 6(1): 95–123.

Wouters, C. (1989b) 'Response to Hochschild's reply', *Theory, Culture and Society*
6(3): 447–50.

Wouters, C. (1992) 'On status competition and emotion management: the study of
emotion as a new field', *Theory, Culture and Society* 9: 229–52.

Part I

Critical perspectives on emotions

1 The sociology of emotion as a way of seeing

Arlie Russell Hochschild

INTRODUCTION

The sociology of emotion is a new, growing field within the larger discipline of sociology,[1] and part of a wider interdisciplinary renaissance in interest in emotion. All of the nineteenth-century founders of sociology touched on the topic of emotion and some did more. As the American sociologist Randall Collins has pointed out, Max Weber elucidates the anxious 'spirit of capitalism', the magnetic draw of charisma, and he questions what passes for 'rationality'. Emile Durkheim explores the social scaffolding for feelings of 'solidarity'. Karl Marx explores alienation and, in his analysis of class conflict, he implies much about resentment and anger.[2] Max Scheler explores empathy and sympathy, and Georg Simmel a rich variety of sentiments. Sigmund Freud calls attention to the primacy of conscious and unconscious emotion (what he called affect), though not to its sociological character.

In the twentieth century, Erving Goffman traces out the complex web of unconscious rules of acting that guide us through a typical day. Goffman also implies, though he draws back from positing, feeling rules, and an emotional actor capable of managing emotions in accordance with such rules. As a whole, current sociology is rich in ethnographic 'thick descriptions', which leak evidence of emotion, on one side, and in theories that imply them, on the other. But missing until recently has been a carefully developed, grounded, sociological theory of emotion. This volume gathers research that forms part of this larger project.

As with any new body of work, the sociology of emotion has generated lively debate, and been quickly subdivided by area, theoretical approach and methodology (Kemper 1989). So it is no easier to speak these days of a 'typical sociologist of emotion' than it is to speak of a 'typical' sociologist. Still, we can ask: what is it like to see the world from the point of view of the sociologist of emotion?[3] Perhaps the best way to convey this point of view is to look very closely at one small episode, and to compare different ways of seeing it. As my episode, my 'grain of sand', I have chosen one young woman's description of her wedding day in 1981, drawn from my book *The Managed Heart*. The young woman says this:

> My marriage ceremony was chaotic and completely different than I imagined it would be. Unfortunately, we rehearsed at 8 o'clock the morning of the wedding. I had imagined that everyone would know what to do, but they didn't. That made me nervous. My sister didn't help me get dressed or flatter me and no one in the dressing room helped until I asked. I was depressed. I wanted to be so happy on our wedding day. . . . This is supposed to be the happiest day of one's life. I couldn't believe that some of my best friends couldn't make it to my wedding. So as I started out to the church thinking about all these things, that I always thought would not happen at my wedding, going through my mind, I broke down and cried. But I thought to myself, 'Be happy for the friends, the relatives, the presents.' Finally, I said to myself, 'Hey, other people aren't getting married, *you* are.' From down the long aisle I saw my husband. We looked at each other's eyes. His love for me changed my whole being from that point on. When we joined arms, I was relieved. The tension was gone. From then on, it was beautiful. It was indescribable.[4]

The sociological view without emotion in focus: the function of a ritual

As Emile Durkheim (1965 [1915]) points out in *The Elementary Forms of Religious Life*, rituals create a circle within which things become extraordinary, amazing, sacred, and outside of which things seem unremarkable. The marriage ceremony makes a profane bond between bride and groom into a sacred one.

But this fretful young woman's wedding was not doing its Durkheimian job. For only when the young bride focuses on herself does the occasion seem to become fully meaningful to her. As she says, 'Finally, I said to myself, "Hey, other people aren't getting married, *you* are."' In a certain sense, the bride reverses Durkheim. She de-ceremonializes the ceremony. She has to remove herself mentally from the collective nature of the ceremony in order to feel her wedding as sacred and to feel herself transformed.

The psychoanalytic view: the bride's narcissistic expectation

What in our bride's tale might catch the psychoanalyst's eye? Dr Christa Rohde-Dachser, a commentator on an earlier version of this chapter (a paper given at the German Psychoanalytic Association in 1995), offered the following interpretation.[5]

The young bride held 'narcissistic expectations of this day'; she expected to feel central, elevated, enhanced. She was therefore disappointed when these expectations were not met. When faced with an inattentive sister, absent friends and bumbling bridesmaids, she grew anxious at having to adopt the 'female depressive solution'; namely to abandon hope of fulfilling her own needs and to focus on the more urgent needs of others. Then she experienced a moment of 'Oedipal triumph', as shown again by the phrase 'people aren't getting married, *you* are'. This is the moment, Rodhe-Dachser argues, in which the young woman leaves the sexual 'white desert' of childhood in which she watches her parents' sexual happiness from the side. Now she may enjoy her own sexual gratification. Why, Dr Rohde-Dachser also asks, does the story end when it ends, at a moment of happy union? Is this a fusion of her narcissistic expectation with her Oedipal triumph, central and united for ever, and do these form a denial of reality?

In looking at our bride in this way, the psychoanalyst relies on the idea of personality structure, itself formed in the course of early psycho-sexual development within the immediate family. This is because psychoanalysis is a body of theory about *individual human development*. Its focus is on those moments in human development when things go wrong, attachments are ruptured, traumas occur. The psychoanalyst thus often dwells upon extreme or pathological emotion, and, as a practice, focuses on healing emotional injuries. Culture enters in as the *medium* in which human development, injury and repair take place.

Like the 'regular' sociologist, the psychoanalyst might not ask how it is that a certain emotion – like anxiety, or feeling 'his love for me' – does or does not stand out from an array of expectable or appropriate feelings. Both might rely on an intuitive notion of appropriate affect, based on a prior notion of a mentally healthy response to this situation in this culture at this time. They might see feeling as a simple matter of instinct or nature, and leave it at that. They would pass over the crucial question of how cultures shape feeling.

THE SOCIOLOGY OF EMOTIONS VIEW

How would a sociologist of emotion approach the same bride? Like the psychoanalyst, the sociologist of emotion notes that the bride is anxious, and links her anxiety with the meanings she attaches to the wedding. But the sociologist of emotion does not usually focus on a person's childhood development *per se*, or on injury and repair, but instead on the sociocultural *determinants* of feeling, and the sociocultural bases for defining, appraising and managing human emotion and feeling.

Three questions arise. Why did the bride feel 'nervous', and 'depressed', as she put it, and break down and cry? How did she define her feelings? And how did she appraise the degree to which they corresponded with what she thought she 'should' feel?

To answer the first question, we would need to discover far more about the bride's prior expectations and her current apprehension of the self-relevance of her situation. I would personally argue that emotion emerges as a result of a newly grasped reality (as it bears on the self) as it clashes against the template of prior expectations (as they bear on the self). Emotion is a biologically given sense, and our most important one. Like other senses, hearing, touch and smell, emotion is a means by which we continually learn and relearn about a just-now-changed, back-and-forth relation between self and world, the world as it means something just now to the self.[6]

Most of us maintain a prior expectation of a continuous self, but the character of the self we expect to maintain is subject to profoundly social influence. To understand the bride's distress, we would need to understand the template of prior expectations she had about herself, as a daughter, a girlfriend, a woman, a member of her community, and her social class. We would need to know how close she felt she 'really was' to the friends who didn't appear at her wedding, to the sister who didn't reassure her. We would need to know just what she picked out to see and absorb as she saw her sister from the dressing-table, and what gestures caught her eye among participants at the rehearsal. From these details we might reconstruct the social aspects of the moment of disappointment and tears. To be sure, the social aspect isn't everything. Emotion always involves some biological component: trembling, weeping, breathing hard. But it takes a social element, a new juxtaposition of an up-until-just-now expectation and a just-now apprehension of reality to induce emotion. That is one aspect of emotion the sociologist of emotion studies.

Second, how does the bride define her feelings? She draws from *a prior set of ideas about what feelings are feel-able*. She has to rely on a prior notion of what feelings are 'on the cultural shelf', pre-acknowledged, pre-named, pre-articulated, culturally available to be felt. We can say that our bride intuitively matches her feeling to a nearest feeling in a collectively shared emotional dictionary. Let us picture this dictionary not as a small object outside herself, but as a giant cultural entity and she a small being upon its pages.

Matching her feelings to the emotional dictionary, she discovers that some feelings are feel-able and others not. Were she to feel sexual and romantic homosexual attraction in China, for example, she would discover that to most people, homosexual love is not simply considered 'bad'; it is considered not to exist.

Like other dictionaries, the emotional dictionary reflects agreement among the authorities of a given time and place. It expresses the idea that within an emotional 'language group' there are given emotional experiences, each with its own ontology. So, to begin with, the sociologist of emotion asks, first, to what array of acknowledged feelings, in the context of her time and place, is our bride *matching* her inner experience, and, second, is her feeling of happiness on her wedding day a perfect match, a near match, a complete mismatch? This powerful process of matching inner experience to a cultural dictionary becomes, for the sociologist of emotion, a mysterious, important part of the drama of this bride's inner life. For culture is an active, constituent part of emotion, not a passive medium within which biologically pre-formulated, 'natural' emotions emerge.

Third, we ask: what does the bride believe she *should* or shouldn't feel? If, on one hand, the bride is matching her emotion to a cultural dictionary, she is also matching it to a bible, a set of prescriptions embedded in the received wisdom of her culture. The bride lives in a *culture of emotion*. What did the bride expect or hope to feel on this day? She tells us a wedding 'is supposed to be the happiest day of one's life'. In so far as she shares this wish with most other young heterosexual women in America, she has internalized a shared feeling rule: on this day feel the most happy you have ever felt. Specifically, the bride may have ideals about *when* to feel excited, central, enhanced, and when not to (around age 25, not 15). She has ideas about *whom* she should love and whom not (a kind, responsible man, not a fierce one) and *how strongly* she should love (with a moderate degree of abandon; not complete abandon, but not too cool and collected either).

Her feeling rules are buttressed by her beliefs concerning *how important* love should be. The poet Lord Byron wrote, 'Man's love is of man's life a thing apart, 'tis woman's whole existence.'

Does love loom larger for our bride than it does for her groom? Or does she now try to make love a smaller part of her life, as men in her culture have tried to do in the past? What are the new feeling rules about the place of love in a modern woman's life? How desirable or valued is the emotion of love or the state of deep attachment?

According to the western 'romantic love ethic', one is supposed to fall 'head over heels' in love, to lose control or come close to doing so. Within western cultures, there are subcultural variations. In Germany, *romantische Liebe* has a slightly derogatory connotation that it lacks in the USA. In many parts of non-western societies, such as India, romantic love is considered dangerous. On the basis of interviews with Hindu men on the subject of love, Steve Derne found that the Hindu men felt that 'head over heels' romantic love was dangerous and undesirable. Such love occurred, but it inspired a sense of dread and guilt, for it was thought to compete with a man's loyalty to his mother and other kinspeople in the extended family. This dread, of course, mixes with and to some extent alters the feeling of love itself.[7]

So we do not assume that people in different eras and places feel 'the same old emotion' and just express it differently. Love in, say, a New England farming village of the 1790s is not the 'same old' love as in upper-class Beverly Hills, California in 1995 or among the working-class Catholic miners in Saarbrucken, Germany. Each culture has its unique emotional dictionary, which defines what is and isn't, and its emotional bible, which defines what one should and should not feel in a given context. As aspects of 'civilizing' culture they determine the predisposition with which we greet an emotional experience. They shape the predispositions with which we *interact* with ourselves over time. Some feelings in the ongoing stream of emotional life we acknowledge, welcome, foster. Others we grudgingly acknowledge and still others the culture invites us to deny completely.

Finally, like any sociologist, the sociologist of emotion looks at the *social context* of a feeling. Is the bride's mother divorced? Is her estranged father at the wedding? And the groom's family? How unusual is it for friends not to attend weddings? How serious were the invitations? Mothers, fathers, siblings, step-parents and siblings, friends: what are the histories of their 'happiest days'? This context also lends meaning to the bride's feelings on her wedding day.

THE MODERN PARADOX OF LOVE

Given the current emotional culture (with its particular dictionary and bible) on the one hand, and the social context on the other, a society often presents its members with a paradox – an apparent contradiction that underneath is not a contradiction but a cross-pressure.

The present-day western paradox of love is this. As never before, the modern culture invites a couple to aspire to a richly communicative, intimate, playful, sexually fulfilling love. We are invited not to hedge our bets, not to settle for less, not to succumb to pragmatism, but, emotionally speaking, to 'aim high'.

At the same time, however, a context of high divorce silently warns us against trusting such a love too much.[8] Thus, the culture increasingly invites us to 'really let go' and trust our feelings. But it also cautions: 'You're not really safe if you do. Your loved one could leave. So don't trust your feelings.' Just as the advertisements saturating American television evoke '*la belle vie*' in a declining economy that denies such a life to many, so the new cultural permission for a rich, full, satisfying love-life has risen just as new uncertainties subvert it.

Let me elaborate. On one hand, the culture invites us to feel that love is more important than before. As the historian John Gillis argues, the sacredness once attached to the Church and expressed through a wider community has been narrowed to the family. The family has become fetishized, and love, as that which leads to families, elevated in importance. Economic reasons for a man and a woman to join their lives together have grown less important, and emotional reasons have grown more important.[9] In addition, modern love has also become more pluralistic.[10] What the Protestant Reformation did to the hegemony of the Catholic Church, the sexual and emotional revolution of the last thirty years has done to romantic love. The ideal of heterosexual romantic love is now a slightly smaller model of love within an expanding pantheon of valued loves, each with its supporting subculture. Gay and lesbian loves can, in some subcultures, enjoy full acceptance; single career women now have a rich cultural world in which a series of controlled affairs mixed with warm friendships with other women is defended as an exciting life. Some of this diversification of love expands the social categories of people 'eligible' to experience romantic love, whereas some of it provides alternatives. But on the whole, the ideal of romantic love has increased its powerful grip by extending and adapting itself to more populations.

Paradoxically, while people feel freer to love more fully as they wish, and to trust love as a basis of action, they also feel more afraid to do so because love often fades, dies, is replaced by a 'new love'. The American divorce rate has risen from about 20 per cent at the turn of the century and stands now at 50 per cent, the highest in the world. Norms that used to apply to American adolescent teenagers in the 1950s, 'going steady', breaking up, going steady again with another, now apply to the adult parents of children. The breakup rate for cohabiting couples is higher still. In addition, more women raise children on their own, and more women have no children.[11]

These combined trends present our young bride with a tease. She is inspired by the image of a greater love, but sobered by its 'incredible lightness of being'.[12] The promise of expressive openness is undercut by the fear of loss. For in order to dare to share our innermost fears, we need to feel safe that the individual we love, the person dearest to us, perhaps a symbol of 'mother' in the last instance, is not going to leave.

NEW DEMANDS FOR EMOTION MANAGEMENT

Faced with this paradox, the bride may resort to one of several strategies for managing emotion. An act of emotion management, as I use this term, is an effort by any means, conscious or not, to change one's feeling or emotion. We can try to induce feelings that we don't at first feel, or to suppress feelings that we do. We can – and continually do – try to shape and reshape our feelings to fit our inner cultural guidelines. These acts of emotion management sometimes succeed; often they are hopeless. But however hopeless they are, such acts provide a clue to who we are trying, inside, to be; an emotional 'strategy' as a larger plan guiding acts of emotion management.[13] What strategies might the young bride pursue? She might try to make love last by unconscious, 'magical' means. In one study of emotional responses to the 'divorce culture', the sociologist Karla Hackstaff discovered that some young lovers who grew up in divorced homes unconsciously warded off the 'evil eye' of divorce in their own love-life by creating a First-Love-That-Fails and a Second-Love-That-Works.[14] Our bride could have met a perfectly nice boyfriend before she met her husband. But because she feels she is destined to suffer a divorce and is eager to avoid that, she projects on to a first lover 'everything bad'. She tries to fall out of love. She leaves. Then she meets a second young man, just like the first, on whom she projects 'everything good'. With him, she tries to stay in love. Through this unconscious magic, our bride makes her first marriage into a symbolic second one, and magically clears away the danger of divorce.

Alternatively, the bride might try to adapt to the disquieting uncertainties of love by protecting herself with emotional armour. She defends herself against 'dangerous' needs – her own and those of others. She becomes a 'cool modern' person who avoids problems by avoiding needs.[15] She tries to expect less. She tries to care less. She tries to feel that no one can hurt her. Ironically, in an era of sexual and emotional liberation, our bride 'trains' herself to be an emotional Spartan. Her emotional armour can be donned in a great many ways. In one recent study of single women, Kim De Costa found that women tried to limit their trust of men; to dampen their fantasies of rich, emotional bonds with men, and to expand their fantasies of great love for children.[16] With children, one could dare to 'fall in love', and could, perhaps, displace on to children the dependency needs one feels one cannot afford to feel with men.

Loss itself is not new. Through the ages, people have lost loved ones through disease and war, and have managed their feelings about the possibility of such loss. But when the defences against uncertainty arise from the *culture of love itself*, when the cultural dictionary elaborates varieties of guarded loves and ex-loves, and when this culture of love is linked to capitalism, we need the best sociological thinking we have to understand it.

What forces are driving the modern paradox of love? The strongest force, I believe, is the runaway horse of capitalism. Capitalism is a culture as well as an economic system. As Anthony Giddens has argued in *Modernity and Self-Identity*, the economy, the state, the mass media have become vast, far-flung empires, 'abstract systems' he calls them, which dwarf, undermine and 'disembed' local cultures.

Giddens (1991) is unclear about precisely how they do this. One mechanism is substitution. We watch television more and talk to each other less. We turn on the radio more, play musical instruments less. Listen to call-in television more, vote less. In these ways, an abstract system, the mass media, comes to 'substitute for' local customs and domestic folkways. But underneath such substitutions, a more pervasive and deep-seated mechanism may be at work: the adaptation of the metaphors of abstract institutions to the local, intimate, more 'traditional' sphere of private life.

Replacing the idea of love, devotion, sacrifice, in our collective unconscious, is the metaphor of emotional capital. This metaphor poses a new set of questions. Do people think of emotion as that which they invest or divest so that the self is ever more lightly connected to feeling? Does emotion itself take on the properties of 'capital'?[17] Can we speak of new emotional investment strategies so that people more easily invest and divest their emotional capital? Is this emotional capital now more 'mobile' across social territory than in previous eras? Can we speak of a deregulation of emotional life, so that it flows across new boundaries according to private notions of emotional profit? If so, how does this affect the emotion management of a young bride? Given that in one American study, half of the divorced fathers of children five years after divorce had not seen their child during the last year, we can also ask: How does it affect children?

I am not arguing that people automatically enter relationships 'more lightly' nowadays than they did thirty years ago, or that they think shallow connections are better than deep ones. I am suggesting, rather, that one strategy of emotion management may be to try to become capable of limiting emotional connection. That emotional strategy fits the uncertain, destabilized intimate life shaken by the flight plan of capitalism. For the uncertain, destabilized intimate life is a life of potential profit and loss. The task of emotion management is to rise to the opportunity, and prepare for the loss. But the stance of emotional entrepreneur is in no way a natural one. We need to feel attached to others, and we dread the loss of attachment in a very pre-modern way. In such late modern times, it requires an extreme degree of emotion work to feel 'normal'. For as we begin each relationship, we are forever practising the end 'just in case'. This is the emotional insurance policy, the emotional hardening required of the postmodern hunter and gatherer of love. Fleeting as they are, magnified moments of emotion management tell a great deal about the brief steps through which we embrace or resist a capitalist culture of intimate life. In the case of mild feelings, acts of self-control also actually help shape the emotion. We may try to alter the expression of our feeling and in doing so actually alter the inward feeling (surface acting). Alternatively, we can verbally prompt ourselves to feel one emotion and not another (one kind of deep acting). Or we can try to enter into a different way of seeing the world (this is the deep acting in which professional actors often engage, the so-called 'method acting'). Whatever the method of emotion management, the emotions managed are not independent of our management of them.

Emotions always involve the body; but they are not sealed biological events. Both the act of 'getting in touch with feeling' and the act of 'trying to feel' become part of the process that makes the feeling we get in touch with what it is. In managing feeling, we partly create it.

We can see the very act of managing emotion as part of what the emotion becomes. This idea gets lost if we assume, as do more organismic theorists such as Charles Darwin and Sigmund Freud, that how we manage or express feeling is extrinsic to the emotion itself. It gets lost if we see emotion as simply 'motored by instinct'. In fact, I believe that culture impinges at many points: at the point of recognizing a feeling, at labelling a feeling, at appraising a feeling, at managing a feeling and expressing a feeling. Thus, an emotional strategy useful in defending oneself against the paradox of modern love, provides not simply an emotional armour, but, to some degree, the feelings that are armoured.[18]

Thus, through how it makes us see relations, define experience and manage feeling, the culture of capitalism insinuates its way into the very core of our being. Weaving together the tatters of a waning tradition, the bride seeks to enter a private emotional bubble, her happiest day. In this light, her wedding is both a holdover and an act of resistance. She wants this day to be the happiest day of her life, but the day is lodged in this wider context, and her wish forms part of a larger paradox of modern love. Ultimately, this may be the source of the bride's unease. This paradox itself is a product of a misfit between old feeling rules (a former emotional dictionary-cum-bible) and a newly emergent social context. But feeling rules change, and so do social contexts. History provides a moving series of paradoxes.

I therefore believe that the important questions for the sociologist of emotion to ask are these. What emotional paradox are we apparently trying to resolve in order to live the life we want to live? By what dialectical interaction between feeling rules and context is this emotional paradox produced? To the historian, we pass the question of what forces have produced shifts between one paradox and the next. In light of these paradoxes, what emotional strategies come to 'make sense'? What kind of emotion work does it demand? And we have not finished the job until we dare to ask the question that begs so many more: what social contexts produce the 'best' ways of feeling?

NOTES

1 This chapter is adapted from a talk given to the German Psychoanalytic Association in Saarbrucken, Germany, 1 October 1995.
2 Randall Collins, 'Emotion as a key to restructuring social theory', paper to be presented to the Australian National University, July 1997.
3 Within American sociology, the sociology of emotions is one of over twenty subfields. It was established in the mid-1980s, and publishes a quarterly newsletter with notes about new articles and books in the field. The British Sociological Association has a 'study group', as does the International Sociological Association. Also in the mid-1980s, the International Association for Research on Emotion was established to bring together sociologists with psychologists and other social scientists interested in emotions. For exposure to a fuller range of perspectives and topics within the sociology of emotions, see Franks and McCarthy (1989) and Kemper (1989).
4 Hochschild (1983: 59). The wording is slightly modified for the sake of coherence.
5 Dr Christa Rohde-Dachser holds the Sigmund Freud Chair in Psychology at the University of Frankfurt and is affiliated with the Institut für Psychoanalyse at the University of Frankfurt, Senchenkergantage 15 (Turm) 60054, Frankfurt, Germany.
6 Here, I draw on my discussion in Appendix A, 'Models of emotion: from Darwin to Goffman' (Hochschild 1983: 205).
7 Steve Derne, 'Hindu men's langues of social pressure and individualism: the diversity of South Asian ethnopsychology', *International Journal of Indian Studies* 2(2) (1992): 40–71.
8 This paradox is parallel to but slightly different from that described by Beck and Beck-Gernsheim. In *The Normal Chaos of Love*, Ulrich Beck and Elisabeth Beck-Gernsheim note a contradiction between individual desires (e.g. for higher education and career) and love and family. I am drawing attention to the emotional dilemma created by cultural support for a strong desire for love (which evokes

trust in feeling), and the modern chanciness of love (knowledge of which evokes a distrust of feeling).

9 Changes in intimate life are part of a long-term decline in the functions of the family as the economy, the state, and the professions and various services have taken over activities and purposes that the family used to fulfil. In addition, the social ecology around the family has become weakened too. Local communities, the Church, the world of volunteers that provided support and control for family life, all have declined. Meanwhile, national and global organizations that in new ways connect human beings together, through time and space, have increased in power and importance. The non-market sector has declined, the market sector risen. Some commentators, such as the English sociologist Anthony Giddens, see in these shifts bracing new opportunities, whilst others, such as the German sociologist Sigmund Bauman, see new dangers. See Anthony Giddens's *Modernity and Self-Identity* (1991; English edition, Cambridge: Cambridge University Press). Also see Zygmunt Bauman, *Legislators and Interpreters* (1989). As Gillis notes: 'The Victorians were the first to make room for a spiritualized home, and create within their homes a series of special family times and places where an ideal family could experience itself free from the distractions of everyday life. Families have become fetishized.' See Gillis (1994).

10 I am indebted to Cas Wouters for this insight (see Chapter 13). Cultural norms have not, of course, remained untouched by history. Romantic love has a long social history. As the historian Denise de Rougemont notes, during the middle to end of the feudal period in Languedoc, France, unemployed knights who had lost their feudal lords came to worship unavailable noblewomen. Towards these women, the romantic lover had an unconsummated, sometimes unrequited love, in which he transferred to the unavailable woman of higher station a worshipful pose he might otherwise have expressed towards his missing employer. The objects of this archetypal romantic love, upper-class married women, were themselves locked into loveless matches which cemented economically useful alliances between families. Today, we seem to be in the midst of a move away from this model of love, as the paper argues.

From this moment in history, one can trace over time the transmutation of this ideal of love – its growing association with sexual expression, with marriage, with procreation and, indeed, with the institution of the bourgeois family. In the United States, this new cultural synthesis of romantic love, with marriage and procreation, came to fullest development in the 1950s when a full 95 per cent of the population married at some point in their lives.

11 The divorce rate has greatly affected the relations between fathers and children; one study found that half of American children, ages 11 to 16, living with their divorced mothers, had not seen their fathers during the entire previous year. An in-depth study of divorcing families in California found that half of the men and two-thirds of the women felt more content with the quality of their lives after divorce, though only one in ten children did. Half of the women and a third of the men were still intensely angry at their ex-spouses ten years after the divorce. Wallerstein and Blakeslee (1989). Arlie Hochschild, 'The fractured family', *American Prospect* (Summer 1991): 106–15.

12 I believe other sociologists miss this point. Niklas Luhmann in *Love as Passion* (1986) suggests that sexuality has become a 'communicative code', a language rather than an experience integrated with a full range of implied social ties and controls. Also see Alberoni (1983).

13 See my book *The Managed Heart: The Commercialization of Human Feeling* (1983).

14 Hackstaff (1991).

15 See Hochschild (1994). Ann Swidler (1986) and Francesca Cancian (1987) argue that commitment plays a diminishing part in people's idea of love, whilst the idea of growth and communication plays a more important part. Data from national opinion polls also document a twenty-year decline in commitment to long-term love.
16 See Kim De Costa, 'Rationalizing love with men, essentializing love of children' (MA paper in progress, University of California, Berkeley). The idea that people have become more guarded in the wake of greater freedoms runs counter to popular notions of the 1970s and 1980s as a period of the 'culture of narcissism', as the historian Christopher Lasch calls it.
17 Larrie Lauren, 'Emotional capital', unpublished paper; Laurie Schaffner, 'Deviance, emotion and rebellion: the sociology of runaway teenagers' (honors thesis, Sociology Department, Smith College, 1994). See Loic Wacquant's use of the term 'bodily capital' in 'The pugilistic point of view: how boxers think and feel about their trade' (*Theory and Society* 24 (1995): 489–535).
18 Hochschild (1983: 18). Also see Appendices A and B.

BIBLIOGRAPHY

Alberoni, F. (1983) *Falling in Love*. New York: Random House.
Bauman, Z. (1989) *Legislators and Interpreters*. Cambridge: MA: Polity Press.
Beck, U. and Beck-Gernsheim, E. (1995) *The Normal Chaos of Love*. Oxford: Polity Press.
Bowlby, J. (1969) *Attachment and Loss*. New York: Basic Books.
Cancian, F. (1987) *Love in America: Gender and Self-Development*. Cambridge, MA: Cambridge University Press.
Coontz, S. (1992) *The Way We Never Were*. New York: Basic Books.
Derne, S. (1995) *Culture in Action: Family Life, Emotion and Male Dominance in Banaras India*. New York: State University of New York Press.
Durkheim, E. (1965 [1915]) *The Elementary Forms of Religious Life*. London: Allen & Unwin.
Elias, N. (1987) 'On human beings and their emotions: a process-sociological essay', *Theory, Culture and Society* 4(2–3): 339–61.
Franks, D. and Doyle McCarthy, E. (eds) (1989) *The Sociology of Emotions: Original Essays and Research Papers. New York: JAI Press.*
Frijda, N. (1988) 'The laws of emotions', *American Psychologist* 43(5): 349–58.
Gergen, K. J. (1994) *Realities and Relationships: Soundings in Social Construction*. Cambridge, MA: Harvard University Press.
Giddens, A. (1991) *Modernity and Self-Identity*. Stanford, CA: Stanford University Press.
Gillis, J. (1994) 'What's behind the debate on family values', plenary session, section on Sociology of the Family, American Sociological Association.
Hackstaff, K. (1991) 'Divorce culture: a breach of gender relations', unpublished PhD dissertation, Sociology Department, University of California, Berkeley.
Hochschild, A. R. (1975) 'The sociology of feeling and emotion: selected possibilities', in M. Millman and R. Kanter (eds) *Another Voice*. Garden City, NY: Anchor.
Hochschild, A. R. (1979) 'Emotion work, feeling rules and social structure', *American Journal of Sociology* 85: 551–75.
Hochschild, A. R. (1983) *The Managed Heart: The Commercialization of Human Feeling*. Berkeley, CA: University of California Press.
Hochschild, A. R. (1990) *The Second Shift: Working Parents and the Revolution at Home*. New York: Viking Press.

Hochschild, A. R. (1994) 'The commercial spirit of intimate life and the abduction of feminism: signs from women's advice books', *Theory, Culture and Society* 112 (2 May): 1–23.

Kemper, T. (ed.) (1989) *Recent Advances in the Sociology of Emotion*. New York: State University of New York Press.

Kohut, H. (1971) *The Analysis of the Self*. New York: International Universities Press.

Lasch, C. (1979) *The Culture of Narcissism*. New York: Norton Press.

Lear, J. (1990) *Love and Its Place in Nature: A Philosophical Interpretation of Freudian Psychoanalysis*. New York: Farrar, Straus & Giroux.

Luhmann, N. (1986) *Love as Passion: the Codification of Intimacy*. Cambridge: Polity Press.

Mahler, M. (1968) *On Human Symbiosis and the Vicissitudes of Individuation*, Vol. 1, *Infantile Psychosis*. New York: International Universities Press.

Smith, T. (1992) *Strong Interaction*. Chicago: University of Chicago Press.

Stern, D. (1985) *The Interpersonal World of the Infant: A View from Psychoanalysis and Developmental Psychology*. New York: Basic Books.

Swidler, A. (1986) 'Culture in action: symbols and strategies', *American Sociological Review* 51: 273–86.

Wallerstein, J. and Blakeslee, S. (1989) *Second Chances: Men, Women and Children a Decade After Divorce*. New York: Ticknor & Fields.

Winnicott, D. (1965) *The Maturational Processes and the Facilitating Environment*. New York: International Universities Press.

Wouters, C. (1998) 'Changes in the "lust balance" of sex and love since the sexual revolution', this volume.

2 Emotion and communicative action

Habermas, linguistic philosophy and existentialism

Nick Crossley

INTRODUCTION

The current trend in theories of social action is towards an intersubjective or communicative approach (Crossley 1996). This model takes social inter-action to be the most basic and fundamental unit of action analysis and understands its structure to be irreducible to the sum of its parts. The earliest pioneer of this approach was George Herbert Mead (1967). Mead formulated the basic notion of the irreducibility of interaction. The major exponent in current theory is Jürgen Habermas (1987, 1991) (cf. also Turner 1988). Habermas adds many insights and innovations to Mead's model and he draws out the implications of the model for more general issues in social theory and philosophy. Two innovations in particular are important. First, Habermas uses the communicative model to replace the Parsonian idea that action is the most basic unit of social analysis and is the mechanism of social integration (Parsons 1951). Interaction is the most basic unit of analysis, he argues, and interaction is the means through which social integration is achieved. Selves, personalities and culture are also said to be reproduced through this mechanism. Secondly, he identifies and investigates the normative framework of interaction and the validity claims that are raised by all of our ordinary speech acts. All speech acts are oriented towards mutual understanding, according to this model, and all can be contested on the basis of 1) their *propositional content*, 2) the *social and moral right* of the speaker to say what he or she has said, and 3) the *sincerity* of the speaker (these are the aforementioned validity claims). This point is important because it stresses the potential defeasibility of social actions and allows us to consider such actions from a normative as well as an analytic position. We can consider the extent to which particular social arenas are regulated by rational agreement[1] and the extent to which the potential for agreement is overridden by, for example, economic and political power.

Habermas's position is impressive. It can be criticized, however, for failing to give sufficient attention to the affective dimension of communicative action.[2] Habermas fails to consider that communication is (or at least can be) more than an exchange of symbols and ideas; that it is a process of mutual affecting in which interlocutors make emotional as well as cognitive appeals. Furthermore, he fails to consider that communications can and do take place within the context of different types of emotional relationship. These ideas are not incommensurable with Habermas's view. They are issues that he has ignored rather than precluded. Nevertheless, his failure to consider them is a serious omission. Not only does it make his approach one-dimensional and incapable of dealing with 'strong interactions' (Smith 1992), it makes it seem weak and implausible. We know from experience that emotions are involved in communicative action and any theory that fails to acknowledge and account for this therefore seems inadequate.

It is the purpose of this chapter to resolve this problem. I will argue both that Habermas's approach can absorb an account of emotional life and be strengthened by it and that emotional life can and should be seen as interwoven with the fabric of communicative rationality, as he describes it. Moreover, in the process of establishing this I will show that emotion plays a constitutive role in social life.

THEORIES OF EMOTION

The most obvious theories to turn to for a 'Habermas-commensurable' account of emotions are the major sources of his own theory of action: Mead, psychoanalysis, linguistic philosophy (e.g. Wittgenstein) and phenomenology. There are problems with each of these theories, however. Mead himself is primarily a cognitivist and lacks an adequate account of emotion. Psychoanalysis, on the other hand, has an account, but it is problematic for our purposes. Psychoanalysis posits theories of emotional life and emotional development but in doing so it takes the nature of emotion itself for granted. It does not offer a philosophical problematization of emotion, or at least, in so far as it does offer such an account, it tends to offer a reifying and mechanistic account which contradicts the hermeneutic turn that Habermas advocates in his work. The third source, linguistic philosophy, is more promising. It provides a starting-point for thinking about emotion. I will outline its positive contribution before I consider its weaknesses.

Linguistic philosophy and emotion

The presupposition of the linguistic approach is that the concepts and structure of our everyday language effectively constitute the limits of our world; that is, the world as we can know and understand it. This necessitates that an investigation of anything, including emotion, must begin with a consideration of the language by which that phenomenon is made meaningful. A very particular conception of language and meaning is employed, however, which is both non-representational and non-atomistic. Linguistic meaning, for philosophers in this tradition, such as Wittgenstein and Austin, derives from the use to which we put words in concrete contexts and the rules or practical 'grammar' which regulate that use. They argue that speech is a form of (social) action which has many uses in addition to reference: e.g. we can order, question, insult, exclaim, etc. These various different uses are referred to as language games and linguistic analysis is an analysis of these language games.

Coulter (1979) has applied this method to the study of emotion. His analysis begins by challenging representational interpretations of expressions of emotion. It is common in everyday discussions of emotion, he observes, for us to talk of 'feelings'. We say that we feel happy, feel sad, feel angry, etc. This has led some philosophers, who assume a representational theory of meaning and thus understand emotional expressions to be subjective reports, to posit that emotions must consist in feelings or sensations. This is a misunderstanding according to Coulter. Expressions such as 'I feel happy' are not subjective reports on states which exist independently of them, he argues. They are exclamations or expressions which are substituted for other, more natural expressions of emotion (such as a shriek). This observation parallels Wittgenstein's (1953) analysis of pain. The expression 'I am in pain' is not a subjective report, on Wittgenstein's account. It is an exclamation, a form of pain behaviour which we have learned to substitute for more natural pain behaviours (such as a scream or 'Ouch!'). The argument which supports this analysis is as follows: sensations are private experiences; we cannot have words which refer to private experiences because linguistic meaning in a public language (which is the only possible type of language) is necessarily tied to public criteria for its use; therefore sensation words must be doing something other than referring; and in this case what they appear to be doing is exclaiming. This first stage of analysis is preparatory. It prevents our investigation of emotion from being misled by the way in which we talk about emotion.

This preparatory exercise puts emotion and sensation on a par. It is one of the central contentions of linguistic philosophy, however, that the rules pertaining to the language game of emotion are different from those of sensation.[3] Coulter identifies three differences. In the first instance, emotions cannot be localized in the way that sensations can. If one were to say that one had a pain, for example, then it would be perfectly reasonable and meaningful to ask 'Where?' The same is not true of emotions. If a person says 'I feel happy' it would be absurd to ask 'Where?' This would show that we do not understand what 'happy' means. Secondly, whilst it is meaningful to say that one 'has' a sensation of some sort, this does not apply to emotions. I can *have* a pain but I can only *be* happy. Again, the rules of the language game are different. Finally, as Ryle (1949) observes, sensations are neither necessary nor sufficient conditions for the application of emotion words. I might say that I was 'happy all day', for example, without that implying that I had a particular sensation all day, or, indeed, that I had a particular sensation at any point in the day.

Having made these points, Coulter further considers the grammar of the language game of emotion. Two observations are noted. First, we have expectations about reasonable and appropriate emotional responses to certain types of situation and we make judgements about the appropriateness and reasonableness of such responses (e.g. it is perfectly appropriate and reasonable to be upset at a funeral but not at a comedy show – unless there are extenuating circumstances). Secondly, we expect in many cases to be able to argue people out of their emotions, particularly if those emotions are deemed either inappropriate or unreasonable. We might say to a person, for example, that he or she has no reason to feel angry and is being silly. These observations, in turn, have three implications. First, they further differentiate emotions from sensations. It would be absurd if we were to try to argue a person out of their toothache, for example, just as it would if we deemed the toothache unreasonable or contextually inappropriate. Secondly, they remove the notion of privacy and mystery from our understanding of emotion. The emotional realm is conceived as public and potentially contestable. It is identified as intersubjective. Finally, emotion is shown to be woven into the structure of communicative rationality, in the sense that it can be judged appropriate or inappropriate and argued over. Emotion does not lie outside of the social world *qua* rational-intersubjective order, at least not necessarily. It is positioned squarely within it. Emotions, like thoughts, beliefs and other cognitive phenomena, can be and frequently are judged rational or irrational according to their relationship to their context.

What makes this intersubjective structuring possible, on Coulter's account, is that the grammar of the emotions language game is tied to what is publicly observable. It applies to actions and circumstances rather than private sensations. Emotions are constituted as meaningful responses to situations. This is not to say that sensations or physiological processes are not involved at all in the sphere of emotion but even where they are, Coulter insists, they are not determinate. He supports this by quoting a series of experiments which demonstrate that identical physiological responses are interpreted differently by those who undergo them, according to the context in which they are experienced. These experiments show that the same physiological change can be interpreted as either anger or euphoria, according to the evidence provided by contextual factors, particularly the behaviour of others.

The final point which we may glean from Coulter's account is that different action contexts demand that actors assume different emotional attitudes. In explaining this Coulter makes reference to Parsons's (1951) argument in *The Social System*, that there is a conventional preference *ceteris paribus* for 'affective-neutrality' in relation to some types or contexts of action. We can add to this that there is a conventional preference for particular emotions in particular situations: e.g. grief at funerals, excitement at sporting events and pop concerts, etc. And we can further add both that these expectations are differentiated according to 'membership categorizations' (e.g. they are differently applied according to the manner in which a person is identified – as a man, a woman, a child, a doctor, a teacher) and that they will change over time; work by Elias and other writers in his tradition, for example, clearly demonstrates historical shifts in the types of emotional display tolerated and expected in specific social situations (Elias 1984; Wouters 1987, 1991). Finally, following Coulter I suggest that appropriateness is a 'moral' matter in so far as the social order is a moral order. Inappropriate emotional behaviour may be likely to offend and it will certainly attract disapproval because there is an 'ought' clause in the language game of emotion: one *should* feel in particular ways. Goffman's (1972) discussion of the potential offensiveness of the 'inappropriate affect' of those we deem insane provides a clear illustration of this.

Linguistic philosophy assessed

The value of this analysis from Habermas's position should be apparent. Coulter presents a linguistically sensitive account of emotion, which ties it into the communicative rationality of the lifeworld as a defeasible and contestable action orientation. Emotions, in this conception, form part of a mutually meaningful, intersubjective interworld and they are accountable. Indeed, it is clear that emotional expressions can be contested in terms of the same three validity claims that Habermas identifies with all other communicative actions: that is, in terms of the facts of the situation (do they warrant the emotion?), the sincerity of the agent (are they *really* sad/happy?) and the moral-social rights of the agent (is their relation to the situation such as to warrant their reaction to it?). In this sense a consideration of emotion can be wholly incorporated into Habermas's account, without unduly disturbing any of the central concepts of his theory. In addition to this it is clear that the account is strong and insightful. It provides a highly innovative alternative to the often expressed view that emotion and reason are exclusive or conflictual terms and it does so on solid philosophical grounds.

Notwithstanding this, however, the account is inadequate. Linguistic analysis, by its nature, only considers the concept of emotion and the manner in which emotions are accounted for in situations. It fails to consider the way in which they are lived and acted out. Consequently it does not provide us with an understanding of emotion, but rather with an understanding of our understanding of emotion.

It might be objected that sociology can do no more than this if it is to remain consistent with a proper understanding of language and the place of language in social analysis. Winch's (1958) arguments on the relation of sociology and conceptual analysis would be one strong position from which to state such a claim. Such an objection would miss the point, however. When Coulter, Wittgenstein or Winch discusses the manner in which we organize our world and our experience by way of language games, they point towards particular types of behaviour. Language games are not just ways of accounting for or organizing behaviour, they are ways of behaving in their own right, and as such they too may manifest an emotional component; language games can be played *with* emotion. Indeed it may be expected that they should be; for example, proposing marriage should be done with some passion and conviction. The point here is that we do not just account for or organize emotions, we account for and organize things emotionally: emotion is an active force in social life and needs to be analysed as such. Failure to recognize and explore this is problematic from a hermeneutic point of view because it denies the possibility that emotional praxes may constitute ways of understanding and interpreting situations in their own right. It is problematic from a sociological point of view (even if we limit ourselves to a sociology of the lifeworld) because it fails to consider the place of emotion in the reproduction of selves, personalities and social order. Emotion is not just something which is known, defined and judged. It is something which variously holds social situations together or pulls them apart (Collins 1990; Smith 1992) and which provides the necessary condition for the reproduction of stable personalities (Benjamin 1991). In short, linguistic philosophy is problematic because it fails to consider that emotion may play a positive role in the constitution of the social world *qua* intersubjectively meaningful interworld, in addition to being constituted within that world.

I am not suggesting that we reject linguistic analysis. On the contrary, it is important and valid. It provides a good starting-point and there will be cause for us to return to it later. Moreover, it provides an important conceptual framework for any subsequent analysis. It defines emotion as it must be defined in any sensitive hermeneutic account; that is, as agents themselves define it in their routine praxes. What is required, however, is a deepening of the analysis, an inquiry into the phenomena that are demarcated and regulated within the language game of emotion. We need a phenomenology of emotion.

This observation brings us to the fourth source of Habermas's theory of communicative action: phenomenology. This tradition provides rich insights into the lived experience of social actors and should, therefore, provide a basis from which to introduce 'lived emotion' into our understanding of communicative action. We cannot accept Habermas's own choice of phenomenological influences, Husserl and Schutz, however, since neither of these cognitive-oriented phenomenologists has much to say on the issue of emotion. Instead I will focus upon the existential-phenomenologists, Sartre and Merleau-Ponty.

There are differences in some of the basic presuppositions of Sartre and Merleau-Ponty. I believe the position of Merleau-Ponty is stronger (Crossley 1993, 1994; Kruks 1990), although Sartre had more to say about emotion. I will therefore take Merleau-Ponty's position as my base position, recasting Sartre's ideas around it.

EXISTENTIALISM AND EMOTION

Sartre and Merleau-Ponty, like the linguistic philosophers, reject the idea that specific emotions correspond with specific sensations or physiological changes and are thus reducible to them. Sensations and physiological processes and changes are usually involved in emotional shifts and states, they contend, but in themselves these processes do not constitute emotions. This view is based upon an examination of studies which show that very different emotions consist, physiologically, in very similar processes. Joy and anger, for example, involve the same basic physiological changes and sensations. The only difference between the two is the extent of the change. Anger is more extensive than joy. This is problematic, as Sartre (1993) argues, because we cannot legitimately regard anger as an intense form of joy. The difference between anger and joy is qualitative, not quantitative. Another example of this is crying. Crying lends itself equally to happiness, sadness and fear and it cannot therefore serve as a marker to distinguish any one of them as a specific emotion. Thus, whilst emotions involve physiological reactions, they are not reducible to them and do not derive their identity from them.

These problems are not solved by suggesting that emotion consists in the perception or interpretation which one forms of specific physiological changes or sensations. Sartre illustrates this by reference to terror. To be terrified, he notes, is quite different from recognizing certain sensations as constitutive of terror – as anybody who has ever been terrified will confirm. When we are terrified the world takes on a whole new complexion and we are quite unaware of the changes taking place in our body. Indeed the only thing that we may be aware of is the thing that we are terrified of.

For Merleau-Ponty and Sartre, this necessitates a shift to a psychological model. Whilst it involves a critique of behaviourist reductions of emotion, the model they recommend is strongly anti-mentalist; that is, it is opposed to the invocation of ghostly inner states. Merleau-Ponty and Sartre understand psychological life to consist in sensuous, embodied, meaningful and engaged human praxis. Furthermore, as such, they argue that psychological life is intersubjective. Our perceptions and actions open us on to the world, Merleau-Ponty (1962) argues, and any 'inner' psychological search must therefore end 'outside' in the intersubjective world – which is another way of saying that there is no inwards or outwards, only being-in-the-world-with-others:

> We must reject the prejudice which makes 'inner realities' out of love, hate or anger, leaving them accessible to one single witness: the person who feels them. Anger, shame, hate and love are not psychic facts

hidden at the bottom of another's consciousness: they are types of behaviour or styles of conduct which are visible from the outside. They exist
on this face or in those gestures, not hidden behind them. Psychology did
not begin to develop until the day it gave up the distinction between mind
and body.

(Merleau-Ponty 1971: 52–3)

A number of points should be noted in this passage. First, Merleau-Ponty
equates emotions with specific ways of behaving. This is not to deny the
role of inner sensations but rather to argue that the same sensations may
be involved in different emotions, as noted above, and that what tie those
sensations to specific emotions are the forms of behaviour that they accompany. This is best expressed by saying that emotion consists neither in
sensation nor conduct but rather in *sensuous conduct*. This claim requires
a few points of elaboration. First, as is clear from the passage, it may be
the style with which a behaviour is performed which constitutes its emotional aspect, rather than the behaviour itself. We can perform the same
behaviours lovingly, angrily, etc., and it is the way that we do it which constitutes the emotional aspect of the behaviour. Furthermore, as Goffman
(1972) has observed, we can accentuate these emotional styles for specific
communicative purposes. Secondly, context is crucial. The nature of an
emotion is revealed in the relation of an action to a particular set of circumstances, not in the act in isolation. Finally, as situated conduct, the nature of
emotion unfolds through time and may appear different according to the
time segment in which it is viewed: e.g. the anger of one person towards
another may start to look like jealousy from within a broader time frame,
and this jealousy might in turn be found to be rooted in love. This temporal
dimension constitutes a further useful argument against both physiological
and mentalistic views because even if we could locate the immediate sense of
anger in a person's physiology or 'inner world', it is much less likely that we
could simultaneously locate the jealousy and love underlying such anger.
This view accords and is consonant with the views of the linguistic philosophers. As I noted above, they too identify emotion with conduct and
context.

A second observation on the passage is that emotion is regarded as an
embodied phenomenon, but that the 'body' involved is a communicative
agent rather than a mechanical being. The corporeal dimension of emotion
is not a third-person physiological process but engaged and expressive
praxis (see Crossley 1994, 1995a, 1995b, 1996, 1997 for an elaboration of
this theme).

Thirdly, following directly from these points, it is clear from the passage
that Merleau-Ponty shares Coulter's concern to emphasize the public nature
of emotion. For him emotions belong, in the first instance, to our shared
interworlds of meaning and communication. This is an important point if
the insights of existentialism and linguistic philosophy are to be combined

in a recasting of Habermas's ideas. We need to be able to understand the place of emotion in intersubjective life and the place of intersubjectivity in the constitution of emotion.

An additional observation which develops this point is that the form of emotional praxes is culture-bound and conventional. This is argued most clearly by Merleau-Ponty in *The Phenomenology of Perception,* where he notes differences in emotional expression between Japanese and European societies: e.g. the Japanese are said to smile in anger, which would be quite inappropriate in Europe. His conclusion to this discussion is that feelings and passion-conduct are 'invented like words' (Merleau-Ponty 1962: 89). Furthermore, he maintains that these differences are more than cosmetic; they constitute different ways of being emotional. This identification of the conventionality of emotion suggests that emotional forms of conduct belong to the forms of life of our societies and thus to the communicative order or lifeworld. Again, this is important if these ideas are to be merged with Habermasian theory.

Having identified emotion as praxis we must next consider the nature of emotion praxes. Sartre's *The Emotions* is most useful here. Sartre begins by considering the work of Janet, who, he argues, poses an interesting problem for the theory of the emotions. For Janet, at least according to Sartre's (1993: 26–33) reading, emotional conduct is an inferior or pathological form of conduct. It is a 'setback behaviour' into which human beings slip when they are unable to sustain a particular course of action; for example, I might become angry if I can't think of an appropriate way to finish this sentence. Sartre is prepared to accept this as a provisional description. It seems clear from experience, he notes, that people can become emotional when normal conduct is difficult or impossible. Moreover, this is supported in psychological studies, which also show that emotional conduct simplifies situations by removing or ignoring some of the codes and conventions that would ordinarily restrict and structure conduct (Sartre 1993: 33–6); for example, if I can't finish my sentence I think, in anger, 'Sod the style, this will do!' There is a confusion in Janet's work, however, as to how best to interpret this phenomenon. He seemingly adopts two quite different interpretations at different times. Sometimes he adopts a mechanistic, passive and negative interpretation. This involves conceptualizing the change in conduct as a diversion of energy within the organism, which reduces tension. In this case, Sartre observes, emotion is more like a mechanical process than praxis. It is not a meaningful response to an event, but rather a dysfunctioning of the personality system. The second interpretation is purposive, active and positive. It suggests that a person 'throws himself [*sic*] into the inferior behaviour in order not to maintain the superior behaviour' (Sartre 1993: 31). Emotion, in this case, purposively masks, rejects or substitutes behaviour that a person is either unable or unwilling to maintain. It is an 'organised system of means aiming at an end' (ibid.: 32). Or again, a 'subterfuge' and 'strategy'; for example, my anger at my unfinishable sentence is a positive strategy which I deploy (albeit without conscious awareness or reflection) as a means of moving beyond my impasse and, indeed, of convincing myself both that there is no impasse and that there is no problem ('Who cares what it reads like? Nobody will read it anyway!'). Sartre clearly prefers this second interpretation and not only because it preserves a sense of persons as purposive beings. The first interpretation cannot explain why there should be so many different types of emotional conduct, he observes, and why the same situation might be responded to in a variety of ways. If emotion were a dysfunction we would not expect it to be so varied or to be capable of situational appropriateness and inappropriateness (e.g. in the manner discussed by Coulter). Finally, the 'dysfunction' model seems more appropriate to complete emotional breakdown, rather than to average and everyday emotions, which often prove quite successful in allowing us to achieve the goals we set for ourselves. Thus Sartre opts, provisionally, for the purposive and functional model, in which emotion constitutes a positive response to a situation.This model is not sufficient for Sartre, however. He develops it by arguing that emotional attitudes are modes of intentionality.

INTENTIONALITY, EMOTION AND MAGIC

The concept of intentionality, as posited in early phenomenology, entails that consciousness is necessarily consciousness 'of' something or other. We cannot be conscious without there being something of which we are conscious, and in phenomenological parlance being consciously aware of something is 'intending' it. In Merleau-Ponty's phenomenology this notion is recast in a more corporeal vein. Consciousness is, for him, an active and sensual relation with alterity, on behalf of an engaged and embodied being (Merleau-Ponty 1962, 1965). Intentionality, in this conception, refers to the sensuous-perceptual and practical-orientational relation which we (*qua* embodied beings) enjoy with our environment. This second version of intentionality is preferable, not least because it admits emotion into the intentional life of the subject. In early phenomenology intentionality was conceived in purely cognitive terms. However, because existential-phenomenologists assumed an embodied conception of the subject, they were able to extend the notion to consider the emotional atmosphere in which our apprehension of the world takes form. Emotion is thus conceived as an embodied manner of intending objects in the world. This is the insight which Sartre develops. Emotion *qua* praxis, he argues, is a way of intending, apprehending and understanding the world; it bestows a value or significance upon things. Thus, to return to the example of my recalcitrant sentence; when I get angry the problem appears under a completely different light and new possibilities for action open up. A change in one's emotions brings about a change in one's conscious apprehension of the world.

The notion of embodied consciousness which is introduced in this account need not entail self-consciousness. Consciousness and intentionality, in the phenomenological sense, concern the way in which we apprehend our world but they entail no necessary apprehension of ourselves. Such reflexiveness is argued to be dependent upon particular relations with others and upon concrete involvement in the world. Thus, for example, someone may be angry and may assume a relation of anger to the world, without being reflectively or consciously aware that they are angry. Indeed, they may be far too concerned with what they are angry about to notice their own state. This point relates to a more general point concerning pre-reflective, pre-reflexive and pre-objective levels of being, as conceived in existential-phenomenology. The intellectual activities ordinarily associated with consciousness, such as reflection, judgement, interpretation and objectification, existentialists argue, presuppose a prior level of meaningful experience. Reflection requires something to reflect upon, interpretation something to interpret, judgement something to judge, etc. This points to the existence of a pre-intellectual level of being-in and intending the world, prior to any cognitive operations that we might discharge. And this implies that *qua* subjects we are never transparent to ourselves. We take a position in the world prior to any (reflective) awareness that we may have of either ourselves or the world. Emotion clearly belongs to this pre-reflective life. Emotional attitudes are meaningful and purposive, but they cannot be reduced to reflective consciousness. We do not reflectively choose or decide our emotions, or, at least, when we try it seems false (Hochschild 1983, 1989; Wouters 1989a, 1989b) and we are not necessarily aware of the emotional states we are in. Emotion is an intentional way of being which underlies our reflective awareness. It is like light: it enables us to see (or make sense) but it is not necessarily seen itself.

This view could be attributed to both Heidegger (1962) and Merleau-Ponty (1962). Sartre adds an interesting twist to it, however, by positing that emotion constitutes a 'magical' attitude. This idea is related to Janet's view of emotion as a simplification of situations. Sartre replaces the notion of simplification, however, with an idea of magical transformation. When we are faced with a difficult situation or one in which we are unable to get what we want, he argues, we imaginatively transform the situation to make it more liveable. Moreover, we live this magically transformed world with strong and true conviction. A few examples will suffice to illustrate the ways in which this 'magic' works.

In cases of envy, where we want an object but do not have it and cannot get it, we may transform it into an object of hatred that we want to destroy. We may try to degrade the object, often publicly. Having been something we once wanted, it becomes something that we detest and we are convinced that we detest it. Likewise with the aforementioned example of anger; my anger has now convinced me, not only that I don't need to finish the sentence but that there is no need to finish the paper at all 'because it's rubbish anyway!' In cases of joy a similar process takes place. Joy, Sartre argues, is intimately related to the achievement of a desired state of affairs. This seems unmagical. The magical aspect of joy is revealed, however, if we consider the temporal process by and through which desired states of affairs are achieved. There is no given moment or point at which particular things are achieved, from an absolute point of view. Or at least, there is no absolute point at which the value of an achievement or end becomes apparent. But joy and the rituals of joy create and mark such a point, punctuating processes and allowing us to consume achievements or ends as wholes. Extreme cases of this edge into hysteria. Sartre discusses some cases of this in relation to Janet's (psychiatric) case material and he posits a couple of examples of his own. The clearest example is of a person who faints at the sight of danger. Even this is a meaningful process, rather than a third-person and mechanical one, for Sartre. It is an extreme denial of the reality of a dangerous situation, an imaginary escape from that reality.

The fainting example is important because it draws us back to the issue of the physiological aspect of emotion. Although, as I have said, there is no one-to-one correspondence between emotional states and physiological states or sensations, for the existentialists, the latter are said to be integral to the former in so far as they transform one's intentional grip upon the world and thereby situate one differently within it; emotional changes, in this respect, involve non-specific organismic changes. Furthermore, the example of fainting also illustrates the pre-reflective dimension of emotional life. Fainting is a response of the whole organism to a situation, affected by way of physiological changes. It is not a response which can be conjured up by reflective choice. This is the case in all emotion according to both Sartre and Merleau-Ponty. A change in emotion is a change in our world by way of the intentional structure of consciousness and this is achieved by way of a pre-reflective change in our physical being. Emotional changes are constituted through an anonymous shift in the manner in which our body situates us in the world.

Both Merleau-Ponty and Sartre use the example of falling to sleep as a comparison to illustrate this. Like the sleeper, the emotional subject can assume the positions and rituals appropriate to the state but, in the final instance, they must wait for it to come over them. The sleeper, Merleau-Ponty notes, assumes the position. They lie down and pull up their knees. They close their eyes and clear their minds: 'But the power of my will or consciousness stops there' (1962: 163). They must wait for sleep to come over them. This is not a process which consciousness can transform since consciousness is itself transformed in the process. So it is with emotion. This is not to deny that subjects can actively and consciously 'put on' emotions, any less than that they can pretend to be asleep (Hochschild 1983, 1989; Wouters 1989a, 1989b). Moreover, Merleau-Ponty and Sartre are quite clear that such impersonations are sometimes sufficient to induce the 'real thing'. The point is, however, that emotions are more than behavioural masks that we can consciously manage: they actually subtend and make possible our conscious grip on the world. Our emotions form part of our point of view on the world; we do not just have them, we exist in and by way of them.

This discussion of the transformation of consciousness and the powerlessness of consciousness with respect to changes is bordering on a psychoanalytic account of the unconscious. Sartre and Merleau-Ponty are both aware of this and offer a mixed response. On the one hand both agree that, in so far as psychoanalysis attempts to understand the meaning or significance of behaviours and responses, it is useful and valuable (even though they would not always agree with the particular interpretations offered). They stress, however, that this concern for meaning cannot be reconciled with an account of unconscious causation, since this would involve a combination of incommensurable levels and forms of analysis. Furthermore, they equally insist, at various points in their work, that we cannot make reference to unconscious 'choices' since this would presuppose that the unconscious was a representational subject (i.e. capable of presenting options to itself) and therefore conscious – which it cannot be by definition. Thus, although the existentialists are prepared to accept that a great deal of what human beings do is done unconsciously, they do not invoke 'the unconscious' as an explanation of action or a centre of agency. Emotional shifts are understood as processes of blind but purposive adaptation on the behalf of the person *qua* organism.

INSTRUMENTAL AND COMMUNICATIVE ACTIONS

Up until this point, Sartre's theory is apparently centred around an instrumental conception of the actor, with emotion representing a magical 'degeneration' of instrumental (means-end) rationality. Towards the end of *The Emotions*, however, he adds a new twist. He posits a distinction between 'social' and 'instrumental' situations and argues that all social situations are rooted in magic, even if an instrumentally rational superstructure is built over the top of this: 'man is always a wizard to man [*sic*], and the social world is at first magical' (Sartre 1993: 84). Thus the magical (emotional) attitude is said to be primordial, with instrumental rationality being a secondary achievement, and emotion-magic is identified as normal (rather than degenerate) in relation to specifically social or intersubjective situations. The social world is magical for Sartre; it is emotionally constituted.

This is an interesting and important twist, in terms of the basic concerns of this chapter, because the split that Sartre makes between instrumental and intersubjective contexts is very similar to the distinction which Habermas draws (throughout his work) between instrumental and communicative actions. The former, for Habermas, involves objectification of our environment (which might include other people) and consists in the attempt to make it controllable and predictable. The latter is oriented towards fellow subjects and consists in the attempt to understand and make oneself understood. Moreover, in some conceptions, it involves a desire for recognition in the Hegelian sense (Habermas 1974; Honneth 1995). Notwithstanding this formal similarity, however, Habermas's characterization of intersubjective or communicative situations has a very different emphasis from that of Sartre. He understands such situations to be (at least potentially) regulated by and based in communicative rationality rather than emotion (and magic). Communicative rationality is different from instrumental rationality. It concerns the pragmatics of human understanding and agreement rather than means–end calculation. Nevertheless it is still rationality. Furthermore, it is essential for the achievement of social integration in Habermas's view. Without the possibility of shared understanding and agreement, which is what communicative rationality enables, there could be no social world. We would be condemned to an extreme version of the anti-social world of Hobbes's (1971) *Leviathan*.

This brings us to the crux of the issue under discussion in this chapter. We have two distinct perspectives on the social world: Sartre's, which emphasizes its emotional constitution, and Habermas's, which emphasizes its rational and cognitive constitution. We must determine whether each is sound and whether the two are mutually compatible.

There can be little doubt, if we examine common experience, that social interactions can be guided by the kind of magical-emotional thinking that Sartre describes. It is perfectly ordinary for people to form magical associations and to constitute the world in accordance with their moods. Human conduct and the bonds of many social relations are precisely magical: people take aversion to things, they idealize things, they like or dislike 'the feel' of things, they are offended and amused, envious and grateful. These are just routine and mundane features of our everyday lifeworld. Moreover, Sartre's description of them as magical is useful. It allows us to grasp emotions as specific ('enchanted') ways of being-in-the-world, open for analysis, and to avoid the tendency to view them negatively as failures in instrumental reasoning – a view which would consign everything, from Platonic love to the passion of a football crowd, to the categories 'pathological' and 'dysfunctional'.

On the other hand, Habermas is right to emphasize the rationality of communicative situations. Numerous interactionist studies have shown how situations are made rationally accountable and how the process of interaction involves the mutual checking and correcting that is necessary for an intersubjective understanding to be reached. Habermas is hardly alone amongst sociologists in believing this to be so. Indeed, much of the history of sociological theorizing, beginning with Durkheim's *Division of Labour*, has involved an attempt to challenge naive utilitarian reductions of the social by demonstrating that the social world is ordered through shared norms or expectations (and thus intersubjective accountability and rationality).

Our question, then, is how it is possible for both of these descriptions to be true. How can our world be constituted both by emotion and by reason? The answer to this question has already been given, when we considered the view of linguistic philosophy. From this philosophy we arrived at the view that emotion is integrated with the order of communicative rationality; that it can be either rational or irrational. We showed that emotional responses raise validity claims which can be challenged or confirmed and that, like any cognitive belief, an emotional response is something that we believe we can talk people out of when they are wrong (i.e. when their emotional response is irrational). Thus there is no reason why our social worlds cannot be simultaneously constituted through emotion and communicative rationality. Indeed, we can say that emotion forms part of the sphere of communicative rationality.

What it means, more precisely, to say that emotions form part of the sphere of communicative rationality is that they can strike us as either appropriate or inappropriate, rational or irrational, that we find them perfectly intelligible when we encounter them in others, that we explain them in terms of reasons rather than causes and that we hold people responsible for them, just as we do for any other of their actions. It is important to add here, moreover, that even many apparently irrational emotional responses are not completely divorced from the rational-intersubjective world. Emotional outbursts do not preclude communicative reasoning, even if they sometimes distort it. Like the sleeper who is awoken by events in the waking world, the emotional subject is (usually) still responsive to calls from 'outside'. We can be argued (and perhaps sometimes dragged) back to intersubjective reality when our responses are at odds with it. And the reason for this is that we never completely leave intersubjective reality, even at our most fraught moments.

There is a distinctly existentialist aspect to this line of argument. It is central to the existentialist position, as I have said, that emotional responses are meaningful, purposive and social structured praxes or social actions, not simply third-person mechanical responses. It is for this reason that they can form part of the communicative order. Like any other human action they open out into a shared interworld, where they assume a significance and call for a response.

EMOTION, ARGUMENT AND SOCIAL ORDER

We can expand this observation further into the territory of communicative action by noting that communicative praxes routinely involve an emotional appeal. Interlocutors often have expectations about the way in which their other should feel about certain issues, for example, and they address them accordingly. Or alternatively, they may try to invoke certain feelings in the other, even taunting them. This poses an important question. What is it that is appealed to when emotions are provoked in argument? What is an emotional appeal? Answering this question will provide further insights into the relationship between emotion and communicative order.

I want to note, as a first step in answering this question, that an emotional appeal (as distinct from a taunt) forms part of the sphere of communicative rationality in so far as it raises validity claims. A person who makes an emotional appeal effectively appeals to what he or she imagines will be the response of the other person to a specific situation or image, which, in turn, he or she believes is a reasonable and justified response, calling upon the other to act in a way which would justifiably follow from that response. The appeal is to a court of common sentiment. For example, scenes of dying children are used in charity appeals because they 'should' invoke more or less uniform responses of sadness, revulsion, anger, etc. This always leaves open the possibility that an interlocutor can respond in a way that is unexpected, or can convey that he or she 'knows what their partner is up to' but believes that there are other factors which need to be considered in relation to the type of response that their partner is calling for. Nevertheless this is true of any type of appeal.

Described thus, an emotional appeal may be likened to an appeal to fundamental beliefs which either are shared or are believed to be shared; it is an appeal to common sense. In this respect an emotional appeal is no different, in principle, from any other communicative appeal. All argument must appeal to what is commonly held to be true – to the assumptions of the lifeworld. This casts at least some doubt on the common assumption that an emotional appeal is, in principle, inferior as a mode of argument – although, of course, magical-emotional thinking can be stirred up as a way of obfuscating the complexity of issues.

A further speculation which can be added to this position is that emotion may sometimes function as a safeguard for many of our more fundamental beliefs. If there is no final ground for our lifeworld assumptions, as we are told by postmodern thinkers, then it must be an element of emotional magic which keeps them in place when they are under threat. Otherwise we would endlessly deconstruct our own beliefs and never make any positive steps forward. What else other than magical sentiment could do this job? Certainly it would seem true to say that our emotions are aroused when our fundamental beliefs or our ways of reasoning are under threat. They are an often used defensive resort. If emotion does play this role then it is clearly of great importance for maintaining social integration and rational interaction (see also Collins 1990).

Some support for this view is provided in Scheff's (1984) analysis of mental illness. Deviance, and particularly the 'residual deviance' of mental illness, tends to provoke strong emotional reactions amongst those who are witness to it, Scheff observes. The reason for this, he contends, is that a violation of norms and taken-for-granted assumptions shatters our socially constructed and intersubjectively shared sense of reality. The apparent rationality of the world is threatened and emotional responses are attempts ('magically') to reassert rational order. Goffman's (1972) analysis of the 'insanity of place' provides a similar notion to this, as does R. D. Laing's (1961) work on 'ontological security'. In all cases we can see emotional responses as attempts to preserve a sense of order and rationality in situations where such rationality or order is challenged. In such cases emotion provides a magical reaffirmation of the sense of rational order and a (magical) negation of the cause of disruption.

It does not follow from this that emotion necessarily fulfils a conservative function in communicative interactions, nor that such functioning is necessarily positive. Emotions may be used to defend reactionary or unacceptable beliefs or to champion new and interesting ways of thinking. Furthermore, emotion may constitute a reaction against the frustration created by distortions, inequalities or a lack of reciprocity in communicative situations: e.g. anger may be a response to the impossible situation created by a 'double bind' (Bateson 1973) or it may be a response to the refusal of one's interlocutors to take one's speech acts seriously. For these reasons we can never pronounce on the politics or functioning of emotion in communicative situations in general. Alternatively, like psychoanalysts, we should see emotion as a signal to be interpreted. And we should be clear that the manner in which we interpret (and evaluate) cannot be decided in advance. What an emotion means will depend upon what it signifies in a particular situation and what it does, and its value will depend upon the value that we attribute to what it is doing. The point in highlighting the positive relation between emotion and order, was simply to challenge the counter-assumption that emotion and rational order are necessarily antagonistic or exclusive. They are not.

These issues and processes are not limited in significance to the microcosm of face-to-face argumentation. They can and do occur at the wider level of society. Emotions reinforce arbitrary conventions and boundaries. They give them a sense of meaning or reality and necessity. And political processes, symbols and rituals function to call up those emotions and utilize them. The political uses of patriotic sentiment would be one good example of this, as would the use of flags, anthems and slogans to 'whip' it up. Sociology has known about this type of phenomenon since Durkheim's (1915) analysis of religious ritual. And it is equally supported in the existentialist literature. Although the existentialists oppose the idea that we can (reflectively) choose our emotional state, they nevertheless acknowledge that rituals might be used to induce certain emotions. Through marches, dances and songs we call up the emotional magic that reinforces and supports our (contingent) ways of acting and thinking. Again, this is important in relation to questions of social integration and order. Although, again, it is equally possible for emotion to have a disruptive effect and to be a motivating force in macro-cosmic change (cf. also Collins 1990).

EMOTION AND PERSONAL HISTORY

Having identified the place of emotion in communicative exchanges it is necessary to make a brief note with respect to the issue of individual personality. In the work of Sartre, both *The Emotions* and more generally (e.g. Sartre 1969), there is a tendency to ahistoricity. Sartre's untenable belief in absolute human freedom leads him to the view that human beings respond to each of their situations anew, constantly re-creating themselves. This, as Merleau-Ponty (1962) observes, runs contrary to what we know of the predictability and regularity of human behaviour and of the apparent stability of human personalities. In contrast to Sartre, Merleau-Ponty posits a notion of the 'institution' of personal history, which is intended to capture the process by which repeated responses and forms of understanding and interpreting become sedimented in our praxes over time, giving rise to stable preferences for certain types of response (Crossley 1994). This extends to the sphere of emotion for Merleau-Ponty. We acquire and develop an individual emotional repertoire, he notes, or, to use another (equally apt) expression, an emotional 'habitus' (Crossley 1994).

This is not to deny the possibility of radical personal change. It is possible that we might 'blow' our sedimented ways of being 'sky-high' (Merleau-Ponty 1962: 442). But it is to suggest that such change is very unlikely or improbable. One example of this which Merleau-Ponty discusses is of an 'inferiority complex' (in the colloquial sense):

> It is improbable that I should at this moment destroy a inferiority complex in which I have been content to live for twenty years. That means that I have committed myself to inferiority, that I have made it my abode, that this past, though not a fate, has at least a specific weight and is not a set of events over there, at a distance from me, but the atmosphere of my present.
>
> (Merleau-Ponty 1962: 442)

These dispositions are not arrived at by the individual in isolation. Like Habermas, Merleau-Ponty recognizes that personalities are produced and reproduced by way of communicative action; that the individual is an abstraction from the group. Our emotional habitus is the result of a shared history.

None of this is new and it is clear that Merleau-Ponty's view raises more questions than it answers. The point in raising it in this chapter, however, is, first, to point out that emotional responses, as they manifest in communicative situations, draw upon a habitus. Thus the significance of any emotional response will not necessarily be reducible to the particularity of an individual's current situation (or role) but will also point backwards to that individual's personal history. Secondly, I raise it to point out that communicative situations and actions can have a relatively permanent effect upon emotional ways of being. Merleau-Ponty's 'inferiority complex' will have effects upon his current and future communicative exchanges. It will be consequential to the attempts at social integration in the arenas that he mixes. But it is equally an effect of his past communicative actions because his history, like any other, is a history of relationships. As the final sentence in *The Phenomenology of Perception* puts it: 'Man is but a network of relationships, and these alone matter to him [*sic*]' (1962: 456).

THE LIMITS OF EXISTENTIALISM

The existentialist view of emotions has many important strengths. In particular it allows us to overcome the tendency to reduce emotion to a series of mechanical or physiological responses (unintelligent sensations) and to see it as an aspect of the purposive and intentional (in the phenomenological sense) life of human beings. We can see emotion as a positive, purposive and meaningful response to situations. More specifically we can see it as a 'magical' way of reasoning about and constituting the world. The description of emotion as magical is particularly persuasive because it captures well the unusual processes of association which accompany emotive thought and the manner in which emotive subjects transform the complexion of the world. Moreover, the general description of emotion as a purposive behaviour opens the door to a sociological treatment of it. It puts emotion within the remit of social theories and studies of interaction. This allows us to join it with the work of Habermas and thus to consider the emotional aspect of communicative action.

Notwithstanding this, however, there are a number of difficulties with the existential position. Two in particular require discussion. In the first instance I would suggest that our concern with the meaningful and purposive nature of emotion should not be allowed to obscure the potential for the alteration of emotional states at the biological level. Mood-altering drugs, from Prozac to Ecstasy, form part of the everyday life of many people in our society. And though the placebo effect of such drugs, combined with the social learning required to experience certain drug effects (Becker 1953), may be strong factors in transforming biological processes into psychological and social experiences, it would be foolish to ignore the role of biology. This is an issue which the existentialists, or at least Merleau-Ponty, recognize. Our organic constitution facilitates meaningful and purposive engagement with the world, he argues, but it is still organic and it is still subject to the vulnerabilities of all organic systems, with the psychological consequences which this entails. Nevertheless, it is a point which needs closer consideration than he affords it, particularly in light of the increasing development and use of bio- and pharmo-technologies. We must recognize the place of artificial (chemical) as well as natural (purposive) emotions in social life.

Another issue which existential theories fail to engage with is the extent to which emotions are reflexively monitored and managed (Hochschild 1983). Emotion is part of the pre-reflective structure of consciousness and it is important to recognize and discuss this (as the existentialists do), but it is equally a key figure in the reflective projects and accounts of social agents (Hochschild 1983; Giddens 1991, 1992). In addition to what I have already said in this chapter, our emotions can be 'things' that we think and talk about and that we put a value upon. Indeed it may be quite fashionable in some circles to talk about emotions (Wouters 1991), as it has been fashionable amongst the middle classes to suffer from 'nerves' in the past (Porter 1990). Furthermore, given this, it is important to recognize that emotional subjects are open to manipulation or interpellation by various psychotherapeutic technologies and the markets in which they operate. Ours is an era that has seen a vast expansion of psy- discourses and practices, which invite and persuade us to inspect, master and control various aspects of our emotional life, or, again, which offer us happiness and emotional fulfilment (Rose 1989; Giddens·1991, 1992; Craib 1995). There are extensive networks and technologies for the inspection, confession, governance and transformation of affect. And they are significant. Within the institutions of psychotherapy and psychology decisions are made about the reasonableness of emotional states, and those deemed unreasonable are transformed into 'technical' problems which require technical solutions (Rose 1989; Craib 1995; Kendall and Crossley 1996). Clearly the operation of such industries should be a concern for sociologists of the emotions, as indeed should the emotional extremes that they sometimes deal with. This is a point of overlap between the sociology of emotions and the sociology of psychiatry and psychotherapy.[4]

It is important to raise this point, in light of the Habermasian concerns of this chapter, because for Habermas the 'colonization of the lifeworld' by expert systems, and the consequent 'cultural impoverishment', is one of the key features of the contemporary social world. He is precisely concerned that communicative action is increasingly less able to function unhindered – which is partly what is at stake in the governance of emotion. This is an issue which we cannot develop here, but it is clearly important and deserves future discussion. Moreover, it is a problem that will necessitate that we go beyond the horizons of the existential approach.

CONCLUDING REMARKS

I began this chapter with the observation that Habermas's theory of communicative action, although at the leading edge of theories of social action, fails to consider the place of emotion in social interaction. The purpose of the chapter, I stated, was to consider how this problem could be corrected. The chapter then considered two approaches to the study of emotion which would enable Habermas to incorporate an understanding of emotion: linguistic philosophy and existential-phenomenology. My argument has been that Habermas must incorporate insights from both of these approaches (and more besides) into his account if it is to be adequate.

Neither approach is adequate on its own. In particular, the linguistic approach deals with the reflexive accountability of emotion, to the detriment of the lived experience, whilst existentialism deals with pre-reflective lived experience, to the detriment of the reflexive accountability. Furthermore, both fail to consider that the reflexive accountability of emotion is bound up, in the contemporary era, with complex discourses and technologies for the observation, regulation and transformation of emotional life – an issue that is important from the Habermasian viewpoint. Despite their differences, however, the linguistic approach and the existential approach both point in a similar direction. Both try to show that emotional life, in principle at least, forms part of the intentional and intersubjective life of human beings, and as such that it falls within the parameters of communicative rationality and the normative order of the lifeworld. The significance of this is that Habermas's theory of communicative action *can* incorporate a concern with emotion, allowing itself to be broadened and strengthened by such considerations, without any fundamental alterations in its basic structure. The lifeworld can be seen to consist in emotional as well as cognitive processes. The full implications of this for Habermas's philosophy and sociology must be considered at another time. For present purposes it is sufficient to have established a space within his work for the emotions.

However, this chapter has not just been about Habermas. Whilst the gaps in his work have formed the framework for my discussion, much of the substantive content of the chapter has addressed the possible contributions of linguistic philosophy and existential-phenomenology to a social theory of emotions. These theories, I have shown, provide a great number of insights into emotional life and its place within the social world. And they overlap at a number of points with other work currently being done in the sociology of the emotions. It is my hope that this will prove sufficient to stimulate further discussion of their work amongst social scientists with an interest in emotions, perhaps independently of the Habermasian moorings that I have adopted here.

NOTES

1 'Rationality' is used here in Habermas's (1994) post-metaphysical sense. In essence it implies that interactions are able to be examined in terms of the intersubjectively shared validity claims discussed in this paper.
2 I have also criticized Habermas for his failure to consider the perceptual subject (Crossley 1996) and for his failure to consider embodiment (Crossley 1997). This reflects my general view that Habermas provides one of the most useful starting-points for contemporary sociology and social theory, but that his work must be broadened to take consideration of existential issues.
3 This line of argument does not preclude the possibility of an overlapping, in practice, of emotions and sensations. For a discussion of such an overlapping, in relation to pain, see Bendelow and Williams (1995). Their paper also draws out the numerous ways in which pain sensations assume meaning and are related to

pain behaviours – a more sophisticated view of sensation than my brief discussion manages.

4 The field of the sociology of psy- sciences is too broad to make any specific references. For a general overview of the field, however, see Pilgrim and Rogers (1994).

BIBLIOGRAPHY

Austin, J. (1971) *How to Do Things with Words*. Oxford: Oxford University Press.

Bateson, G. (1973) *Steps to an Ecology of Mind*. St Albans, Herts: Granada.

Becker, H. (1953) 'Becoming a marihuana user', *American Journal of Sociology* 59: 235–42.

Bendelow, G. and Williams, S. (1995) 'Pain and the mind–body dualism: a sociological approach', *Body and Society* 1(2): 83–103.

Benjamin, J. (1991) *The Bonds of Love*. London: Virago.

Collins, R. (1990) 'Stratification, emotional energy, and the transient emotions', in T. Kemper (ed.) *Research Agendas in the Sociology of the Emotions*. New York: State University of New York Press, pp. 27–57.

Coulter, J. (1979) *The Social Construction of Mind*. London: Macmillan.

Craib, I. (1995) *The Importance of Disappointment*. London: Routledge.

Crossley, N. (1993) 'The politics of the gaze: between Foucault and Merleau-Ponty', *Human Studies* 16(4): 399–419.

Crossley, N. (1994) *The Politics of Subjectivity*. Aldershot, Hants: Avebury.

Crossley, N. (1995a) 'Merleau-Ponty, the elusive body and carnal sociology', *Body and Society* 1(1): 43–63.

Crossley, N. (1995b) 'Body techniques, agency and intercorporeality: on Goffman's *Relations in Public*', *Sociology* 29(1): 133–49.

Crossley, N. (1996) *Intersubjectivity: The Fabric of Social Becoming*. London: Sage.

Crossley, N. (1997) 'Corporeality and communicative action: embodying the renewal of critical theory', *Body and Society* 3(1): 17–47.

Durkheim, E. (1915) *The Elementary Forms of Religious Life*. London: Allen & Unwin.

Durkheim, E. (1964) *The Division of Labour*. New York: Free Press.

Elias, N. (1984) *The Civilizing Process*. Oxford: Blackwell.

Giddens, A. (1991) *Modernity and Self-Identity*. Cambridge: Polity Press.

Giddens, A. (1992) *The Transformation of Intimacy*. Cambridge: Polity Press.

Goffman, E. (1972) *Relations in Public*. Harmondsworth, Mx: Penguin.

Habermas, J. (1974) 'Labour and interaction: remarks on Hegel's Jena *Philosophy of Mind*', in *Theory and Practice*. London: Heinemann, pp. 142–69.

Habermas, J. (1987) *The Theory of Communicative Action*, Vol. 2, *System and Lifeworld*. Cambridge: Polity Press.

Habermas, J. (1991) *The Theory of Communicative Action*, Vol. 1, *Reason and Rationalisation*. Cambridge: Polity Press.

Habermas, J. (1992) *Knowledge and Human Interests*. Cambridge: Polity Press.

Habermas, J. (1994) *Postmetaphysical Thinking*. Cambridge: Polity Press.

Heidegger, M. (1962) *Being and Time*. Oxford: Blackwell.

Hobbes, T. (1971) *Leviathan*. Harmondsworth, Mx: Penguin.

Hochschild, A. (1983) *The Managed Heart: The Commercialization of Human Feeling*. Berkeley: University of California Press.

Hochschild, A. (1989) 'Reply to Cas Wouters' review essay on *The Managed Heart*', *Theory, Culture and Society* 6(3): 439–47.

Honneth, A. (1995) *The Struggle for Recognition*. Cambridge: Polity Press.

Kendall, T. and Crossley, N. (1996) 'Governing love: on the tactical control of counter-transference in the psychoanalytic community', *Economy and Society* 25(2): 178–94.

Kruks, S. (1990) *Situation and Human Existence*. London: Unwin Hyman.

Laing, R. (1961) *The Divided Self*. Harmondsworth, Mx: Penguin.

MacMurray, J. (1962) *Reason and Emotion*. London: Faber & Faber.

Mead, G. (1967) *Mind, Self and Society*. Chicago: University of California Press.

Merleau-Ponty, M. (1962) *The Phenomenology of Perception*. London: Routledge.

Merleau-Ponty, M. (1965) *The Structure of Behaviour*. London: Methuen.

Merleau-Ponty, M. (1971) *Sense and Non-Sense*. Evanston, IL: Northwestern University Press.

Merleau-Ponty, M. (1988) *In Praise of Philosophy and Themes from the Lectures at the Collège de France*. Evanston, IL: Northwestern University Press.

Parsons, T. (1951) *The Social System*. New York: Free Press.

Pilgrim, D. and Rogers, A. (1994) 'Something old, something new: sociology and the organisation of psychiatry', *Sociology* 28(2): 521–38.

Porter, R. (1990) *Mind-Forg'd Manacles*. Harmondsworth, Mx: Penguin.

Rose, N. (1989) *Governing the Soul*. London: Routledge.

Ryle, G. (1949) *The Concept of Mind*. Harmondsworth, Mx: Penguin.

Sartre, J-P. (1969) *Being and Nothingness*. London: Routledge.

Sartre, J-P. (1993) *The Emotions: Outline of a Theory*. New York: Citadel.

Scheff, T. (1984) *Being Mentally Ill*. New York: Aldine.

Smith, T. (1992) *Strong Interaction*. Chicago: University of Chicago Press.

Turner, J. (1988) *A Theory of Social Interaction*. Cambridge: Polity Press.

Williams, S. and Bendelow, G. (1996) 'Emotions and sociological imperialism', *Sociology* 30(1): 145–55.

Winch, P. (1958) *The Idea of a Social Science*. London: Routledge & Kegan Paul.

Wittgenstein, L. (1953) *Philosophical Investigations*. Oxford: Blackwell.

Wittgenstein, L. (1969) *On Certainty*. Oxford: Blackwell.

Wouters, C. (1987) 'Developments in the behavioural codes between the sexes: the formalisation of informalisation in the Netherlands 1930–85', *Theory, Culture and Society* 4(2–3): 405–28.

Wouters, C. (1989a) 'The sociology of emotions and flight attendants: Hochschild's managed heart', *Theory, Culture and Society* 6(1): 95–124.

Wouters, C. (1989b) 'Response to Hochschild's reply', *Theory, Culture and Society* 6(3): 447–51.

Wouters, C. (1991) 'On status competition and emotion management', *Journal of Social History* 24: 699–717.

3 The limitations of cultural constructionism in the study of emotion

Margot L. Lyon

INTRODUCTION

The following chapter explores limitations of the cultural constructionist approach to emotion.[1] It does so through a reading of sources drawn primarily from anthropology. Although narrow in a disciplinary sense, the concentration on the anthropological literature is valuable, in that it allows a more direct consideration of how the culture concept itself is directly implicated in the limitations of constructionist treatments of emotion so influential in both anthropology and sociology.[2]

It is in anthropology, beginning with early psychoanalytic anthropology and with culture and personality studies, that the question of the influences of culture on emotion received its earliest discussion, although emotion was not itself the main object of study. And it is in anthropology that the culture concept takes its most self-conscious and forceful form. Anthropology is thus an ideal locus for the consideration of how the treatment of emotion is shaped in reference to this concept and its impact on cultural constructionism more generally. With a greater understanding of the logical foundations of cultural constructionism and the problems inherent within it, the value of a larger perspective on emotion should be manifest. Such a perspective should make possible the consideration of more fundamental questions in the study of emotion, including the place of the body in social agency.

CULTURAL CONSTRUCTIONISM AND EMOTION

The concept of culture continues to dominate knowledge production in contemporary anthropology. It has considerable importance in sociology as well, and, partly through the burgeoning field of cultural studies, has had increasing impact in the social sciences and humanities more generally. Culture is typically represented as a complex system of symbols, meanings, categories, models, or schemata that structure experience and action. The terms used are various but all place emphasis on questions of meaning and order, which in turn inform our discourse whatever our particular subject-matter. Cultural anthropology and 'cultural sociology' continue to give emphasis to the study of systems of meaning, and to see culture, through these, as generating both meaning and structure in social life.

In this way, culture is seen to mediate social processes and is construed as the source of real phenomena, that is, as determining the very structure and substance of human existence. Within the cultural constructionist approach, our categories of thought (and thus the ideas we have), how we talk (and thus what we say), our experiences and feelings, and what we express and do, are primarily determined by the culture in which we live. From this perspective, culture is seen as the primary source and the locus, to use a more sociological language, of the norms, values and rules, the internalized 'guidelines', in terms of which we live.

The conceptualization of culture through the construct of symbol dates most forcefully from the 1960s, stemming from C. Geertz's (1973 [1966]) pathbreaking formulation of culture as a symbolic system, as well as the work of others such as V. Turner (1967) and Schneider (1968). Although it has many variants (Ortner 1984), the concept of symbol has come to represent the range of 'nonrational ideas (presuppositions, cultural definitions, declarations, arbitrary classifications) and their verbal and nonverbal means of expression' (Shweder 1984: 45). Symbols are seen as vehicles for representations which in turn create or constitute the systems of meaning that 'make up' culture. The forms these representations take are seen to vary enormously in different contexts and different cultures. Symbols are further seen as capable of determining how different aspects of life are conceptualized and experienced by participants in a culture, that is, how individuals in that culture construct their worlds. The main idea of a symbolic anthropology, says Shweder, 'is that much of our action "says something" about what we stand for' (Shweder 1984: 45). The elaboration of some form of the symbolic as analytic has provided the basis for the enrichment and refinement of the culture concept.

The limitations of the anthropological application of the concepts of culture and symbol become most apparent in the treatment of emotion. Emotion – including feelings, sentiments, motivation, expression, and their representations – is seen from this perspective to be the product of cultural construction through an individual's socialization and his or her continuing experience in a particular sociocultural context. Typically, this emotion is accessed through a particular culture's language categories, its 'vocabularies of emotion' (H. Geertz 1959; Davitz 1969) as examined in cultural context. Words are seen to be premier symbols.

From the constructionist point of view, almost any aspect of being may be conceived of as a cultural production, and it is this process of production which is the subject of much of cultural anthropology. The self, for example, is perceived as primarily a cultural production, as are the concepts of person and other (Levy 1984). An enriched notion of culture is seen to underpin an increased understanding of such concepts and their interrelationships (M. Rosaldo 1984). Emotion, too, is understood as a cultural production, and is seen to take its place alongside other constructs in anthropological inquiry. When so placed, emotion is often treated in terms of its implications for the construction of self or person in a particular cultural context. Indeed, the growing interest within a 'postmodern' anthropology in the concept of self and person has fuelled a resurgence of interest in emotion, but an interest that continues to operate largely within the constructionist frame.

Marcus and Fischer addressed the interrelationships of person, self and emotion in their work on anthropology as cultural critique (1986: 45–76). The authors saw the new concern with cultural 'conceptions of personhood – the grounds of human capabilities and actions, ideas about the self, and the expression of emotions' as a means to reveal cultural differences while cutting through 'the apparent homogenization of contemporary institutional forms of social life, particularly now that there seems to be a withering away of publicly enacted traditions' (1986: 45). According to Marcus and Fischer, anthropologists must now 'resort to cultural accounts of less superficial systems of meaning' (1986: 45) in the context of postmodernity where the relationship between private meaning and public symbol is problematized. The focus on the concepts of person, self and emotion, then, is seen as a means of seeking and accessing a more authentic cultural domain. The authors go on to provide a review of a number of works in anthropology which treat the cultural account of personhood and related themes in differing ways (Marcus and Fischer 1986: 45–76).

In the context of postmodernity as they define it, cultural tools may indeed reveal cultural differences. But the problems put in perspective by Marcus and Fischer are also useful in clarifying the limitations of the constructionist approach to emotion – not only in conventional ethnography but in anthropological accounts of contemporary society. One must go beyond constructionism if one aims, for example, to understand the role of contemporary institutional contexts in the generation and development of cultural difference. This holds as well for the generation, experience and expression of emotion. By going beyond purely cultural accounts, one can more directly address the problematic relationship between private meaning and public symbol (or action) to which Marcus and Fischer draw attention.

In a truly social account, the relationship between public and private domains is the very point. That is, it is important to consider the social conditions which make problematic the relationship between a person's place in a particular social-structural context and his or her subjective experience of that place, including interpretations arising from it. This theme recalls Mills's (1959) notion of the 'sociological imagination' through which the connections between private experience and public issues may come to be understood. Individuals 'in the welter of their daily experience, often become falsely conscious of their social positions', for 'within that welter, the framework of modern society is sought, and within that framework the psychologies of a variety of men and women are formulated' (1959: 5).

The sociological imagination 'enables its possessor to understand the larger historical scene in terms of its meaning for the inner life and the external career of a variety of individuals' (1959: 5).

What does anthropology typically do when it addresses emotion? Anthropological understandings of emotion have generally been achieved, whatever their individual differences, through more detailed and refined cultural analysis.[3] A number of these have raised issues fundamental to the anthropological analysis of emotion. Here, at least initially, I shall briefly draw on a few sources only, among them Michelle Rosaldo's 'Toward an anthropology of self and feeling' (1984) and Lutz's discussion of the cultural construction of emotion in *Unnatural Emotions* (1988). Other sources will be introduced for the purposes of the clarification of particular points. I have placed Rosaldo's work in the foreground because she is one of the first authors directly to formulate key issues in the cultural construction of emotion, and many of these formulations have in one form or another been followed by others. I would ask the reader to note here that the critique that is the subject of this chapter refers to certain dominant perspectives in the cultural construction of emotion; it is not intended as a critique of any individual author's exploration of emotion in the diverse cultural contexts in which he or she worked. Indeed, much of what constitutes differences between particular cultural accounts of emotion seems to be the result of the use of variants in the culture concept. This looks like an attempt to overcome problems in the treatment of emotion, problems that are, in fact, more fundamental than can be resolved in this fashion.

The cultural anthropological study of emotion seeks at base to understand 'the ways that innerness is shaped by culturally laden sociality' (M. Rosaldo 1984: 140). This view, Rosaldo says, closely follows the work of Geertz in its insistence 'that meaning is a public fact, that personal life takes shape in cultural terms, or better yet, perhaps, that individuals are necessarily and continually involved in the interpretive apprehension (and transformation) of received symbolic models' (M. Rosaldo 1984: 140). Lutz, too, follows Rosaldo's emphasis on viewing emotions 'as forms of symbolic action' (Lutz 1988: 6). For Rosaldo, and for others concerned with its cultural construction, emotion is construed as part of an inner and, by implication, psychological life, which is both produced by culture and subject to cultural influence that acts on the individual, whatever finer differences are put on it. Affects are, says Rosaldo, 'cognitions – or more aptly, perhaps, interpretations – always culturally informed, in which the actor finds that body, self and identity are immediately involved' (M. Rosaldo 1984: 141).

Following Rosaldo, Lutz frames her discussion of emotion in terms of 'how emotional meaning is fundamentally structured by particular cultural systems and particular social and material environments' (1988: 5). Emotion has 'value as a way of talking about the intensely meaningful as that is culturally defined, socially enacted, and personally articulated' (Lutz 1988: 5).

The social world for Rosaldo and for most constructionists is subsumed, through the person, to culture just as is emotion: 'Society . . . shapes the self through the medium of cultural terms' (M. Rosaldo 1984: 150). The emphasis on the concept of self has been regarded as an advance because it is seen as taking the consideration of emotion out of a psychobiological realm that is not accessible to conventional anthropological analysis. It also goes beyond the psychoanalytic focus on the individual psyche to regard the individual in a context, although this is still clearly a psychological approach.

The cultural constructionist approach to emotion has real limitations. I say this because emotion is more than a domain of cultural conception, more than mere construction, and thus cannot be treated merely as parallel to constructions such as self and person in the sense that they are used in most cultural anthropology. Person and self seem to function as intermediate constructs in anthropology, as 'surrogate symbols' or complexes thereof, which often function to mystify the relationships they are meant to encompass. To treat these purely as domains of cultural inquiry (self, person and emotion), or as different sets of ethnographic information each of which may inform the construction of meaning in the other, seems a form of chasing one's tail. In such an approach, emotions simply become subsumed to the concept of person as this is culturally constructed. The defining of one subject in terms of others within the same cultural context does not just risk circularity; it restricts our ability to ask more fundamental questions about the subjects of concern including their basis in different social and bodily forms. Culture itself is not, of course, self-sustaining; it has a basis in social organization and practices, and is subject to change. Nor is it, in itself, capable of producing identifiable effects independent of its rootedness in social structure and social praxis.

While accepting that the cultural dimensions of emotion are an important subject of inquiry, wholly constructionist approaches can obscure our view of the phenomenon of emotion in the larger sense, that is, the understanding of the importance of emotion not only in culturally produced and mediated experience, but in social and bodily agency as conceived in terms of its foundation in social structure. One might contrast, for example, Shweder's (1984: 45) statement that 'much of our action "says something" about what we stand for' with Mills's understanding of the situating of actions in reference to vocabularies of emotion, or 'motive' to use Mills's terms. Mills shows that what is 'said' through our action is often less about *what* we stand for than *where* we stand. That is, the vocabulary of motive (actions, words) varies also according to a person's place in society: '[t]he variable is the accepted vocabulary of motives, the ultimates of discourse, of each man's dominant group about whose opinion he cares' (Mills 1940: 910). Motives, for Mills, 'stand for anticipated situational consequences of questioned conduct. Intention or purpose . . . is awareness of anticipated consequence; motives are names for consequential situations, and surrogates for actions leading to them' (1940: 905). The study of motives is thus about the nature of the 'groups, their location and character', which determine them (Mills 1940: 910). While the repertoire of words and actions that help to shape the 'vocabulary of motive' is culturally grounded, the sociological focus helps take inquiry about emotion beyond the question of cultural forms and its associated emphasis on psychological models, and thus beyond questions of personhood and self.

IDEATIONAL BIAS IN THE CULTURAL CONSTRUCTION OF EMOTION

Implications of the overall ideational bias of constructionism are frequently underacknowledged. This is a crucial matter in the case of emotion. In constructionist treatments, emotion is generally understood in primarily ideational terms, i.e. as a cognitive or mental phenomenon which is subject to cultural production. The apprehension of emotion in this sense is seen to be achieved through an understanding of cultural categories of emotion and expression. This is not to deny the importance of culture in the experience of emotion, through its conceptual and expressive forms, and in behaviour; it is to say that the exploration of the influence of culture in these is neither the beginning nor the end of the matter. The notion of cultural *construction* might even be seen as a misnomer in that cultural information does not actually 'construct' anything; rather, it is important as it arises as part of the shaping of the organizational possibilities of interacting parties (Kemper 1978a, 1981).

In anthropology, the treatment of emotion becomes a function of the conception of culture that is held and of the 'units' of culture under study. This takes a number of forms. Emotion may be ignored or excluded, as in utilitarian or practical approaches to causal explanation in cultural domains (for example, in economics and models of cultural change), or as in the treatment of culture as pure knowledge (in structuralism and much of earlier cognitive anthropology). It may be treated as part of the realm of symbolic forms that are seen as concerned with meaning and order and thus harnessed to the concept of symbol or related concepts. Or, it may be regarded primarily as an aspect of the individual psyche, however the relationship of this psyche to action may be seen, such as in various psychodynamic or psychoanalytic approaches. The first two types exclude the affective dimension and emphasize reason and rationality in human cognitive functioning. The third, through the concept of symbol, seeks to combine both cognitive and affective components, although the way in which this is done is not always explicit. Psychological forms of explanation may take emotion into account through its functioning in the psyche or through some form of psycho-cultural explanation. All of the above tend to be ideational in orientation (Keesing 1974). The concern in this chapter is primarily with symbolic anthropology and its difficulties in specifying the relationship between cognitive and affective components and the consequent limitations on its treatment of emotion.

In cultural analysis, to reiterate some earlier points, emotion is most frequently examined in terms of what are seen to be its major symbolic forms and their expression. For example, one sees the representation of emotion through the symbols of language, within classification systems, in the socialization process, in ritual and so forth, that is, in terms of ideas about emotion which are seen to determine its expressive and active forms. Yet, the concept of symbol is used both to *represent* an emotion or feeling aspect and as something that can *engender* emotion in actors (C. Geertz 1973 [1966]). Symbols, as the vehicles of cultural representations and therefore culture, are seen to contain somehow or represent the feeling and expressive dimensions of culture, as well as to function in ways that arouse and establish emotion states. This dual aspect, this dual function that is made to be served by the concept of symbol, is partly a result of the ideational emphasis in cultural analysis.

The inchoateness of the symbol concept gives rise to contradictions which become ramified in the analysis of emotion. This is not least because, while one can deal with the cultural representation of emotion in various domains, it becomes impossible to deal directly and explicitly with the human embodiment of emotion – the 'guts' of feeling which are a necessary part of its experience. It is also impossible within the symbolic domain to deal adequately with the importance of social relations in the genesis of emotion. The duality of the concept of symbol needs to be made manifest and faced directly if we are to go beyond the limitations of the constructionist approach in the understanding of emotion.

UNRESOLVED CONTRADICTIONS IN THE CONCEPT OF SYMBOL

As noted above, the concept of symbol in cultural anthropology may be characterized in terms of its emphasis on 'nonrational ideas (presuppositions, cultural definitions, declarations, arbitrary classifications) and their verbal and nonverbal means of expression' (Shweder 1984: 45). Culture, to quote Shweder again, is seen to be rational as well as a manifestation or realization of a 'nonrational, extra-logical, arbitrary partitioning of the world' (Shweder 1984: 45). In so far as cognition and emotion as received categories are both encompassed within the concepts of culture and symbol, each may be viewed as forms of rational as well as non-rational phenomena without considering the problematic of the relationship between them. The inchoateness of the concept of culture acts to maintain and leave unquestioned the conventional distinction between emotion and cognition.

This inchoateness also acts to hinder transcendence of the distinction between the rational and irrational. Terms such as non-rational and extra-logical attempt to overcome in lexical form the problem of the irrational/rational distinction that underlies so many categories in social science. However, though such terms apparently step outside it, they also serve to acknowledge and maintain it, albeit in a modified form, and thus in themselves do little to obviate it. In effect, this approach seems simply to place the concepts of culture and symbol on top of conventional western thought categories that at base are grounded in such distinctions, and therefore serve to mystify them by including both aspects within the one concept. Under this regime, emotion, when considered within the symbolic approach (whether or not mediated through the notion of non-rational), may continue to be identified with the irrational as it is in western folk categories (Leeper 1948) and in psychoanalytic approaches (Spiro 1984). The concept of symbol applied to emotion makes it difficult to 'unpack' or clarify emotion, for it cannot be fully explicated using terms such as rational, irrational, non-rational; yet such terms encourage the continuance of discourse on emotion in reference to them. It further reinforces the treatment of emotion primarily as a mental process, and thus contributes to the avoidance of a confrontation with any of its material implications.

The distinction made between the irrational and the rational reflects and parallels many other oppositions in Anglo-western thought, such as those of subjectivity and objectivity, body and mind, the ideational and the material, culture and biology, and so forth. Such dualisms became embodied in the categories of the social sciences during the period of their intellectual organization in the late nineteenth and early twentieth centuries, when an increasingly rigid division was drawn between natural and non- or anti-naturalist sciences (Benton 1991). And, they persist today. Over time, in both anthropology and sociology the respective emphases on the cultural and the social as autonomous domains increased the separation of these fields from the natural sciences, leading to further restriction in the scope of inquiry.

The persistence of such contradictions places the treatment of emotion in anthropology in a curious position. There is the emphasis on the culturally influenced ideational aspects of emotion, aspects that via the concept of symbol as non-rational simultaneously include what are seen to be irrational and rational dimensions. This ideational emphasis also involves the treatment of emotion in a way that is discontinuous with its material and bodily dimensions. Further, emotion as an aspect of culture is seen as located simultaneously within individual minds and within cultural phenomena as a whole. Embedded in this position are the same tensions regarding the 'locus' of emotion as in arguments about the locus of culture more generally, that is, how does one treat emotion as simultaneously of the individual and the group in a way that is both dynamic and capable of clarifying the relationship between the two? And, what is its relationship to social forms?

The problem of the 'location' of emotion

So 'where' is emotion? If it is seen to lie primarily in the symbolic domain, it is therefore subject to the ideational bias and other limitations of the symbolic approach. If it is seen as a function of the individual psyche and therefore primarily a psychological construct, the question of the relation of emotion in this 'inner' sense to emotion as a cultural construct becomes central. This tension between the locating of emotion in culturally constituted phenomena or in individual psyches has led to a tendency in the anthropology of emotion to talk about emotion as though it is sometimes a creation of culture (which primarily inheres in the individual through socialization processes) and sometimes outside of cultural or societal restraints and so part of the irrational impulses of the individual psyche. Spiro, for example, addresses this tension and argues that emotion is properly considered outside the conception of culture (Spiro 1984: 324). Whatever the means of resolution, a cultural constructionist perspective entails the persistence of the problem of the relationship between 'inner' mental representations and 'outer' cultural representations, and thus the dominance of a psychological frame.

There is the additional and, to some degree, parallel question of how the bodily component of emotion can be introduced without treating it primarily as a cultural construct and thus 'inside' culture, or as a physical entity 'outside' of culture (and the mind). How can the bodily aspects of emotion be represented both in reference to individual bodies and in reference to the collective organization of bodies without being forced into a sort of Cartesian loop of movement between body and mind, between physicalist and idealist perspectives?

In sociology, emotion has traditionally been considered to inhere in individuals and to be outside social rules, thus to be a function of some asocial part of human nature, a view currently challenged by a new sociology of emotion (Thoits 1989). Anthropology, on the other hand, embraced emotion in terms of how its conception and expression were subject to cultural production. Yet the tensions in the two are in some ways parallel, for the problem of emotion's locus in the individual remains. Michelle Rosaldo states, for example: 'In anthropology, as in psychology, the cultural/ideational and the individual/affective have been construed as theoretically, and empirically, at odds' (M. Rosaldo 1984: 139).

More importantly, the problem of an individual versus a social-relational locus of emotion is compounded by the tendency to collapse analytically the distinction between culture and social relations (and thus, culture and society). In cultural anthropology, particularly, the former tends to be treated as somehow prior to the latter. This was of course a chief axis of tension between British and American anthropology up to the 1960s, and remains a source of tension in cultural constructionist versus materialist approaches to social life. There continue to be a number of forms of analysis in contemporary anthropology which give emphasis to the societal, e.g. studies of colonialism, peasant resistance, the effects of global capitalism (see Roseberry 1988 for a review). However, in so far as such studies are truly sociological, their explanatory models are to some degree independent of or superordinate to cultural constructionism. The collapse between culture and society remains and indeed seems to have been reinforced within current cultural anthropology (see Roseberry 1989 for a critique). In the case of emotion, such a position makes it difficult fully to address the question of the social-relational *ontology* of emotion which, as shall be seen, provides an alternative and more encompassing approach to the understanding of emotion. Emotion is thus more effectively approached in terms of how it organizes behaviour (Kemper 1978a; de Rivera 1984).

When the conceptual boundaries of the cultural-ideational framework become clear, and the limitations of cultural constructionist explanation are reached, it is evident that emotion remains conceptually inchoate and inner in form. The bodily dimensions of emotion remain underacknowledged except as they may be seen to be culturally and therefore conceptually defined, mobilized, or repressed. When the bodily, especially the physiological, dimensions of emotion *are* addressed directly in anthropology, the dominance of ideational perspectives often means that they are placed outside culture in a way which involves a partial reassertion of a physicalist (and causal) perspective; for example, in 'biogenetic structuralism' as applied to the analysis of ritual experience (Aquili *et al.* 1979). In the case of studies of emotion, such an approach tends to cast it in terms of how its manifestations are a function of particular physiological states modified in the context of culture. This remains close to the position of seeing emotion as associated with the primitive or irrational, even if ritual may be seen to shape and channel these manifestations.

The disappearing body

Within the cultural constructionist perspective, attention to the body is primarily through its representations, such that both the body and emotions 'take their shape from what one's world and one's conceptions of such things as body, affect, and self are like' (M. Rosaldo 1984: 143). Thus, body, self and affect are seen in terms of how they are mediated by their appropriate cultural conceptions. Michelle Rosaldo uses the phrase 'felt ideas' to harness the body to the cultural constitution of being: 'Emotions are thoughts somehow "felt" in flushes, pulses, "movements" of our lives, minds, hearts, stomachs, skin. They are *embodied* thoughts' (1984: 143). Emotions, like ideas, are located in the self and thus the two, emotion and cognition, are linked: emotions can be seen 'as cognitions implicating the immediate, carnal "me" – as thoughts embodied' (M. Rosaldo 1984: 138). Emotions 'are about the ways in which the social world is one in which *we* are involved' (M. Rosaldo 1984: 143). Emotion, for Rosaldo as well as for

Lutz (1988: 4, 63–4), comes into being when the self is engaged – an engagement which is partly mediated through the body. Attached to the concept of cognition is thus an implicate bodiliness.

Yet it is difficult to reconcile this with the limitations of the concept of culture: '[O]ur feeling that something much deeper than "mere" cultural fact informs the choices actors make may itself be the product of a too narrow view of culture' (M. Rosaldo 1984: 140). It remains that the bodily engagement in such accounts is seen to have to be mediated by culture, and that this mediation is via individual choices played out through interpretation and action in the context of culture. Culture makes a difference not only in what we think but how we feel about it, says Rosaldo, because 'through "interpretation", cultural meanings are transformed. And through "embodiment", collective symbols acquire the power, tension, relevance, and sense emerging from our individuated histories' (1984: 140–1). Thus, one is returned to the domain of symbols and meaning, with the power of collective symbols given their force through individual interpretation and the involvement of the body in this process.

There is, here, an acknowledgement of the bodily dimension; but in the overall context of the study of emotion, its cultural implicitness is troublesome. The bodily component remains 'hedged', harnessed closely to culturally mediated thought. It is so partly because it is caught up in the ideational bias of the concepts of culture and symbol. But the implication of this culturally implicate bodiliness, mediated through 'selves' acting in culture, also bears within it a view of the physical components of emotion as something beyond culture and so potentially disruptive. This dilemma and the confusion it creates are reflected in Rosaldo's own statements. For example, she states that '[i]t may well be that we require psychologies – or physiologies – or "energy" to fully grasp the ways in which symbolic forms are shaped, and given sense, through application to "embodied" lives'. She continues: '[B]ut then . . . it seems that insofar as they are culture-bound, psychologies lose their energetic force; whereas, when culture-free, accounts of psychic energies are, at best, provisional' (1984: 141). Such statements highlight the inability of purely cultural accounts to encompass and make sense of emotion in lived existence. The dilemma is made apparent again by Rosaldo's retreat to a restatement of the opposition between crude physicalist and symbolic accounts, when she states: '[F]eelings are not substances to be discovered in our blood but social practices organised by stories that we both enact and tell. They are structured by our forms of understanding' (M. Rosaldo 1984: 143).

The importance of the bodily dimension of emotion is acknowledged in Renato I. Rosaldo's 'Grief and a headhunter's rage: on the cultural force of emotions' (1984), an article which is frequently cited in connection with the critique of narrow cultural constructionism. R. Rosaldo states that cultural analysis is not sufficient to account for the power of feelings. It cannot make plausible such acts as severing a head (1984: 178). Using the terms 'emotional force' and the 'cultural force of emotion', Rosaldo attempts to reinsert the force of actual lived experiences into the cultural domain: 'The concept of force calls attention to an enduring intensity in human conduct which can occur with or without the dense symbolic elaboration conventionally associated with cultural depth' (1984: 192). But what is this 'force' and what is its relationship to the body and to culture? *How* does emotion assert a 'cultural force'? In undefined form, and particularly as it is glossed with culture, it seems to represent some notion of an irreducible core of strong feeling which somehow may underlie cultural forms, 'showing through', like the passions, somewhere in between M. Rosaldo's 'substances in the blood' and 'social practices'.

The point here is not to take either of these authors to task but to explore ways in which one might transcend the posing of category oppositions such as 'blood' and 'stories', and yet be able to deal with emotion in ways which make possible the understanding of its 'force'. The persistence of such oppositions is, as we have noted, at least partly a function of the limitations of the culturalist perspective itself, an echo of the culture/nature or material/ideational dichotomies embedded within it. Emotion is simultaneously treated as a primal force inhering in individuals by virtue of their bodily being, and yet constructed through cultural categories which also act upon our bodies. What must be considered are the processes by which collective symbols or anything else acquire power, not merely as they emerge from individual histories (within any given culture) but as they emerge from explicitly *social* ones. This, as we will see, provides a means to transcend the limitations of treating emotion as merely a function of culture or of individual psyches within a culture. Further, this emphasis permits the acknowledgement of the bodily dimensions of emotion through the understanding that social relationships are necessarily bodily: social processes are not just given being through ideas, rules, custom.

To make emotion a special form or case of cognition (Lutz 1988; M. Rosaldo 1984) contributes to the maintenance of the boundaries between biological being and the cultural world, and thus to the maintenance of category oppositions such as the immaterial or ideal versus the material. This persistence in anthropology (and social science generally) of theoretical tension between ideal approaches and those considered materialist or positivist has been noted above (Benton 1991; Ingold 1990). Its persistence in anthropology has been strengthened by more recent reactions to positivism in related fields such as the extreme relativism of postmodernism (Frank 1990). This axis of tension between the positivist and constructionist parallels the general bias in western philosophical traditions toward the opposition of body and mind, rationality and emotion, etc. To attempt to talk about the body within social science tends to result in one's discourse being directed into either a purely physicalist mode, or a cognitively biased mode which assigns 'mind priority over body, and severs it from its embodied form' (Freund 1988: 839). Hence, the dominance in anthropology of approaches which deal only 'with the meanings that cultures "bestow" on bodies' (Scheper-Hughes and Lock 1987), or with how the physical body constitutes a screen for projection of cultural and social concerns (Douglas 1970). An expanded inquiry into the body and embodiment would directly address the relevance of the physical body for the social order and, therefore, the search for a better understanding of the agency of the body in the social world (Freund 1988).

There have been a number of calls for an expanded study of the body in anthropology. One of the earliest was that of Blacking, who commented on 'the need to study the biological and affective foundations of our social constructions of reality' (1977: 1). Others include Jackson (1983), Scheper-Hughes and Lock (1987), and Csordas (1990). Further examples could be drawn from the literature of medical anthropology. Most of these draw directly on the phenomenological tradition, giving emphasis to the place of the body in human experience. Michael Jackson, for example, using Merleau-Ponty's concept of the 'lived body', as well as Bourdieu, calls for the development of 'a grounded and common-sense mode of analysis which lays emphasis on patterns of bodily praxis in the immediate social field and material world' (1983: 327). Culture, through the notion of the superorganic, has served, he says, 'as a token to demarcate, separate, exclude and deny; and although at different epochs the excluded "natural" category shifts about among peasants, barbarians, workers, primitive people, women, children, animals and material artefacts, a persistent theme is the denial of the somatic' (Jackson 1983: 328).

Other arguments for taking account of direct bodily experience which might be included here are those that emphasize the material bases of the formation of cognitive categories, such as the studies of the linguist Lakoff (1987) and the philosopher Johnson (1987). Their work on conceptual categories and key metaphors demonstrates the grounding of cognitive and cultural factors in bodily experience. Drawing on the work of Rosch on prototypes and basic-level structures, Lakoff presents a view of human cognitive categorization central to which is the notion that 'cognitive models are directly embodied with respect to their content, or else they are systematically linked to directly embodied models' (1987: 13). The primacy of basic-level categories is linked to bodily capacities, and their demonstrable grounding in the body provides support for his argument. Lakoff cites, for example, the work of Ekman *et al.* (1983) on facial and autonomic system correlates of a limited set of basic states associated with emotions which we name as anger, fear, sadness, happiness, etc. Taking the example of anger, Lakoff shows that metaphorical understandings of anger as heat and internal pressure correlate with particular bodily changes when anger is experienced. Thus, Lakoff, building on the work of Ekman *et al.*, suggests 'that our concept of anger is embodied via the autonomic nervous system and that the conceptual metaphors and metonymies used in understanding anger are by no means arbitrary; instead they are motivated by our physiology' (Lakoff 1987: 407). While Lakoff's concern here is with the nature of conceptual categories, an extension of Lakoff's work would be possible through the consideration generally of the place of emotion in processes of (cultural) categorization using, for example, sources on the role of emotion in learning and memory (for example, LeDoux 1989). Work on the psychoevolutionary ontology of emotion – such as that of Reynolds (1981) and Plutchik (1984) – could also be mentioned here. Reynolds, for example, shows how the affective and instrumental dimensions of human action are both evolutionarily and functionally intertwined and how human evolution, including cultural variation, involves the elaboration of these mechanisms (Reynolds 1981).

EMOTION, SOCIETY AND THE RE-EMBODIMENT OF SOCIAL SCIENCE

It is through the study of emotion that anthropology, and social science more generally, may best be fully 're-embodied'. But it can be so only through an understanding of emotion that goes beyond the ideational bias of most constructionist accounts of emotion, accounts which 'culturalize' emotion, extracting or alienating it from both societal and bodily domains. This expanded understanding of emotion must take account of the body *qua* body not simply as it is mediated by 'mind' but as part of the conception of emotion itself. Such an approach need *not* give priority to an innate biology of being. Biologies themselves are socialized, as Mauss, for example, argued in his account of 'techniques of the body' (1973 [1935]).

The study of emotion can provide an expanded understanding of the place of the body in society through a consideration of the agency of the body. Emotion has a central role in bodily agency, for by its very nature it links the somatic and the communicative aspects of being and thus encompasses both social and cultural domains. The body is the means by which we experience and actively apprehend the world (Merleau-Ponty 1962); through its agency we know the world and act within it. This 'being-in-the-world', this grounding in reality, is fundamentally linked to the material aspects of our bodies.

Our bodily existence means also that we exist in relationship to other material entities, that is, to other bodies and to the environment. An understanding of the agency of the body in society thus comes through its inter-communicative and active functions. Human emotional capacities are closely linked to sociality and thus have an important place in this agency. Action in the world is necessarily bodily, but it is also complex, for movements are never simply individual ones; they are always associative and therefore communicative, a process in which emotion is ever implicated (Lyon and Barbalet 1994: 48). Awareness of the somatic dimensions of action has been foregrounded in many areas in the social and natural sciences; for example, the importance of the body in social interaction (e.g. Goffman 1959), physiological sociology (e.g. Barchas 1976), medical sociology (B. Turner 1992, 1996), medical anthropology (e.g. Hahn and Kleinman 1983; Kleinman and Good 1985), behavioural medicine and immunology (e.g. Ader and Cohen 1975; Lyon 1993), as well as in phenomenological accounts as already mentioned.

But while the phenomenological position, for example, gives emphasis to the sensory interface between the body and the world that is experienced through it, the affective component in this process, the *felt* sense, the 'guts', is not fully represented. Nor is the way in which the body is implicated in larger social forms represented. The phenomenological perspective requires further extension through the consideration of emotion and its bodily and social dimensions. It is this that can lead us towards a more complete account of the body in society.

A richer view of emotion can be achieved by attending to the multiple facets of emotion all of which are implicated in its foundational role in social relations. Scherer (1984), for example, views emotion in terms of a series of aspects or components that function in the relationship of the individual to his or her social and material environment. These components include the evaluation of experience, physiological correlates, expression, a motivational component including intention or readiness, and subjective feeling states (Scherer 1984: 294). In this view, and indeed in any full approach to emotion, the bodily components are as much a part of the understanding of emotion as any other (Papanicolaou 1989).

Emotions are central to the understanding of the communicative and associative functions of the body (and thus the embodied person). Emotions activate bodies in ways that are attitudinal and physical and that have implications for the way individuals together create a common (though ever-changing) design, purpose, or order (Lyon and Barbalet 1994: 48; Lyon 1994). The activation occurs always in a social-relational context. Thus, emotion cannot be conceived as entirely separate from either psycho-physiological *or* social phenomena. Even from the perspective of neuro-anatomy, the neocortex and the limbic system, which are both involved in the experience and expression of emotion and the assessment of cognitive input, are also centrally associated with social behaviour (Pribram 1984).

A number of writers have shown that irrespective of culture, social-relational patterns – for example, relations of power and status – are productive of particular emotions (Kemper 1978a; de Rivera 1977). Thus, all other things being equal, it could be said, for example, that any action by one person or group of persons that is interfered with by another person or group can give rise to anger. Such a relational perspective takes us beyond the conceptualization of emotion as merely internal states whose experience and expression may be studied, depending on the discipline, through verbal, facial, autonomic, or other manifestations; it moves us towards the study of emotions as social phenomena. From the social-relational perspective, 'emotional behaviour is always relative to an *other*' (de Rivera 1984) and must be seen in reference to the social context. A truly sociological theory of emotion 'requires a sociological model of the conditions that may vary so as to induce emotions', for it is the case that 'an extremely large class of human emotions results from real, antici-pated, imagined, or recollected outcomes of social relationships' (Kemper 1978b: 32). For Kemper, culture has an important role in determining the nature of the power and status rights of actors in relationships within any given occasion, including ritual ones; in this way culture is implicated in the generation and experience of emotion (Kemper 1981: 355). M. Rosaldo, too, says that emotion has to do with the *sense* that something is at stake in which *we* are involved, but, as in much of the cultural constructionist work, the social and bodily bases of this sense are not – indeed cannot easily be – given prominence and so remain largely unexplored.

This is not to say that social-relational or social-structural bases of emo-tion are not addressed in the cultural anthropological literature. They are, of course. But social relations tend to be acknowledged primarily in terms of how they are part of the ethnographic context, the cultural circumstances which give emotions their expressive forms and their meaning, rather than as foundational in the genesis of emotion. The relationships between social-structural forms and emotion have rarely been acknowledged for their import in theorizing emotion cross-culturally (beyond the culture–individual axis). The descriptions of the social-relational contexts in which emotions are experienced among the Baining, the Ifaluk, the Kaluli and the Balinese, for example, as given in Fajans (1983), Lutz (1988), Schieffelin (1983) and Wikan (1990), respectively, are detailed and informative. Such accounts inform the reader of the specific cultural contexts encompassing particular patterns of relations. However, the very basis of the relationship between patterns of social relations and patterns of experience and expres-sion of emotion are not often explicitly examined. Thus, the relevance of social structure to the generation and organization of emotion is not given due attention. The rich material presented in such accounts would, however, lend itself to reworking in reference to the social-emotional approach advocated here.

Some anthropological accounts come closer to a social approach than others. Wikan (1990), for example, locates her account of Balinese fear of black magic in the discussion of wider social-structural issues. Myers, in his work on the Pintupi (1979, 1988), although still constructionist in orien-tation, takes pains to locate emotion in reference to explicit social-structural forms and strategies. Following Solomon (1976), he treats emotions as forms of judgement and logic, in the Kantian sense of 'those basic judgments and concepts through which . . . we constitute the world of our experience' (Solomon 1983 [1976]: 251). The emotions of anger and compassion, for example, separately and in a dialectical relation to one another, play an important role in the construction of political and kinship-based entities. While he sees these emotions in terms of how they are given specific cultural meanings, he also wishes to see them in terms of how they are grounded in a universal 'logic' of relations. The concept of 'logical forms' is thus used to embody both the idea of types of social relations and the conceptual structures possible in those social-relational contexts. While this is a step beyond narrower culturalist accounts, the concept of logical forms itself remains tied to cognitive or conceptual domains and does not give scope for how the body is implicated, that is, how it is activated in social-relational contexts.

An important implication of a truly social-relational perspective on emotion is to see not only how emotion has social consequences but how social relations themselves generate emotion. Emotion has a social ontology. That is, the experience of emotion, which involves both physical and phenomenal dimensions, has also a social-relational genesis. And what is subject to social relations is not merely the cognitive faculties but living human bodies, for society is also bodies in relation. Examples of accounts of the role of emotion in sociality in its various aspects, such as group formation and integration, and social differentiation, can be found, for example, in the work of Scheff (1988) and Collins (1984, 1990), as well as Kemper (1978a, 1984, 1990b).

This larger perspective should ultimately extend and refine the exploration of the semantic dimensions of emotion, as well as do so in a way less likely to fall back on standards of value and categories of meaning drawn from the dominant culture (a chief argument advanced in favour of cultural constructionist approaches). This applies as much to our intellectual categories as to our common-sense ones. As already noted, the ideational and psychological bias of much of the anthropology of emotion is a function of particular forces in the development of anthropology and the social sciences more generally. An expanded understanding of emotion and its social *and* biological ontology is required to move beyond the limitations of cultural constructionism. We must seek to take account of the formal social relations, such as power and status, which function in a structural manner irrespective of given differences in cultural context, in regrounding our study of emotion in society. And, we must overcome our fear of biology and thus seek to re-embody anthropology. There is nothing to prevent social scientists from studying embodied subjects in order to find ways better to comprehend human experience and behaviour, including social, religious and political phenomena, health and healing, and so forth. The study of emotion, in that it represents a bridging of social and somatic domains, is a most productive avenue for this.

56   *Margot L. Lyon*

NOTES

1 This chapter is a revised version of an article that appeared in *Cultural Anthropology* 10(2) (May 1995) under the title 'Missing emotion: the limitations of cultural constructionism in the study of emotion'. Reproduced by permission of the American Anthropological Association. Not for further reproduction.
2 There is a significant overlap between sociology and anthropology in the constructionist enterprise, fed partly by the growing influence of 'cultural studies' in each discipline (see McCarthy 1994 for consideration of the influence of culture theory on the social construction of emotion). The dominance of constructionism in sociology also has its roots, partly at least, in the influence of symbolic interactionism (Kemper 1990b: 16) (see Denzin 1987 for an interactionist perspective on culture and emotion). The sociology of emotion literature, taken in its broadest sense, tends to be more theoretically diverse than the anthropological literature. For a constructionist-orientated view review that gives emphasis to cross-cultural considerations, see Brakel (1994).
3 For example, in the informative work of anthropologists such as Abu-Lughod (1985, 1986), Briggs (1970), Epstein (1992), Fajans (1983), Feld (1982, 1990), H. Geertz (1959), Heider (1991), Keeler (1983), Lebra (1983), Levy (1973, 1984), Lutz (1988), Myers (1979, 1986, 1988), M. Rosaldo (1980, 1983, 1984), R. Rosaldo (1984), Schieffelin (1976, 1983), White (1985) and Wikan (1990), to name but a small selection of authors.

BIBLIOGRAPHY

Abu-Lughod, L. (1985) 'Honor and the sentiments of loss in a Bedouin society', *American Ethnologist* 12(2): 245–61.
Abu-Lughod, L. (1986) *Veiled Sentiments: Honor and Poetry in a Bedouin Society*. Berkeley, CA: University of California Press.
Ader, R. and Cohen, N. (1975) 'Behaviourally conditioned immunosuppression', *Psychosomatic Medicine* 37: 333–40.
Aquili, E. d', Laughlin, C. and McManus, J. (eds) (1979) *The Spectrum of Ritual: A Biogenetic Structural Analysis*, with Tom Burns, Barbara Lex, G. Ronald Murphy, SJ and W. John Smith. New York: Columbia University Press.
Barchas, P. (1976) 'Physiological sociology: interface of sociological and biological processes', *Annual Review of Sociology* 2: 299–333.
Benton, T. (1991) 'Biology and social science: why the return of the repressed should be given a (cautious) welcome', *Sociology* 25(1): 1–29.
Blacking, J. (1977) 'Toward an anthropology of the body', in John Blacking (ed.) *The Anthropology of the Body*. London: Academic Press, pp. 1–27.
Brakel, J. van (1994) 'Emotions: a cross-cultural perspective on forms of life', in W. M. Wentworth and J. Ryan (eds) *Social Perspectives on Emotion*, Vol. 2. Greenwich, CT: JAI Press, pp. 179–237.
Briggs, J. (1970) *Never in Anger*. Cambridge, MA: Harvard University Press.
Collins, R. (1984) 'The role of emotion in social structure', in K. R. Scherer and P. Ekman (eds) *Approaches to Emotion*. Hillsdale, NJ: Lawrence Erlbaum Associates, pp. 385–96.
Collins, R. (1990) 'Stratification, emotional energy, and the transient emotions', in T. D. Kemper (ed.) *Research Agendas in the Sociology of Emotions*. Albany, NY: State University of New York Press, pp. 27–57.
Csordas, T. (1990) 'Embodiment as a paradigm for anthropology', *Ethos* 18(1): 5–47.

Davitz, J. (1969) *The Language of Emotion*. New York: Academic Press.

Denzin, N. (1987) *On Understanding Emotion*. San Francisco: Jossey-Bass.

Douglas, M. (1970) *Natural Symbols: Explorations in Cosmology*. New York: Pantheon Books.

Ekman, P., Levenson, R. and Friesen, W. (1983) 'Autonomic nervous activity distinguishes among emotions', *Science* 221(4616): 1208–10.

Epstein, A. L. (1992) *In the Midst of Life: Affect and Ideation in the World of the Tolai*. Berkeley, CA: University of California Press.

Fajans, J. (1983) 'Shame, social action, and the person among the Baining', *Ethos* 11(3): 166–80.

Feld, S. (1982) *Sound and Sentiment: Birds Weeping, Poetics and Song in Kaluli Expression*. Philadelphia, PA: University of Pennsylvania Press.

Feld, S. (1990) 'Wept thoughts: the voicing of Kaluli memories', *Oral Tradition* 5(2–3): 241–66.

Frank, A. (1990) 'Bringing bodies back in: a decade review', *Theory, Culture and Society* 7: 131–62.

Freund, P. (1988) 'Bringing society into the body: understanding socialized human nature', *Theory and Society* 17: 839–64.

Geertz, C. (1966) 'Religion as a cultural system', in Michael Banton (ed.) *Anthropological Approaches to the Study of Religion*. ASA Monograph No. 3. London: Tavistock. [Reprinted in Geertz (1973).]

Geertz, C. (1973) *The Interpretation of Cultures*. New York: Basic Books.

Geertz, H. (1959) 'The vocabulary of emotion: a study of Javanese socialization processes', *Psychiatry* 22: 225–36.

Goffman, E. (1959) *The Presentation of Self in Everyday Life*. New York: Doubleday Anchor.

Hahn, R. and Kleinman, A. (1983) 'Belief as pathogen, belief as medicine: "voodoo death" and the "placebo phenomenon" in anthropological perspective', *Medical Anthropology Quarterly* 14(4): 16–19.

Heider, K. (1991) *Landscapes of Emotion: Mapping Three Cultures of Emotion in Indonesia*. Cambridge: Cambridge University Press.

Ingold, T. (1990) 'An anthropologist looks at biology', *Man* (N.S.) 25(2): 208–29.

Jackson, M. (1983) 'Knowledge of the body', *Man* (N.S.) 18(2): 327–45.

Johnson, M. (1987) *The Body in the Mind: The Bodily Basis of Meaning, Imagination, and Reason*. Chicago: University of Chicago Press.

Keeler, W. (1983) 'Shame and stage fright in Java', *Ethos* 11: 152–65.

Keesing, R. (1974) 'Theories of culture', *Annual Review of Anthropology* 3: 73–97.

Kemper, T. (1978a) *A Social Interactional Theory of Emotions*. New York: Wiley.

Kemper, T. (1978b) 'Toward a sociology of emotions: some problems and some solutions', *American Sociologist* 13: 30–41.

Kemper, T. (1981) 'Social constructionist and positivist approaches to the sociology of emotions', *American Journal of Sociology* 87(2): 336–62.

Kemper, T. (1984) 'Power, status, and emotions: a sociological contribution to a psychophysiological domain', in K. R. Scherer and P. Ekman (eds) *Approaches to Emotion*. Hillsdale, NJ: Lawrence Erlbaum Associates, pp. 369–83.

Kemper, T. (1990a) 'Social relations and emotions: a structural approach', in T. D. Kemper (ed.) *Research Agendas in the Sociology of Emotions*. Albany, NY: State University of New York Press, pp. 207–37.

Kemper, T. D. (ed.) (1990b) *Research Agendas in the Sociology of Emotions*. Albany, NY: State University of New York Press.

Kleinman, A. and Good, B. (eds) (1985) *Culture and Depression: Studies in the Anthropology and Cross-Cultural Psychiatry of Affective Disorder*. Berkeley, CA: University of California Press.

Lakoff, G. (1987) *Women, Fire, and Dangerous Things: What Categories Reveal about the Mind*. Chicago: University of Chicago Press.

Lebra, T. (1983) 'Shame and guilt: a psychocultural view of the Japanese self', *Ethos* 11(3): 192–209.

LeDoux, J. (1989) 'Cognitive-emotional interactions in the brain', *Cognition and Emotion* 3: 267–89.

Leeper, R. (1948) 'A motivational theory of emotion to replace "emotion as disorganized response"', *The Psychological Review* 55(1): 5–21.

Levy, R. (1973) *Tahitians: Mind and Experience in the Society Islands*. Chicago: University of Chicago Press.

Levy, R. (1984) 'Emotion, knowing, and culture', in R. A. Shweder and R. A. Levine (eds) *Culture Theory: Essays on Mind, Self and Emotion*. Cambridge: Cambridge University Press, pp. 214–37.

Lutz, C. (1988) *Unnatural Emotions: Everyday Sentiments on a Micronesian Atoll and Their Challenge to Western Theory*. Chicago: University of Chicago Press.

Lyon, M. L. (1993) 'Psychoneuroimmunology: the problem of the situatedness of illness and the conceptualization of healing', *Culture, Medicine and Psychiatry* 17(1): 77–97.

Lyon, M. L. (1994) 'Emotion as mediator of somatic and social process: the example of respiration', *Social Perspectives on Emotion*, Vol. II. Greenwich, CT: JAI Press, pp. 83–108.

Lyon, M. and Barbalet, J. (1994) 'Society's body: emotion and the "somatization" of social theory', in T. J. Csordas (ed.) *Embodiment and Experience: The Body as Existential Ground of Culture*. Cambridge: Cambridge University Press.

McCarthy, D. (1994) 'The social construction of emotions: new directions from culture theory', in W. M. Wentworth and J. Ryan (eds) *Social Perspectives on Emotion*, Vol. 2. Greenwich, CT: JAI Press, pp. 267–79.

Marcus, G. and Fischer, M. (1986) *Anthropology as Cultural Critique: An Experimental Moment in the Human Sciences*. Chicago: University of Chicago Press.

Mauss, M. (1973 [1935]) 'Techniques of the body' (trans. Ben Brewster), *Economy and Society* 2(1): 70–88.

Merleau-Ponty, M. (1962) *The Phenomenology of Perception*. London: Routledge & Kegan Paul.

Mills, C. (1940) 'Situated actions and vocabularies of motive', *American Sociological Review* 5: 904–13.

Mills, C. Wright (1959) *The Sociological Imagination*. New York: Grove Press.

Myers, F. (1979) 'Emotions and the self: a theory of personhood and political order among Pintupi Aborigines', *Ethos* 7(4): 343–70.

Myers, F. (1986) *Pintupi Country, Pintupi Self: Sentiment, Place, and Politics among Western Desert Aborigines*. Washington, DC: Smithsonian Institution Press.

Myers, F. (1988) 'The logic and meaning of anger among Pintupi Aborigines', *Man* 23: 589–610.

Ortner, S. (1984) 'Theory in anthropology since the sixties', *Comparative Studies in Society and History* 26: 126–66.

Papanicolaou, A. (1989) *Emotion: A Reconsideration of the Somatic Theory*. New York: Gordon & Breach.

Plutchik, R. (1984) 'Emotions: a general psychoevolutionary theory', in K. R. Scherer and P. Ekman (eds) *Approaches to Emotion*. Hillsdale, NJ: Lawrence Erlbaum Associates, pp. 197–219.

Pribram, K. (1984) 'Emotion: a neurobehavioral analysis', in K. R. Scherer and P. Ekman (eds) *Approaches to Emotion*. Hillsdale, NJ: Lawrence Erlbaum Associates, pp. 13–38.

Rivera, J. de (1977) *A Structural Theory of the Emotions*. New York: International Universities Press.

Rivera, J. de (1984) 'The structure of emotional relationships', in Phillip Shaver (ed.) *Review of Personality and Social Psychology: Emotions, Relationships, and Health*. Beverly Hills, CA: Sage, pp. 116–45.

Reynolds, P. (1981) *On the Evolution of Human Behaviour: The Argument from Animals to Man*. Berkeley, CA: University of California Press.

Rosaldo, M. (1980) *Knowledge and Passion: Ilongot Notions of Self and Social Life*. Cambridge: Cambridge University Press.

Rosaldo, M. (1983) 'The shame of headhunters and the autonomy of self', *Ethos* 11: 135–51.

Rosaldo, M. (1984) 'Toward an anthropology of self and feeling', in R. A. Shweder and R. A. Levine (eds) *Culture Theory: Essays on Mind, Self and Emotion*. Cambridge: Cambridge University Press, pp. 137–57.

Rosaldo, R. (1984) 'Grief and a headhunter's rage: on the cultural force of emotions', in S. Plattner and E. Bruner (eds) *Text, Play, and Story: The Construction and Reconstruction of Self and Society*. Washington, DC: American Ethnological Society, pp. 178–95.

Roseberry, W. (1988) 'Political economy', *Annual Review of Anthropology* 17: 161–85.

Roseberry, W. (1989) 'Anthropologies and histories', *Essays in Culture, History, and Political Economy*. New Brunswick, NJ: Rutgers University Press.

Scheff, T. (1988) 'Shame and conformity: the deference-emotion system', *American Sociological Review* 53: 395–406.

Scheper-Hughes, N. and Lock, M. (1987) 'The mindful body: a prolegomenon to future work in medical anthropology', *Medical Anthropology Quarterly* 1(1): 6–41.

Scherer, K. R. (1984) 'On the nature and function of emotion: a component process approach', in K. R. Scherer and P. Ekman (eds) *Approaches to Emotion*. Hillsdale, NJ: Lawrence Erlbaum Associates, pp. 293–317.

Schieffelin, E. (1976) *The Sorrow of the Lonely and the Burning of the Dancers*. New York: St Martin's Press.

Schieffelin, E. (1983) 'Anger and shame in the tropical forest: on affect as a cultural system in Papua New Guinea', *Ethos* 11(3): 181–91.

Schneider, D. (1968) *American Kinship*. Englewood Cliffs, NJ: Prentice-Hall.

Shweder, R. (1984) 'Anthropology's romantic rebellion against the Enlightenment, or There's more to thinking than reason and evidence', in R. A. Shweder and R. A. Levine (eds) *Culture Theory: Essays on Mind, Self and Emotion*. Cambridge: Cambridge University Press, pp. 27–66.

Solomon, R. (1983 [1976]) *The Passions*. Notre Dame, IN: University of Notre Dame Press.

Spiro, M. (1984) 'Some reflections on cultural determinism and relativism with special reference to emotion and reason', in R. A. Shweder and R. A. Levine (eds) *Culture Theory: Essays on Mind, Self and Emotion*. Cambridge: Cambridge University Press, pp. 323–46.

Thoits, P. (1989) 'The sociology of emotions', *Annual Review of Sociology* 15: 317–42.

Turner, B. (1992) *Regulating Bodies*. London: Routledge.

Turner, B. (1996) *Body and Society*. London: Sage.

Turner, V. (1967) *The Forest of Symbols*. Ithaca, NY: Cornell University Press.

White, G. (1985) 'Premises and purposes in Solomon Islands ethnopsychology', in G. M. White and J. Kirkpatrick (eds) *Person, Self and Experience: Exploring Pacific Ethnopsychologies*. Berkeley, CA: University of California Press, pp. 328–66.

Wikan, U. (1990) *Managing Turbulent Hearts: A Balinese Formula for Living*. Chicago: University of Chicago Press.

4   The sociogenesis of emotion
A historical sociology?

Tim Newton

INTRODUCTION

This chapter will draw on the work of Norbert Elias and Marjorie Morgan
in order to place our understanding of emotion within a sociohistorical
context. Attention is paid to the implications of this work for our current
theorizing around emotional labour, informalization, and gender and emotion. Some critical consideration is also given to limitations in the work of
Elias, particularly in regard to the metanarratival ambitions evinced in his
work.

The chapter will attempt to further our understanding of emotion through
a consideration of the development of emotion codes from the sixteenth to
the nineteenth centuries in France and England. Such emotion codes will be
explored through the historical analysis of their inscription within the social
practices of civility, manners and etiquette. The argument to develop this
kind of analysis follows directly from that supportive of social/cultural constructionist perspectives, and their emphasis upon the plasticity of emotion
and its lack of an essential universal vocabulary. For once one acknowledges
that emotion is socially constructed one is also implicitly drawing attention
to the historical, based on the simple argument that the social and cultural
are historically formed (Abrams 1982). In other words, how can we really
claim to know the social or the cultural if we are inattentive to the relations
surrounding their development? More specifically in relation to this book,
how can we aim to understand contemporary issues in emotion without
exploring the historical context in which they have evolved?

Many current writers on emotion would not take exception to such arguments. In consequence, it remains surprising how little detailed analysis has
been undertaken that relates *both* the historical and the social to emotion.
Even writers who are sensitive to the need for history still appear either to
thinly sketch the historical context, or to provide an historical account
that is unintegrated with their analysis of emotion. An example of the
former comes from James who drew on the 'historical perspective' of
Elias in order to argue for the commonality of emotional regulation and
restraint (James 1989: 18). But in her own analysis of the association

between emotional labour and gender, there is very little historical development beyond noting how emotional expression presents a 'particular problem for capitalism' since it may interrupt 'the mode of production' (1989:
24). Catherine Lutz (1988) gives an example of the latter in her interesting
account of the variance of emotional vocabulary across cultures, based on
her study of the 'Ifaluk' (a people who live on a coral atoll in the south-
west Pacific). Lutz provides some detail to her historical account of the
Ifaluk, examining the archaeological evidence and their historical relation
to the 'Yapese' empire, and to Europe and North America. Yet this history
is not related in any direct manner to the experience of emotion among the
Ifaluk. It is largely treated as 'background' material rather than something
which is closely involved in 'explaining' emotion.

Neither James nor Lutz is atypical, except in so far as they do actually pay
some attention to the relevance of history to the social construction of emotion. However, if we look beyond the sociology of emotion to wider influences within social theory, we can witness a growing interest in questions
of history and sociology (as illustrated by the vigorous debates in this
area such as those provided by Goldthorpe 1991, and the series of replies
to him in Hill and Rock 1994). This chapter will attempt to develop such
work by providing an account which is attentive to the argument that
both social relations and our subjectivity are socially created and historically
variable (Burkitt 1991; Newton 1996a). At the same time it will use this
account to question our current theorizing of emotion, particularly in relation to arguments concerning emotional labour, gender and emotion, and
the informalization of emotion codes. First, however, there is a need to
consider the extent to which we can assume any historical continuity in
our subjectivity.

HISTORICAL CONTINUITY?

What I wish to outline below resembles a history more than a Foucauldian
genealogy to the extent that it assumes *some* continuity across time. It does
not assume that history represents a linear development with one historical
'building block' placed neatly upon another. As Arditi argues, 'to the extent
that there is [historical] continuity, it is one punctuated by breaks, by non-
linearity, by unpredictability' (1994: 179). Yet this kind of acknowledgement does not necessarily imply an acceptance of a significant tenet of
Foucauldian genealogy, namely that 'accidents . . . accompany *every* beginning' (Foucault 1984: 80, my italics). Rather, following Elias, social
relations are seen as developing haphazardly, since within any figuration
there is the 'interweaving of countless individual interests and intentions'
(1994: 389). The fact that this interweaving is socially translated from one
moment to the next means that there is some likelihood of continuity.
For example, tacit codes of verbal and non-verbal expression are unlikely

just to disappear overnight, nor are they likely to change merely as the result of an 'accident'.

The work of Elias also has the advantage of developing a history which stresses both the social and the agential, a stress which again provides a point of contrast with Foucauldian genealogies. For though the work of Foucault and Foucauldians is significant in furthering our understanding of the history of the subject, their historicism is often achieved at the expense of a one-dimensionality in their treatment of the social wherein it becomes something 'invented by history and cathected by political passions' (Rose 1996: 3). Yet the Foucauldian dissection of the supposedly long dead body of the social (Baudrillard 1983) runs the risk of never really engaging with the ways in which people may have made sense of themselves and the social in an agential sense, since this dissection tends to take place on the lofty plane where the social is but another series of discursive constructs (Newton 1994, 1996a, 1996c; Findlay and Newton 1997).

While Elias's work does provide a point of distinct contrast, it is not one that is without its particular sins. In particular, his work appears at first sight to be difficult to square with any degree of postmodern sympathy (Newton 1996b), given his concern to develop a seeming metanarrative, and one that is more than occasionally given to the defence of universalistic statements. Though it is beyond the scope of this chapter to present a more general critique of Elias, further limitations with his approach will be considered below.

Elias

A very brief account will be outlined below, focusing on Eliasian concepts such as 'figuration' and 'courtly rationality' which appear particularly relevant to a sociohistorical analysis of emotion.

Elias argues that from the moment we are born we enter into a complex *figuration* of social interdependencies (Elias 1991). These interdependencies have evolved slowly through the changing social and political structures of particular epochs. They reflect the 'underlying regularities by which people in a certain society are bound over and over again to particular patterns of conduct and very specific functional chains, for example as knights and bondsmen, kings and state officials, bourgeois and nobles' (1994: 489). Elias stresses that these sociopolitical structures are in no sense fixed, and that power relations are rarely those of total dominance but reflect the changing balances between individuals and groups. In addition, Elias argues that there is unlikely to be any simple relation between a particular 'strategy' and a particular 'outcome' since within any figuration there is the 'interweaving of countless individual interests and intentions' (1994: 389). In consequence, 'something comes into being that was planned and intended by none of these individuals, yet has emerged nevertheless from their intentions and actions' (1994: 389). Analysis of such 'coming into being' is necessarily a study of processes since social figurations are continually in flux, never static or easily predictable.

In *The Civilizing Process*, Volumes 1 and 2, Elias explores the relation between changing figurations and the sociohistorical construction of codes of emotional display (Burkitt 1991, 1993). As Burkitt (1991) and Kuzmics (1991) illustrate, this aspect of his work has some parallels with the work of Goffman, except that Elias avoids the stasis of Goffman's analysis through linking historical changes in the presentation of the self to changes in power and social relations. For example, he argues that individuals in the Middle Ages could take open pleasure in acts of violence that would be greeted with repugnance today, and further suggests that people were subject to rather limited emotional and behavioural restraint in comparison with that which applies in western society today. He argues that this relatively unrestrained subjectivity changed as physical power became increasingly concentrated in the hands of individual monarchs (rather than being geographically dispersed amongst rival chieftains). He attempts to illustrate how within this new figuration of stable monarchies, the aristocratic classes became the new servants of a centralized power, rather than the defendants of individual fiefdoms. He suggests that one major consequence of the monopolization of the means of violence within individual monarchies was that those immediately subject to this power had to show a far greater civility than before. The emotional displays of this new civility are symbolized by *courtly society*, wherein courtiers beg favour of the king or queen, whilst others beg access to the court. Violence and aggression are replaced by politeness and the careful display of emotions as a tacit understanding of political process. Within the new royal courts

> the coarser habits, the wilder, more uninhibited customs of medieval society with its warrior upper class, the corollaries of an uncertain, constantly threatened life, were 'softened', 'polished' and 'civilized'. The pressure of court life, the vying for the favour of the prince or the 'great'; then, more generally, the necessity to distinguish oneself from others and to fight for opportunities with relatively peaceful means, through intrigue and diplomacy, *enforced a constraint on the affects, a self-discipline and self-control, a peculiarly courtly rationality.*
>
> (Elias 1994: 268, my italics)

Elias thus attempts to show how affective and behavioural constraints were associated with the courtly society, and the need of courtiers to show appropriate restraint to their 'betters' (reflected in current words such as 'courtly', 'civility', 'delicacy'). Through much of this analysis, the social self is not portrayed as static, but rather is seen to develop within the context of broad figurational changes.

REREADING THE SOCIOLOGY OF EMOTION THROUGH ELIAS

Amongst 'Eliasians' it is particularly Cas Wouters (see Chapter 13) who has attempted to reframe work on the sociology of emotions, most notably in his rereading of Arlie Hochschild's *The Managed Heart*. Wouters accuses Hochschild of falsely contrasting contemporary emotional labour with a supposed pre-industrial age where emotion management was a 'private act' (Hochschild 1983: 186), and where demands for emotional labour were considerably reduced (if not eliminated). As Wouters argues: 'such an ideal society never existed. Emotion management was never only a private act, nor were rules of feeling ever only privately negotiated' (Wouters 1989: 105). Yet one can question the degree to which this critique can be applied, particularly in the accusation that Hochschild's analysis is reliant on a vision of some former emotional utopia. For instance, Hochschild does appear sensitive to the way in which our present desire to regain an authenticity of feeling is conditioned by our history. She suggests that the image of the pre-industrial self contained in Rousseau's Noble Savage seems both savage and noble to us because he has an 'utter absence of calculation' (1983: 194) and 'he simply felt what he felt, spontaneously' (1983: 192). She argues that our attraction to the Noble Savage is the result of mid- to late twentieth-century capitalism and its 'commercialization of human feeling'. As she puts it, 'the more the heart is managed, the more we value the unmanaged heart' (1983: 192).

The problem from an Eliasian perspective, however, is that her analysis presents us with a rather foreshortened history. For Elias, the Rousseauian desire for a simpler self is primarily conditioned not by twentieth-century capitalism, but by the legacy of courtly society:

> It will not be possible to understand Rousseau and his influence, the possibility of his success even with the *monde*, unless he is seen as expressing a reaction to courtly rationality and to the suppression of 'feeling' in court life.
>
> (Elias 1983: 113)

This argument can be illustrated through extending the reference which Elias makes to the seventeenth-century observer of French court society, La Bruyère, who both describes the false self of the courtier, and laments the loss of a more sincere and true self:

> An accomplished courtier is master of his gestures, his eyes, his face; he is deep and impenetrable; he can dissemble when he is doing an ill turn, smile on his enemies, restrain his temper, disguise his passions, act contrary to his feelings, speak against his conviction, *and all this only to polish a vice we call falsehood, and is sometimes of as little use to the courtier as candour, sincerity, and virtue.*
>
> (La Bruyère 1890: 112, my italics; part quoted, though with a different translation, in Elias 1994: 476)

This quotation supports the argument that, contrary to Hochschild, the conflict between the sense of a false and a supposed true self was *pre*-industrial and *pre*-capitalist, and may have received a significant 'spur' with the development of court society. The projection of an 'appropriate' self was critical since 'behaviour at any time and every day could decide a person's place in society, could mean social success and failure' (Elias 1983: 115; cf. Elias 1994: 476). In such a society, courtiers performed emotional labour almost as a matter of course. Indeed the courtier appears subject to a style of observation that evokes the architecture of the panopticon, except that courtly rationality referred to a more socialized form of observation (e.g. courtiers knew their observers).

The lack of historical relativity in Hochschild's analysis results in theorizing which can appear limited in its depth of social analysis. For example, Hochschild observes that

> If it is women, members of the less advantaged gender, who specialize in emotional labour, it is the middle and upper reaches of the class system that seem to most call for it.

> (1983: 20)

Hochschild's explanation of this state of affairs is that

> In general, lower-class and working-class people tend to work more with things, and middle-class and upper-class people tend to work more with people.

> (1983: 21)

But the problem with this explanation is not just that it presents a rather stereotyped view of class, but that it lacks any analysis of why variances in emotion management might have historically developed between different social classes.

The need for a more sensitive historical analysis is not just confined to the work of Hochschild, but is also apparent with other writers looking at emotion and gender. For example, Jean Duncombe and Dennis Marsden (1993, 1995) have furthered James's attention to the association between gender, emotion and the public/private by arguing that women's domestic emotional labour is central to the support of traditional heterosexuality. Like James though, they allude to but do not really develop an historical account of heterosexual gender roles. And though some writers have historicized gender and emotion through reference to, say, Marxist or feminist theory (e.g. Hearn 1987), this has generally been accompanied by rather limited historical analysis.

The problems of cursory historical analysis are further underscored by writers who have tried to promote new kinds of emotion rules. For example, Putnam and Mumby draw on Hochschild's work in order to argue that the negative associations of emotional labour need to be replaced with more positive 'work feelings', where such feelings are 'spontaneous' and 'emergent rather than organizationally prescribed behaviour' (Putnam and Mumby 1993: 52), and express 'interrelatedness' rather than feelings as commodities (Putnam and Mumby 1993: 51; Mumby and Putnam 1992: 477). Their assumption is that through, for example, 'employee manuals and training programs' (Mumby and Putnam 1992: 478), employees can be encouraged to move away from the 'negative' commercialization of feeling towards a 'positive' rediscovery of 'real', 'spontaneous' feeling. Aside from problems with the allusion to a Rousseauian/true self which this entails, what is remarkable about Mumby and Putnam's prescription is their audacious attempt to rewrite history. It seems that with the aid of company training programmes a few centuries of emotional restraint can be conveniently swept aside. The consequence will be that

> As individuals share emotional experiences, their initial sense of anonymity gives way to feelings of community through the development of mutual affect, cohesion, and coherence of purpose.
>
> (Mumby and Putnam 1992: 478)

Such humanist prescriptions for organization development are not new, and can be traced from 1920s human relations onwards (Rose 1990; Hollway 1991). Even so, it seems a wondrous project that can rewrite historically conditioned patterns of western emotional restraint through devices such as employee manuals and training programmes. At the same time, it seems incredible that such a project can be advanced in the absence of any detailed consideration of the relation of present-day organizational life to the historical development of gendered labour markets, professionalization, the divorce of public and private, and so on. They appear to assume that this history, and its possible relation to emotion work, can just be rewritten without any detailed analysis of the social and power relations that may surround it.

EXPLAINING AHISTORICISM

The relative ahistoricism of work on the sociology of emotion is hardly unique to this area of study. Nevertheless, it can appear as more salient because work on emotion has traditionally been undertaken within psychology and social psychology. Given that these latter areas are often studiously ahistorical (Newton *et al.* 1995), it might have been expected that work by sociologists would have applied some corrective. Yet while sociologists of emotion exhibit a far greater sensitivity to context than that traditionally displayed by psychologists, it remains the case that the historical context of emotion and subjectivity is relatively unexplored in their work. For example, with a seeming sensitivity to context, Denzin argued that 'many of the feelings people feel and the reasons they give for their feeling are social, structural, cultural, and relational in origin' (1984: 53). Furthermore, he states that

> The study of emotionality is necessarily *historical* (Sartre, 1981). That history will be part family, part sexual, part educational, part occupational, and part friendship, both adult and child.
>
> (1984: 53, my italics)

But, like some psychologists, the historical context Denzin appears to be concerned with here is that of child and adult development. The fact that the child is born not into a vacuum, but into a rich, historically formed social world, does not appear to be considered here. Yet 'family', 'sex', 'education', 'occupation', 'norms' of 'friendship' (referred to above) are all historically formed, with the consequence that we need to be concerned with what happens *before* the birth of the child, as much as if not more than with what happens after.

Elsewhere, however, Denzin does show historical sensitivity beyond that of the developing child/adult, as in his interesting work examining the postwar relation between Hollywood, television and emotion (e.g. Denzin 1990). Yet, following Elias, there remains a need to adopt a much broader timescale. For instance, Denzin argues that the popular culture of Hollywood and television 'contributes to the deep-seated violence that rests at the core of the American society' (1990: 106). But if we follow Elias, such a statement needs to be historically relativized by acknowledging that it is only comparatively recently that western society has moved away from a widespread acceptance of the open celebration and enjoyment of violence (especially by men). In this sense, the fact that 'forms of violent emotionality are valued' in Hollywood needs to be seen in more than just the context of postwar popular media. Rather, if we accept Elias, it needs to be related to the argument that we have had a restraint on violence subsequent to the monopolization of violence in monarchic states, not its elimination. Following such an argument, one could also add a sort of social-psychoanalytic adjunct in suggesting that the success of Hollywood violence is a reflection of this restraint, and the desire for release through film fantasy (cf. Elias 1994: 452–3). Such arguments are in no way suggested as an excuse for male violence, but rather to note that (particularly) men have a long-standing historical relation to violence.

In sum, once we assume that the 'delivery' of a blow, a smile, a grimace or a tear is variant across cultures (elicitation depending on the particular cultural context), then we are acknowledging that even the seemingly 'basic' non-verbal aspects of our practical consciousness have been strongly historically conditioned. As Elias argues:

> The behaviour patterns of our society, imprinted on the child from early childhood as a kind of second nature . . . are to be explained . . . not in terms of general, ahistorical human purposes, but as something which

has evolved from the totality of western history, from the specific forms of behaviour that develop in its course and the forces of integration which transform and propagate them.

(Elias 1994: 518)

It seems as though many writers on the sociology of emotion implicitly point to the relevance of history, whilst some actively theorize history (e.g. Hearn 1987). The step that has not generally been taken, though, is to engage in historical analysis. Equally, there is almost no cross-reference to work undertaken by social historians, even though some recent work in this area has touched on issues directly related to emotion, sensibility and subjectivity. As a step in this general direction, an attempt will now be made to develop an historical sociology of emotion by working from the Eliasian analysis of courtly society towards a consideration of the emotional economy of the eighteenth- and nineteenth-century bourgeoisie. In so doing I will draw further on Elias, and then on the work of the social historian Marjorie Morgan.

FROM COURTLY SOCIETY TO THE BOURGEOISIE

As noted above, for Elias courtly society marked a critical period in relation to emotional and social codes in the west. In his later writing, Elias developed this analysis by paying greater attention to the movement from courtly society to 'salon culture' and to the development of the nineteenth-century professional bourgeoisie. He notes that, though there were changing power relations and interdependencies throughout this time, there was also some continuity in terms of emotional and behavioural codes. He first argues that the circumference of the 'good society' associated with the court gradually expanded. For example, in France after the death of Louis XIV, the notion of good society moved beyond high court nobility to include the residences of non-princely court aristocrats (the so-called '*hôtels*'), and it then spread out to include the houses or *salons* of both nobles *and* non-aristocratic financiers. Yet Elias argues that the model for 'salon culture' in France remained that of the court of Louis XIV (1983: 79). The concern in salon culture was to attain 'the perfection of pleasing forms, by refinement, courtesy, delicacy of manners. . . . Appearance and behaviour, gestures and etiquette were exactly fixed by "good society"' (Elias 1983: 62, quoting the description, by de Goncourt and de Goncourt (1877), of the salon of the Maréchale de Luxembourg).

In *The Court Society*, Elias contrasts both courtly and 'good' society with the development of the 'professional bourgeoisie' (1983: 92). He argues that courtly life represents 'one of the early stages and preconditions' of the professional bourgeois (1983: 92). More generally he suggests that 'many of the forms [of] the court society . . . live on in the nineteenth and twentieth centuries' (1983: 113). Yet what is critically different from the eighteenth century onwards is the separation of public and private spheres as the need for affective and behavioural constraint becomes gradually a matter of the individual's 'public' face. For example, within the social life of the developing merchant and professional classes, a *man* could withdraw *him*self from the 'glare of public life' (1983: 115). In consequence, if we follow Elias it is not simply that 'men created . . . the private realm' (O'Brien 1981: 56, quoted in Hearn 1987: 79), or that the public/private differentiation is a simple consequence of a gendered labour market, but that the industrial revolution and the market economy enabled a physical separation of a public workplace from a private home.[1]

According to Elias, the consequence of this is that by the time of 'bourgeois mass society', '*the professional sphere is the primary area in which social constraints and formative tendencies impinge on people*' (1983: 115–16, original italics). Elias also argues that another critical difference associated with the nineteenth- and twentieth-century professional bourgeois is that value is no longer chiefly defined by social rank and prestige, but rather 'utilitarian and economic interests mingle with prestige-values' (1983: 103). He illustrates how money and wealth were important in court society only as a means of access to this society since 'anyone who cannot maintain an appearance befitting his rank loses the respect of his society' (1983: 67). In contrast, the professional bourgeoisie had a strong need for *économie*, the subordination of expenditure to income, and the limitation of consumption in the interest of saving. The attainment of higher prestige depends on a 'saving-for-future-profits ethos' (1983: 67), so that wealth creation becomes an end in itself (1983: 60) rather than a means of access to the 'good society'. Nevertheless the emotional and social restraint associated with the 'good society' ('manners', appearance, etiquette, civility) continues to operate to some reasonable extent amongst the professional bourgeoisie. The critical difference is that prestige came to be increasingly reflected in symbols of wealth such as salary, rather than in the 'older' symbols of social rank.

In *The Court Society* Elias thus explores the continuities *and* discontinuities between courtly society and bourgeois life, attempting to show how the latter differed from the former. Yet his arguments with respect to the bourgeoisie are open to criticism since they are not supported by the same detail of analysis as that which he applied to courtly society. As Bogner (1987) and Kuzmics (1991) note, Elias's work was principally concerned with analysing courtly society of the seventeenth and eighteenth centuries, especially that relating to France. And though writers such as Kuzmics (1991) and myself (Newton 1996a) have examined the similarities between courtly rationality and twentieth-century organizational life, we nevertheless lack analyses which explore the developing emotional economy of urban-industrial society. Fortunately some detailed attention to this issue has recently been provided by the work of the US social historian Marjorie Morgan, in her analysis of bourgeois emotional life within the early English industrial period.

FROM COURTLY TO INDUSTRIAL SOCIETY

Morgan's work reflects a growing concern amongst social historians, a concern with issues related to subjectivity. To this extent it represents a departure from the more 'traditional' work of social historians of the nineteenth century, who have tended to focus on the development of institutions and social classes rather than analysing how such developments relate to changes in subjectivity. For example, one central debate in English social history concerns the question of which class was dominant in the nineteenth century, that of the aristocracy, or the growing middle classes (e.g. Perkin 1989). Another examines the argument that an attachment to pre-industrial aristocratic values in nineteenth-century England (reinforced by public schools) was responsible for English economic and industrial decline through the twentieth century (e.g. Wiener 1981; Perkin 1989). These analyses do occasionally touch on issues related to subjectivity. Thus Perkin echoes Elias's references to *économie* (discussed above) in arguing that middle-class subjectivity was affected by an 'all-pervading sense of [economic] insecurity' (1989: 95). But in general, issues of subjectivity remain a minor concern. In contrast, though Morgan's work remains situated within social history debates, it extends them by examining how (in sociological terms) changing power relations are interwoven with changes in subjectivity. It is therefore of particular interest because of the way in which she not only extends the arguments of social historians who have attended to issues relating to subjectivity (such as Halttunen 1982), but also places them within a context that is of particular relevance to sociological analysis.

The vehicles for Morgan's analysis are three forms of writing, the so-called 'courtesy', 'conduct' and 'etiquette' books. Through contrasting these three distinct forms of literature, Morgan begins to trace out the significance of the last of the three, etiquette, and its relation to emotion work among the middle and upper classes of the early English industrial period. Etiquette books blossomed in the 1830s, and maintained particular popularity during that decade and the 1840s. Like Arditi (1994), Morgan argues that they were principally characterized by the way in which, in contrast to courtesy and conduct books, they largely divorced manners from morals: 'Etiquette writers' overwhelming concern was to codify and dispense the proprieties requisite for performing comfortably and successfully in social or public settings' (1994: 23). The social codes they so dispensed derived from a particular social set, namely 'the polished, fashionable aristocratic members of London "Society" who dictated the courtesies of life composing etiquette' (1994: 24).

Morgan attempts to explain why the etiquette book eclipsed the influence of more moralistic literature (particularly 'conduct' books), and continued to influence social codes throughout the Victorian era. Echoing Elias, she first notes how they represented some continuity with courtly rationality, since the London 'Society' codes they advocated themselves represented a fashioning of courtly etiquette and values. At the same time, she argues even more strongly than Elias that 'Society' codes had a pervasive influence, at least in early to mid-Victorian England: 'It was this elite [London Society] to which the [English] nation deferred for dictates regarding what to wear and how to behave in social settings' (1994: 24). The hub of 'Society' life was the English drawing-room, and within its walls careful control and display were the order of the day. By way of illustration, Morgan quotes from the central character in Bulwer-Lytton's novel about the 'Adventures of a Gentleman', *Pelham*:

> The distinguishing trait of people accustomed to good society, is a calm, imperturbable quiet . . . they eat in quiet, move in quiet, live in quiet, and lose their wife, or even their money, in quiet.
>
> (Bulwer-Lytton 1840: 8–9)

The desire for civility in courtly society and for etiquette in London 'Society' had a similar effect, being designed to conceal real feelings and to maintain an appropriate appearance and gentility. According to one authority on etiquette, the drawing-room was designed to 'produce harmony and effect' (Douglas 1849, quoted in Morgan 1994: 96), aided by good manners and the 'emotionally repressive quality known as tact' (Morgan 1994: 97).

Morgan argues that the 'emotion-curbing conventions' of etiquette were gradually diffused amongst the developing middle classes of urban-industrial English society (1994: 99). She provides a number of reasons as to why etiquette 'triumphed' in this way as a code for public social intercourse. First, there was the increasing loosening of time and space constraints (Giddens 1984), with a far greater social mobility occasioned by wealth and technological feasibility. Morgan argues that 'writers of etiquette books assumed that their readers were rising from the humbler ranks to wealth and higher station' (1994: 20), and the rules of etiquette provided the 'oil' that allowed people to be more effective social climbers by making it appear that a certain status was more naturally theirs. She further suggests that external appearance and one's public persona were increasingly important because of the 'psychological association of purchasable things with personal worth and competence' (1994: 104), particularly in urban society where people lack personal knowledge of each other. For instance, she gives the example of doctors who needed the trappings of wealth such as an 'equipage' before they would be trusted by their clients. Writers of etiquette books aided such commercialization of the self by providing advice on how to 'massage' one's personal appearance. In particular, they provided a code through which social climbers might '*puff*' themselves up, and 'succeed': 'etiquette augmented individuals' social value by associating them with the fashionable set who determined its qualities' (1994: 117).

Through this kind of argument, Morgan comes close to Hochschild in associating etiquette with emotional restraint, and both with 'the growing commercialization of . . . personal identity' (1994: 117). The difference, however, is that she provides a detailed historical analysis which situates this commercialization process within the early nineteenth century rather than the twentieth century and, like Elias, relates the development of etiquette codes to a much earlier courtly society.

Morgan also argues that etiquette was of significance because of the widespread changes in social relations within nineteenth-century English urban-industrial society. As Giddens notes, 'In most pre-modern contexts . . . trust relations were localised and focused through personal ties' (1991: 189). In contrast, among modern urban dwellers 'the notion of "stranger" loses its meaning' (Giddens 1991: 152), since communication is no longer based largely on local personal ties and people have to interact with all manner of acquaintances. In Eliasian terms, the developing market economy witnessed a much greater complexity of social interdependencies, and Morgan stresses how the impersonality of these interdependencies occasioned an emotional restraint. Just as 'courtiers ideally concealed their true emotions behind a repertoire of stylised behaviours' (1994: 95), so

> [p]eople artificially reinforced the naturally impersonal nature of the more urban, market-regulated society by their self-conscious attempt to remain, at least in public, emotionally detached.
>
> (1994: 97)

In sum, Morgan's analysis suggests that the emotional economy of the Victorian English classes was based on a development of courtly social and emotional codes within the constraints of a market economy. Such codes provided an ordered detachment appropriate to the increasing impersonality of the age, as well as an avenue for social climbing, a means for '*puffery*' of a more commercialized self. Her analysis can be seen to broadly extend Elias's argument that the nineteenth-century middle class inherited aspects of courtly rationality, yet combined this with a concern for money not as a means to an end, but as an end in itself.

THEORIZING EMOTION: FROM INDUSTRIAL TO CONTEMPORARY SOCIETY

Given that we lack work integrating social histories of the twentieth century into an analysis of the historical sociology of emotion, any attempt to extrapolate from Elias and Morgan to the present day must remain somewhat tentative. Nevertheless, given that this book is in large part concerned with contemporary issues in emotion, I will close this chapter by examining some theoretical questions which their work raises in relation to present-day emotion codes.

It would be difficult to explore contemporary issues without referencing the work of Cas Wouters who has done much to extend Elias's theorizing to twentieth-century analysis (see Chapter 13). Wouters (1977) draws on Elias to argue that the twentieth century has been marked by an 'informalization' of social and emotional codes, presenting a contrast to hitherto formal codes such as those of etiquette. Rather than a lessening of self-restraint, however, this informalization has been associated with a restraint more reliant on internal self-discipline than on external rules such as those of etiquette, an internalization which Wouters explains (in part by drawing on Elias) through a kind of strengthening of the super-ego (Wouters 1977, 1986). Central to Wouters's work appears to be the argument that the 'lessening of power inequalities is conducive to greater informality' (1977: 447), and he has explored this thesis in the context of postwar Europe, especially the period from the 1960s to the present within his native Holland (e.g. Wouters 1977, 1986, 1989). However, though Wouters provides some interesting propositions, questions do remain in relation to the conjectures he presents, which at times appear idealized and limited in depth of historical analysis. For example, Wouters argues that the 1960s and 1970s represented a period both of heightened social equality and of informalization. He asserts that 'For many people, it became more and more difficult to picture any kind of unequal relation as being harmonious' (1986: 7). Yet this appears as a highly idealized image of the 1960s and 1970s since it can be argued 1) that such views reflected those of a minority rather than a majority, and 2) that social *practice* deviated widely from this ideal with, for example, little sign of gender relations, domestic or otherwise, being characterized by equality – even in the Netherlands where, as Mennell argues, the 'social transformations of the 1960s and 1970s were perhaps more dramatic' (1989: 241). Some of Wouters's related assertions also appear open to question, such as his argument that the 1980s were characterized by the association of greater inequality with an increase in the formalization of emotional and social codes (Wouters 1986, 1989). Yet within countries such as Britain which have experienced marked increases in wealth inequality, there has been little clear evidence of increases in formalization (such as a return to more formal etiquette, or other formalization of social codes). Finally, one can question the extent to which twentieth-century informalization has been accompanied, as Wouters asserts (following Elias), by an increasing internalization of restraint rather than a conformity to external 'rules'. Instead, what may have changed is the need for an external 'show' of restraint, through the lessening of one's ability, say, to appropriate a class 'act'. Etiquette allowed one to 'exhibit' one's internal restraint, one's civility and decorum, to show, for example, the sort of gentleman one was. It was the ability to perform *and* play around this act that was significant as an arbiter of one's social standing. But this does *not* necessarily imply either that internalization of restraint has increased, or that etiquette 'functioned' as an 'external' restraint. Just because you can successfully perform a surface act does not mean that you rely on that act to maintain your self-restraint.

Despite such criticisms, some of Wouters's arguments do receive support within the work of Elias and Morgan. For instance, in drawing on Elias, Wouters suggests that a key factor in informalization has been the increasing material security of the west (1986: 3). Returning to Elias's work in order to develop this point, one might argue that 1) the desire for *économie* and the significance of prestige values (Elias 1983) are likely to decrease with both increasing wealth and wealth equality, and that 2) the significance of social and emotional codes *associated* with wealth and economic security might similarly reduce. In terms of Morgan's work, it seems likely that the display of formal codes such as etiquette would be less important as a means of social 'puffery' since there is less of a need to 'puff' oneself up and climb the socioeconomic ladder in conditions of increased wealth and wealth equality. Yet at the same time, the need for emotional and behavioural restraint remains. We still live in a world of strangers characterized by the kind of impersonality which Morgan attributes to nineteenth-century England. But drawing on Elias, Morgan and Wouters, one can argue that greater economic security and equality mean that there is no longer such a need for a 'class act' (as was apparent in the mid- to late nineteenth-century England; Perkin 1989), and in consequence there is a lessening of a desire for the *formality* that went with this act.

Yet a question that remains is that of whether it is rather reductionistic to equate a loss of faith in the need to assimilate aristocratic codes *solely* with increasing economic security or equality. For example, it seems likely that other issues are equally, if not more, relevant, such as universal suffrage, the perception of an open, democratic and meritocratic society (the American dream, etc.), and the general feeling that skill and talent will be rewarded (never mind whether social reality actually fits that expectation). For example, to the extent that one feels that promotion at work is, *or* should be, related to reliable and meritocratic assessment, then what matters is one's skill and experience, rather than social puffery and the creation of a 'seeming' appearance. At the same time, economic security may be important, but not simply in the sense implied by Elias (1983). Rather it may be that welfarism has critically reduced the threat of destitution, and in so doing also enabled people to reject the need to ape their betters. Western individualistic pride, constituted in notions of democratic and human rights, and divorced from anxieties over penury, seems more likely to reject social climber pretensions, or the need to 'conform' to a hierarchically approved social code.

Such arguments highlight the relevance of the Foucauldian project since they suggest a need to relate changing socioemotional codes to power/ knowledge relations, and the role of developing democratic, medico-psychiatric, economic and social science discourse. Yet Elias's work can also be seen as relevant to such an analysis. For example, elsewhere I have explored the relation of medico-social discourse and emotion, arguing that much medico-psychiatric and social science discourse encourages public emotional restraint and the privatization of emotion (Newton *et al.* 1995). Thus, though psychoanalytic and 'stress' discourse problematizes emotion, it does not suggest any radical disruption in codes of socioemotional display. Catharsis on the street is not recommended, and individuals are generally encouraged to 'relieve' their feelings in private settings through psychotherapy, stress management, group-work, and so on. But loosely following Elias, there are good reasons why the display of emotional restraint still makes sense within social figurations of the late twentieth century. It may be unwise to let out your feelings, especially at work where 'outbursts' may have negative effects on your job security, or your prospects of promotion. Any medico-social science writer/practitioner who advanced unrestrained emotionality on the street or in the workplace would be ignoring social and economic realities, since street catharsis is still associated with lunacy and work catharsis may cost you your job. Elias thus draws our attention to the continuing relation between emotion and social figuration, and to the way in which discourse is *established* within the constraints of such figurations (Newton *et al.* 1995).

Such arguments, however, are not meant to suggest a predominant continuity in emotion codes through the twentieth century, since it is possible to locate examples of seemingly interrelated changes in figuration and emotion. One such derives from the increasing debate over the emotion codes stereotypically assigned to women and men. Contrary to the impression created by the research of Duncombe and Marsden (1995), traditional gender asymmetry in emotional expression may be changing (especially amongst the more economically independent middle classes). In some heterosexual relationships it may be the woman who is more emotionally detached, and the man who appears more 'needy'. Again, contrary to Duncombe and Marsden (1995), one explanation (loosely informed by Elias) is that such developments reflect a lessening of some women's economic dependency. Admittedly this is to use a crude socioeconomic equation, that women's lessening financial 'neediness' may encourage less emotional 'neediness', but it would be surprising if gendered emotional stereotypes remained static unless broader gender relations are also static. For example, let us say, developing from Elias (1983), that the stereotypical association of women with emotionality and men with emotional restraint/ inadequacy bears some historical relation to an association of women with the private, domestic and subservient roles and men with public, employment and professional roles. To the extent that this is the case, gendered emotionality appears likely to change *if* such roles change. Change, however, may not be simple, as witnessed by the struggles of heterosexual feminists to change both their emotions and their sexuality in relation to male partners (Wilkinson and Kitzinger 1993). In addition, there is unlikely to be a simple linear relation between materiality and emotion. Yet the above example illustrates the potential relevance of changes in figuration to changes in emotion codes.

REFRAMING ELIASIAN ACCOUNTS OF EMOTION

This chapter has attempted to illustrate the potential of historicizing of emotion through particular reference to the theoretical perspectives of Elias and the analyses of Morgan. Though any analysis of this kind is clearly an effect of representation, it can offer the promise of greater understanding of the development of emotion codes. The aim has not been to try to suggest that there is any exact relation between the emotion codes of courtly rationality and those of the present day. The prospect of such invariant subjectivity in the face of changing sociopolitical relations runs counter to the thesis of Elias. Rather, mischievously to paraphrase Foucault (1981), current codes of emotion may lie partly in 'the shadow of the court' since, following Elias, the court symbolized a critical development in power relations in parts of western Europe which encouraged changes in subjectivity, particularly the show of emotional and behavioural restraint.

Yet though the work of Elias and Morgan is supportive of this general argument, neither presents detailed analysis of developments in the twentieth century. In consequence, tracing possible continuities and discontinuities in emotion codes in western Europe is still based on rather limited analysis. In addition, there are criticisms which can be applied to the approaches of Morgan and Elias. Like Wouters's work, that of Morgan is open to the charge that she presents an overly mechanistic view of external rules such as etiquette, since she tends to portray them as the means by which individuals maintained emotional restraint. However, etiquette may have been a means not to maintain, but to *show* emotional restraint, a way of publicly signalling that one was capable of civil behaviour in polite society. Etiquette may have allowed the acting out of an *already* existent internalization of self-restraint within the nineteenth-century bourgeoisie, not some kind of mechanical external censor of 'internal' emotions. This criticism of Morgan and Wouters, of course, also points to a similar difficulty with the work of Elias, since courtly rationality may not have represented a radical change in the internalization of restraint, but instead heralded the need to 'exhibit' publicly the finesse of one's skills in restraint. It does seem unlikely that people suddenly learned the internalization of restraint within the 'hothouse' of courtly society, and it also seems questionable as to whether medieval knights were as wild and unfettered as Elias claims. Again, courtly rationality may have been about changes in tacit rules of emotional display and the general decorum one should appropriate, rather than about some suddenly learnt self-regulation. Such arguments point once more to the advantage of applying a Goffmanian framework to Elias (Kuzmics 1991), albeit one that needs to be cognizant of the clash between the static and the dynamic in the work of Goffman and Elias.

Another critical difficulty with Elias has already been alluded to, namely the strongly metanarratival ambitions of his overall project. For instance, in his writing he was given to rather sweeping universalistic statements, as in his strident assertion that the 'monopolization of the means of violence . . . plays no less a part as a source of power than the monopolization of the means of production' (Elias 1987a: 230). The implicit claim here seems to be that in terms of metanarrative, Elias saw himself more or less as on a par with Marx. Such stridently metanarratival desires, however, may be capable of some accommodation if one views Elias from a far more relativistic position than he allowed; for instance, accepting that the monopolization of violence may *not* represent a universalistic trend that is always associated with emotional restraint and the 'civilizing' process. More generally, the arguments of 'Eliasians' might be more seductive were their propounders not quite so staunch in their defence of Elias and if they acknowledged, for example, that some of Elias's rhetoric does appear somewhat essentialistic and substantialist (Maso 1995) wherein, to the extent that he follows Freud, he may have continued to retain vestiges of an essentialistic 'id', if not an essentialistic 'ego' or 'superego' (e.g. see Elias 1994: 492–4 and Elias 1995: 9–11). Similarly, acceptance that his arguments may be culturally relative (Mouzelis 1995) appears more persuasive than a staunch defence against such relativization (e.g. Mennell 1989). Elias's work has *some* consistency with a more relativistic approach if only because he continually reaffirmed how our desires and our emotions are not fixed in stone, but rather are, at least to some reasonable extent, historically variant. Acceptance of historical variance implies cultural variance, provided one can move beyond universalistic arguments about the significance of the monopolization of violence, etc. Such implicit historical/cultural relativism also means that it is perhaps a little too easy to dismiss Elias because he presents a singularly modernist and 'positivist creed' (Pels 1991: 181). The more challenging task may be to try to reframe his work within a more relativistic perspective, whether epistemological or cultural (Newton 1996b).

NOTE

1 Some corrective, however, is needed to Elias's portrayal of the industrial revolution as creating the possibility of escape from the public sphere, with its implicit suggestion that this was a *voluntarily* sought escape. Many men were forced into a greater separation between their public and private worlds since they had little choice but to work away from home, whilst women's activities were simultaneously privatized and marginalized through their reconceptualization as domestic activities (see, for example, MacDonald 1995: 127).

BIBLIOGRAPHY

Abrams, Philip (1982) *Historical Sociology*. Shepton Mallet, Somerset: Open Books.

Arditi, Jorge (1994) 'Hegemony and etiquette: an exploration of the transformation of practice and power in eighteenth-century England', *British Journal of Sociology* 45(2): 177–93.

Baudrillard, Jean (1983) *In the Shadow of the Silent Majorities, or The End of the Social and Other Essays*. New York: Semiotext(e).

Bogner, Artur (1987). 'Elias and the Frankfurt School', *Theory, Culture and Society* 4: 249–85.

Bulwer-Lytton, Edward (1840) *Pelham, or Adventures of a Gentleman*. London: Routledge.

Burkitt, Ian (1991) *Social Selves*. London: Sage.

Burkitt, Ian (1993) 'Overcoming metaphysics: Elias and Foucault on power and free- dom', *Philosophy of the Social Sciences* 23(1): 50–72.

Burkitt, Ian (1994). 'The shifting concept of the self', *History of the Human Sciences* 7(2): 7–28.

de Goncourt, E. and de Goncourt, J. (1877) *La femme au XVIIIe siècle*. Paris.

Denzin, Norman K. (1984) *On Understanding Emotion*. San Francisco: Jossey-Bass.

Denzin, Norman K. (1990) 'On understanding emotion: the interpretive-cultural agenda', in Theodore D. Kemper (ed.) *Research Agendas in the Sociology of Emo- tions*. Albany, NY: State University of New York Press.

Douglas, A. E. (1849) *The Etiquette of Fashionable Life*. London: Simpkin, Marshall.

Duncombe, Jean and Marsden, Dennis (1993) 'Love and intimacy: the gender divi- sion of emotion and emotion work', *Sociology* 27(2): 221–42.

Duncombe, Jean and Marsden, Dennis (1995) '"Workaholics" and "whingeing women": theorising intimacy and emotion work – the last frontier of gender inequality', *Sociological Review* 43(1): 150–69.

Elias, Norbert (1978) *The Civilizing Process*, Vol. 1, *The History of Manners*. Oxford: Blackwell.

Elias, Norbert (1982) *The Civilizing Process*, Vol. 2, *State Formation and Civilization*, Oxford: Blackwell.

Elias, Norbert (1983) *The Court Society*. Oxford: Blackwell.

Elias, Norbert (1987a) 'The retreat of sociologists into the present', *Theory, Culture and Society* 4(2–3): 223–47.

Elias, Norbert (1987b) 'On human beings and their emotions: a process-sociological essay', *Theory, Culture, and Society* 4(2–3): 339–61.

Elias, Norbert (1991) *The Society of Individuals*. Oxford: Blackwell.

Elias, Norbert (1994) *The Civilizing Process*, Vols 1 and 2. Oxford: Blackwell.

Elias, Norbert (1995) 'Technization and civilization', *Theory, Culture and Society* 12: 7–42.

Findlay, Patricia and Newton, Tim (1997) 'Reframing Foucault', in Alan McKinlay and Ken Starkey (eds) *Foucault, Management and Organization Theory: From Panopticon to Technologies of Self*. London: Sage.

Foucault, Michel (1979) *Discipline and Punish*. Harmondsworth, Mx: Penguin.

Foucault, Michel (1981) *The History of Sexuality*, Vol. 1. Harmondsworth, Mx: Penguin.

Foucault, Michel (1982) 'Afterword: the subject and power', in H. F. Dreyfus and Paul Rabinow (eds) *Michel Foucault: Beyond Structuralism and Hermeneutics*. Brighton: Harvester Press.

Foucault, Michel (1984) 'Nietzsche, genealogy, history', in Paul Rabinow (ed.) *The Foucault Reader*. Harmondsworth, Mx: Penguin.

Giddens, Anthony (1984) *The Constitution of Society*. Cambridge: Polity Press.

Giddens, Anthony (1991) *Modernity and Self-Identity*. Cambridge: Polity Press.

Goldthorpe, John (1991) 'The uses of history in sociology: reflections on some recent tendencies', *British Journal of Sociology* 42(2): 211–30.

Grey, Chris (1994) 'Career as a project of the self and labour process discipline', *Sociology* 28(2): 479–98.

Halttunen, Karen (1982) *Confidence Men and Painted Women: A Study of Middle-Class Culture in America, 1830–1870*. New Haven, CT: Yale University Press.

Hearn, Jeff (1987) *The Gender of Oppression: Men, Masculinity and the Critique of Marxism*. Brighton: Wheatsheaf.

Hill, Stephen and Rock, Paul (1994) 'The uses of history in sociology: a debate', *British Journal of Sociology* 45(1): 1–2.

Hochschild, Arlie (1983) *The Managed Heart: the Commercialization of Human Feeling*. Berkeley, CA: University of California Press.

Hollway, Wendy (1991) *Work Psychology and Organizational Behaviour*. London: Sage.

James, Nicky (1989) 'Emotional labour: skill and work in the social regulation of feelings', *Sociological Review* 37: 15–42.

Kuzmics, Helmut (1991) 'Embarrassment and civilization: on some similarities and differences in the work of Goffman and Elias', *Theory, Culture and Society* 8: 1–30.

La Bruyère, Jean de (1890) *The Morals and Manners of the Seventeenth Century, Being the Characters of La Bruyère*, trans. Helen Stott. London: David Stott.

Lutz, Catherine A. (1988) *Unnatural Emotions: Everyday Sentiments on a Micronesian Atoll and Their Challenge to Western Theory*. Chicago: University of Chicago Press.

MacDonald, Keith M. (1995) *The Sociology of the Professions*. London: Sage.

Maso, Benjo (1995) 'The different theoretical layers of *The Civilizing Process*: a response to Goudsblom and Kilminster & Wouters', *Theory, Culture and Society* 12: 127–45.

Mennell, Stephen (1989) *Norbert Elias*. Oxford: Blackwell.

Morgan, Marjorie (1994) *Manners, Morals and Class in England, 1774–1858*. Basingstoke, Hants: Macmillan, and New York: St Martin's Press.

Mouzelis, Nicos (1993). 'The poverty of sociological theory', *Sociology* 27(4) (November): 675–96.

Mouzelis, Nicos (1995) *Sociological Theory: What Went Wrong?* London: Routledge.

Mumby, Dennis K. and Putnam, Linda L. (1992) 'The politics of emotion: a feminist reading of bounded rationality', *Academy of Management Review* 17(3): 465–86.

Newton, Tim (1994) 'Discourse and agency: the example of personnel psychology and "assessment centres"', *Organization Studies* 15(6): 879–902.

Newton, Tim (1996a) 'Resocialising the subject: a re-reading of Grey's "Career as a Project of the Self"', *Sociology* 30(1): 137–44.

Newton, Tim (1996b) 'Postmodernism and action', *Organization* 3(1): 7–29.

Newton, Tim (1996c) 'Agency and discourse: recruiting consultants in a life insurance company', *Sociology* 30(4): 717–39.

Newton, Tim, with Handy, Jocelyn and Fineman, Stephen (1995) *'Managing' Stress: Emotion and Power at Work*. London: Sage.

O'Brien, Mary (1981) *The Politics of Reproduction*. London: Routledge & Kegan Paul.

Pels, Dick (1991) 'Elias and the politics of theory', *Theory, Culture and Society* 8: 177–83.

Perkin, Harold (1989) *The Rise of Professional Society: England since 1880*. London: Routledge.

Putnam, Linda L. and Mumby, Dennis K. (1993) 'Organizations, emotions and the myth of rationality', in Stephen Fineman (ed.) *Emotion in Organizations*. London: Sage.

Rose, Nikolas (1990) *Governing the Soul*. London: Routledge.
Rose, Nikolas (1996) 'The death of the social?: re-figuring the territory of government', paper presented at a History of the Present meeting, London School of Economics, 13 March 1996.
Sartre, Jean-Paul (1981) *The Family Idiot, Gustave Flaubert*, Vol. 1, *1821–1857*. Chicago: University of Chicago Press.
Wiener, Martin (1981) *English Culture and the Decline of the Industrial Spirit 1850–1980*. Cambridge: Cambridge University Press.
Wilkinson, Sue and Kitzinger, Celia (eds) (1993) *Heterosexuality: A Feminism and Psychology Reader*. London: Sage.
Wouters, Cas (1977) 'Informalisation and the civilising process', in Peter Gleichmann, Johan Goudsblom and Hermann Korte (eds) *Human Figurations: Essays for Norbert Elias*. Amsterdam: Amsterdams Sociologisch Tijdschrift.
Wouters, Cas (1986) 'Formalization and informalization: changing tension balances in civilizing processes', *Theory, Culture and Society* 3(2): 1–18.
Wouters, Cas (1989) 'The sociology of emotions and flight attendants: Hochschild's *Managed Heart*', *Theory, Culture and Society* 6: 95–123.

Part II

The mediation of emotional experience

5 'Bored and blasé'

Television, the emotions and Georg Simmel

Keith Tester

In his *Farewell to European History*, Alfred Weber attempted to make some kind of sense of the convulsions which had sped through Europe and thereafter much of the world during the first forty-five years or so of the twentieth century (the English translation of Alfred Weber's book appeared in 1947). He also tried to make sense of his own emotional responses to the world. He was sure that the twentieth century represented something unique in history because it stood on foundations which were themselves remarkable. Weber did not reduce the history of Europe to technological developments, but he made the point that certain technological and scientific transformations had taken place which simply demand to be taken into account by anyone who seeks to understand the present and its emotional life. He wrote that

> ever since the scientific and technological discoveries of modern times we have been living no longer on our dear, familiar old earth of wide-open spaces and infinite variety. Instead we have come to live, 'on a new star which in some remarkable manner combines the old geometrical extension with foreshortenings and shrinkings and permanent world-contacts, thus completely altering all life upon it'.
>
> (Weber 1947: ix)

Weber went on to say that 'Formerly we used to hear some six months after the event, that "they were having a war far away in Turkey"; now, every day, we are immediately involved by ear in the struggles of nations for power, their world-spinning battles, their plans and actions, all running in tempo'. He continued: 'Everything that is done, no matter where, is served up to us piping hot a moment later wherever we may happen to be, as though it were going on in the same town, almost in the same room. In short, we live in a world made great and small at once by the conquest of space' (Weber 1947: ix).

For Alfred Weber, the conquest of space which was accomplished and spread throughout the globe by the development of the radio, meant that the individual could never be entirely alone ever again. The old barriers of practices, emotions, imaginations and property which protected the private individual from the outside world had been breached by the technology which, on the one hand, made the individual an informed and knowledge-able 'citizen of the world' but which, on the more terrible other hand, made that individual suffer from what amounted to a surfeit of conscious-ness about the world. But the world was not just a single place in this spatial manner. Running through Weber's comments is a sense that technology like the radio has made the world a single place in a temporal sense as well. All the battles and all the disasters in the world are made to run according to the same clock. Consequently, radio broadcasts of events from around the world are instalments in the story of the great train of history from which the individual is never able to extricate him- or herself.

It is very tempting to try to explain how and why it was that listening to the radio caused all of these problems for Alfred Weber, by referring to the work of Anthony Giddens. In terms of his expressed anxieties at least, it is reasonable to identify Weber as a prime exemplar of Giddens's account of modernity if not, indeed, of what Giddens calls 'high' or 'late' modernity. According to Giddens: 'In high modernity, the influence of distant happen-ings on proximate events, and on intimacies of the self, becomes more and more commonplace.' This is considerably due to 'the media, printed and electronic' (Giddens 1994: 4). In these terms, it can be proposed that Weber is a typical subject of high or late modernity because he knows that 'The "world" in which we now live is in some profound respects . . . quite distinct from that inhabited by human beings in previous periods of history' (Giddens 1991: 4). Following Giddens's terms, it might be proposed as an initial hypothesis that Weber had discovered what it feels like to experience the processes of disembedding: 'Disembedding mechanisms depend on two conditions: the evacuation of the traditional or customary content of local contexts of action, and the reorganizing of social relations across broad time–space bands' (Giddens 1994: 85). This chapter uses the case of Alfred Weber to question and offer an alternative to Giddens's account of modernity and its emotional character. It is an exploration of the relationships between media and the emotional constitution of indi-viduals within the world of contemporary social and cultural relationships. The specific problem which runs through the chapter is: why were so many people so talkative about little Jamie Bulger being murdered by two boys, and why were so many seemingly so indifferent towards mass rape and genocide in the Balkans?

For Giddens, disembedding means that the individual is pulled out of the relationships of trust, certainty and confidence which local tradition nurtures. According to Giddens, tradition can be defined in a somewhat schematic way: 'Tradition . . . is bound up with memory . . . [it] involves ritual; is connected with what I shall call a formulaic notion of truth; has "guardians": and, unlike custom, has binding force which has a combined moral and emotional content' (Giddens 1994: 63). Alfred Weber found him-self in a situation where all of this was thrown into doubt by the way the radio had challenged all of the old understandings and constructions of the social and cultural worlds. Weber could not remember ever knowing these things before (and his contemporaries provided no storehouse of memories to help him); the truth that some places and events matter more than others was turned upside down, because now Turkish wars mattered in Germany; the old guardians of the truth seemed to be as confused as, if not in fact more confused than, everyone else (after all, was not Alfred Weber such a supposed guardian?); and thus moral and emotional verities had question marks put against them.

Giddens contends that the media disembed the individual and, more broadly, play a part in the process of detraditionalization, which is more or less identical with modernity, in two ways. The media do this through their way of operating as 'modalities of reorganising time and space' (Giddens 1991: 26). First, there is what Giddens calls the collage effect: 'Once the event has become more or less completely dominant over location, media presentation takes the form of the juxtaposition of stories and items which share nothing in common other than that they are "timely" and consequential' (Giddens 1991: 26). Second, there is what Giddens refers to as 'the intrusion of distant events into *everyday* consciousness' (Giddens 1991: 27, original emphasis). He explains that 'Many of the events reported on the news, for instance, might be experienced by the individual as external and remote; but many equally enter routinely into everyday activity.' Furthermore: 'Familiarity generated by mediated experience might perhaps quite often produce feelings of "reality inversion": the real object and event, when encountered, seem to have a less concrete existence than their media representation.' Giddens continues: 'Moreover many experiences that might be rare in day-to-day life (such as direct contact with death and the dying) are encountered routinely in media representations; confrontation with the real phenomena themselves is psychologically problematic' (Giddens 1991: 27).

The case of Alfred Weber has two significant implications for the validity of Giddens's account of disembedding and detraditionalization. First, it casts doubt on the viability of the historical process which is implicit to Giddens's analysis. Second (and reflecting the problem of the historical validity of the process of detraditionalization), Giddens's account tends to lead to the conclusion that, in so far as we listen to or watch the news, we are all like Alfred Weber, desperately struggling to come to terms with the worlds we inhabit and experience. But I want to suggest that Alfred Weber is so very interesting precisely because he is so remarkably unlike most of us. The overwhelming point about Alfred Weber is that with all his expressed anxiety and confusion, Alfred Weber could not possibly be one of our contemporaries. Alfred Weber is struggling to understand what it means to be what Kevin Robins has nicely called a 'consumer of suffering and terror' (Robins 1994: 458). Robins sees this as a general problem for all consumers of the media (and especially television). Robins says that we all see quite awful suffering on the screen and that 'the viewer should be devastated by the intense shock of such realities'. But: 'for the most part, at least, this is not what seems to happen. Audiences appear to be relatively unscathed by their encounters with the violence of war . . . they are able to escape the emotional and moral consequences of seeing and knowing' (Robins 1994: 458). It is precisely in this ability to escape the emotional and moral consequences of seeing and knowing that Alfred Weber actually ceases to be one of our contemporaries. He was not possessed of the emotional resources which enabled him to escape knowing so much. But we are; we can witness horror and feel next to nothing.

Kevin Robins has offered his own account of how this ability dully to witness horror through the television has developed. He tries to explain how 'such sights could be tolerated, and tolerated on such a continuous and repetitive basis' (Robins 1994: 458). Robins turns around the model of the rational consumer of the television, which tends to imply that individuals watch television in order to achieve some rational goal which they either have set for themselves or have had set for them by social and cultural pressures. Robins contends that it is possible that the television pictures of horror elicit quite another response and are consumed for quite other reasons: 'We take for granted the desire to know . . . we generally do not take account of, or even recognize the existence of, the equally strong desire to not know, to evade knowledge' (Robins 1994: 459; see also Robins 1993). In other words, because we watch and consume pictures of war and violence, this does not in itself mean that we are thereby making ourselves rationally informed spectators of the world – we could, instead, just be making ourselves aware of what we need to avoid knowing about. After all, 'it may be the case that knowing about such things would entail making some change in ourselves. And because such change would be painful to both the individual and the social group, defensive organizations may be formed to resist and refuse knowledge and its consequences' (Robins 1994: 459). Robins identifies psychological foundations of these defences. He also suggests that 'the medium through which such images are viewed and consumed might also be implicated in defusing their painful reality' (Robins 1994: 459). He says that through the television, the quantity of information which is available to the individual increases but the quality of knowledge is inhibited. As such: 'What is achieved is a condition in which exposure to the world's events is maximized, whilst, at the same time, exposure to their consequences is minimized. The screen that provides us with information about the world's realities, is also a screen against the shock of seeing and knowing about those realities' (Robins 1994: 460). In all, then, Robins's thesis is that we consume television pictures of horror and, in so doing, become quite anaesthetized to any emotional impact they might have upon us. He says that 'we may . . . consider these technologies in terms of sensory distraction and sensory involvement in compensatory realities, that is to say, in terms of the intoxication of phantasmagoria' (Robins 1994: 463).

Certainly, Robins is able to explain how it is that images of war and violence tend to leave their viewers unmoved and, indeed, frequently quite unconcerned. This is because television domesticates and captures the very insecurities which the images might inspire. Robins contends that we use our freedom to consume television not just in order to gain knowledge, not just in order to be entertained, but also in order to enter into a world of televised and therefore reduced yet fantastic horror which can compensate for the fears and dangers of 'a reality and a real world that has become increasingly dangerous and difficult to manage' (Robins 1994: 466). In Robins's terms then, it would probably be argued that Alfred Weber was worried about what he heard from around the world precisely because he existed in a time and place which had not yet generated the necessary defence mechanisms against what it had become possible for individuals to know.

But I want to suggest that Robins takes a wrong turn when he psychologizes his account of the consumption of television pictures and reports of horror, war and violence. The problem with any psychologization of responses to televised images of horror is not just that it always implicitly assumes a degree of functional rationality (after all, even the irrationality identified by Robins is, in itself, quite rational – it is rational to avoid knowledge if knowledge is going to raise unanswerable existential dilemmas). By this psychological account Alfred Weber would simply be a more or less psychotic version of us. But the point is that Alfred Weber is not distant from us because of emotional constitution; he is distant from us because of the social and cultural moment in which he was writing. He was writing at a specific moment when the fabric of credibility had been worn to shreds if not, indeed, torn apart by the media, and we are looking back to him from a vantage point within which the fabric has been sewn back together again by the media. In the specific context of the emotions elicited in individuals to stories of wars and horrors in other places, the media have turned out to be the solutions to the problems which they once created.

Weber was face to face with the emotional crisis of the detraditionalization which the radio represented and expressed. But for us, here and now, televised pictures of horror have been rendered quite banal and boring because we are the subjects of a tradition about what those pictures can and might imply. With this claim that we are the subjects of a tradition I am suggesting that for us, as not for Alfred Weber, it is possible to identify in an ensemble of historical memories, biographical memories and shared practices over time, a series of practices and customs about the media and indeed about television which possess an aura of being relatively long established and which are most certainly experienced at least in part as having been handed down from one generation to another. I am claiming that we are able to tell stories about the media, about television, and that in the currency and commonality of those stories is tradition.

The pictures of horror are banal because of two main aspects of what might be termed the traditionalization of television. First, there is the question of the simple size of the pictures which are available for us to see and consume. However large and technically advanced the television set might be, it is nevertheless the case that the technologies of viewing relatively reduce the size and impact of what they represent. Quite simply, a television is not all-encompassing and neither is it a stark and overwhelming monolith which is presented to the consumer as a world sufficient unto itself. Television might purport to present a world picture, but there is also a world surrounding the picture. Moreover, the pictures are desensualized representations of events and circumstances which are otherwise redolent with smell and touch. The technologies of media consumption, and especially the technologies of viewing, push everything into an aesthetic milieu within which emotional issues are likely to be only contingently present. But, second, pictures of war and violence are unlikely to move us because they are presented to us in the context of a tradition of narrativity.

According to Giddens, of course, television turns the world into a collage. He stresses this coming together of the coincidental but timely, this 'juxtaposition of heterogeneous items of knowledge or information in a text or format of electronic communication' (Giddens 1991: 242). But he also says that this collage is itself a kind of story of the world. Giddens says that the collage is a kind of story because 'the separate "stories" which are displayed alongside one another express orderings of consequentiality typical of a transformed time–space environment from which the hold of place has largely evaporated' (Giddens 1991: 26). He continues to say that these separate stories 'do not, of course, add up to a single narrative, but they depend on, and also in some ways express, unities of thought and consciousness' (Giddens 1991: 26). Even though a genre such as television news might have little or no organizing principle other than the consequentiality and timeliness of what it reports, that organizing principle is extremely powerful. Narrativity, and the tradition of narrativity in television, means that any given image, indeed any single story of horror, is turned into something which is not important in itself, but which is important only in relation to the other things which have happened today. And this also means that today's news will have to restake its claim to newsworthiness tomorrow and that yesterday is continually erased and superseded by today. Consequently, any given image or report is not important in a way which makes either the news or indeed the consumer stop in their tracks. As Otto Kallscheuer has very nicely said about media images of suffering others: 'Between ourselves and the people struggling for survival there is another and none less brutal (Darwinian) battlefield, where information and actuality (and first of all pictures) are fighting for their survival in the evening news and the morning papers' (Kallscheuer 1995: 110). Kallscheuer continues to point out that the finiteness of news broadcasts and publications means that 'The informational market is a zero-sum game: each event or cause or picture that "makes it" to the headlines eo ipso inevitably "kills" countless other possible newsworthy items.' These dead items themselves offered now unrealizable 'possibilities for viewers and readers to be touched by compassion for this or that cause in our worldwide neighbourhood' (Kallscheuer 1995: 111). Narrativity means that pictures of great horror become quite impermanent, fleeting and of only temporary relevance: they do not last.

Some of the terminology I have used almost certainly betrays the debt all of my formulations owe to the sociology of Georg Simmel. Indeed, I want to propose that Simmel's work on the emotional implications of modern cities and the modern money economy contains themes and insights which can be directly pertinent for any study of the emotional dimensions of the consumption of television representations of horror (see Simmel 1950, 1990). Simmel can be employed in order to help us understand precisely why and how it is that the frequently dreadful images invariably have such a very minimal impact upon us. Simmel's work enables us to generate that kind of appreciation while attending to specificities and situations of social and cultural relationships and arrangements, and without having to move into psychology. Just as Simmel makes it plain that certain modes of being in the world with others are historically and situationally specific to the metropolis and the money economy, so it can be suggested that certain kinds of emotional responses to the consumption of images of the insults and injuries suffered by relatively distant others are also historically and situationally specific. Indifference and banality are responses which are specific to those social and cultural situations in which the media in general and the television in particular are accorded the status of being intrinsic and traditional aspects of the everyday life of individuals. As such, the kinds of responses I am exploring are presently specific to North America, western Europe and parts of the Pacific Rim. Only in these places have the media become utterly ordinary and eternally at-hand properties of the everyday. Only in those places would individuals be completely and utterly lost if they were not able to watch evening news broadcasts, just as the inhabitant of Simmel's modern metropolis is quite lost if left in the country for any period longer than a few weeks' holiday.

An explicit connection between television and the city has been made by Zygmunt Bauman, drawing on Henning Bech's neologism *telecity*. Just as we meet strangers on the city streets, so we meet strangers on the television. Yet there is a crucial difference between these two categories of others. Unlike the physically proximate strangers on the streets, the strangers on the television are kept emotionally distant (even though they might come physically close): 'There is, comfortingly, a glass screen to which their lives are confined.' Building on Bech and recalling Simmel, Bauman identifies for these strangers on the screen, the reduction of their existential mode to pure surface. As such they cease to be emotionally compelling: 'In the telecity, strangers are sanitized and safe, like sex with condoms . . . and thus enjoyment need not be spoiled by fore- or after-thought, care may be forgotten, no thought of consequences needs to stir the conscience or poison the pleasure' (Bauman 1993: 178). Indeed, in the telecity, the strangers are 'infinitely close as objects; but doomed to remain, happily, infinitely remote as subjects of action'. Bauman continues to say that: 'In the telecity, the others appear solely as objects of enjoyment, no strings attached. . . . Offering amusement is their only right to exist – and a right which it is up to them to confirm – ever anew, with each successive "switching on"' (Bauman 1993: 178).

Especially important for this tentative Simmelian approach to television and the emotions is Simmel's conception of the blasé attitude of the modern city dweller. Simmel identifies this attitude as a general psychological reaction to the surfeit of stimuli and sensations which the individual is forced to experience simply by virtue of her or his living in the city with all its noises, sights, smells and passing strangers (the blasé attitude is a social and cultural phenomenon which has psychological effects, not psychological causes). In his essay 'The metropolis and mental life' Simmel says that: 'There is perhaps no psychic phenomenon which has been so unconditionally reserved to the metropolis as has the blasé attitude' (Simmel 1950: 413). The city dweller becomes blasé simply because the city has too much to offer; it promises too many pleasures and 'A life in boundless pursuit of pleasure makes one blasé because it agitates the nerves to their strongest reactivity for such a long time that they finally cease to react at all' (Simmel 1950: 414). Just like the city the television too offers a rapidly changing series of impressions which we have to make meaningful and to which we have to learn how to react. Just like the city, the television offers so much that our powers of discrimination actually cease to be able to work effectively, and so instead of conscious engagement with stimulations we simply tend to sit back and let them wash over us.

In *The Philosophy of Money*, however, Simmel shifts the terrain of the blasé attitude away from the city and rather more towards the effects and requirements of the money economy. In his massive book, Simmel argues that the blasé attitude means that the individual 'has completely lost the feeling for value differences. He experiences all things as being of an equally dull and grey hue, as not worth getting excited about, particularly where the will is concerned' (Simmel 1990: 256). Instead of measuring things in terms of intimations of value, the blasé person – and of course 'the blasé attitude is rightly attributed to satiated enjoyment because too strong a stimulus destroys the nervous ability to respond to it' (Simmel 1990: 256) – measures things in terms of the amount of time and effort which is invested in securing them: 'the kind and amount of practically necessary endeavours to acquire them often determines the depth and liveliness of their attraction for us' (Simmel 1990: 256). And, when all is said and done, little time and little effort has to be spent to gain access to television pictures of horror and suffering. Walter Benjamin quotes Paul Valéry, who pointed out that 'Just as water, gas, and electricity are brought into our houses from far off to satisfy our needs in response to a minimal effort, so we shall be supplied with visual or auditory images, which will appear and disappear at a simple movement of the hand, hardly more than a sign' (Valéry quoted in Benjamin 1970: 213). For Simmel, 'the more the acquisition is carried out in a mechanical and indifferent way, the more the object appears to be colourless and without interest' (Simmel 1990: 257). Consequently, the blasé attitude means that instead of identifying the world as a terrain of action or concern to be engaged with, the individual comes to see it as a dull problem out there to be observed from afar; the world with its sufferings and horrors becomes an abstraction.

This is the basis of the general indifference and lack of concern which television consumers tend to demonstrate towards all of the stories that are seen and heard about such events as ethnic cleansing, genocide and rape in other parts of the world. Indeed, Stjepan Mestrovic has sought to draw direct connections between themes from Simmel and the emotional responses of television consumers to coverage of the deeds which were carried out in the Balkans War. Writing as the ethnic cleansing was being prosecuted and as the pictures appeared on the television, Mestrovic said of coverage of the war in the Balkans, 'the news media in general and television media in particular convey hyper-abstract, rational images of reality that lead to the blasé attitude' (Mestrovic 1994: 84). The world is presented as an 'out there' to be looked at as if from a safe distance, with horror in the Balkans as little more than one of its local attractions: 'after all, there exist air pollution monitors, blood glucose monitors, baby monitors, carbon dioxide monitors, and all sorts of monitors up to and including human rights abuse monitors in the Balkans'. And the product of all this blasé and highly specialized, routinized, watching? Mestrovic says that 'In the end, one reacts to the findings of human rights abuse much as one reacts to the finding that there is too much smog over Los Angeles – with indifference' (Mestrovic 1994: 84).

Simmel says that even though the blasé person becomes indifferent and unconcerned about almost everything, nevertheless 'his membership of the human species demands the attractions of life that his individual condition makes intangible for him' (Simmel 1990: 257). The blasé attitude means that things and even other people cease to matter to us but, precisely because we are here in this world, those things have to matter to us if we are going to be able to stand any chance of personal satisfaction and happiness. We might not care about them very much, but they are the only tools of our chance of satisfaction which are ready to hand. And so: 'Out of this there emerges the craving today for excitement, for extreme impressions, for the greatest speed in its change – it is one of the typical attempts to meet the dangers or sufferings in a situation by the quantitative exaggeration of its content' (Simmel 1990: 257). In the precise case of television, this argument would imply that owing to their formal properties of speed and transience as well as their implication in the tradition of narrativity, television pictures or reports of suffering overstimulate the senses and thereby produce in the individual the blasé attitude. But precisely because we cease to be shocked or stimulated by what we see and hear we seek out more and more images of horror in the hope that they at least will stir us a little and be able to prove to us that, perhaps, we remain human. We are unconcerned about why these dreadful images stimulate us, so long as they do stimulate us. As Mestrovic suggests, 'the blasé attitude thrives on cruelty and callousness' (Mestrovic 1994: 84); that is, when it allows individuals to be bothered enough to be stirred and moved by anything at all. Yet, Simmel believes: 'The satisfaction of such cravings may bring about a temporary relief, but soon the former condition will be re-established, though now made worse by the increased quantity of its elements' (Simmel 1990: 257). (David Riesman identified a similar allure with sex: 'Even when we are consciously bored with sex, we must still obey its drive. Sex, therefore, provides a kind of defense against the threat of total apathy . . . the other-directed person . . . looks to it for reassurance that he is alive' (1950: 146).)

But the blasé attitude does not stand alone. In his work on the psychological reactions of individuals to the city and the money economy, Georg Simmel stresses that the blasé attitude is not the only consequence of the superabundance of stimuli. He also emphasizes the importance of the attitude of reserve. It would be somewhat tenuous to propose that television creates reserve amongst its viewers; here the point I want to make is that watching television is not the sole activity of men and women (a lot of media sociologists seem to forget this, or they simply reduce it to what amounts to a methodological pattern variable). The individuals and the groups who spend some of their time watching television news reports from the killing-fields of the world also spend quite a considerable amount of their time in urban environments in which they not only have to come to meaningful terms with the potentially overwhelming sensations of the city but they also have to make some kind of meaningful sense of the experience of meeting and sometimes even bumping into complete strangers. Simmel writes that the individual's 'self-preservation in the face of the large city demands from him a . . . negative behavior of a social nature. This mental attitude of metropolitans toward one another we may designate, from a formal point of view, as reserve' (Simmel 1950: 415). Through reserve, we emotionally withdraw from others even as our physical proximity to them increases. According to Simmel, only in this way can the city dweller retain a sense of individual identity in the face of 'continuous external contacts with innumerable people' (Simmel 1950: 415). As Simmel depicts it, reserve can be appreciated as having significant implications: 'Indeed, if I do not deceive myself, the inner aspect of this outer reserve is not only indifference but, more often than we are aware, it is a slight aversion, a mutual strangeness and repulsion, which will break into hatred and fight at the moment of a closer contact, however caused' (Simmel

1950: 415–16). As such, we are either indifferent towards others or openly hostile towards them.

The implication of the arguments I have been developing is that television, and especially television pictures of horror, are consumed by individuals more or less alone and indifferently. Alone because television consumers are also inhabitants of the city and therefore emotionally reserved in relationships with others. Indifferently, because television representations are too fast and fleeting; all we can do is adopt a quite blasé attitude if we are going to be able to survive the surfeit of sensation. The implication of all this is that television leaves us as monads, unprepared and unwilling to talk with one another about all that we have seen and heard. But of course, it is quite wrong to say that no public discussion is occasioned by the pictures and the stories broadcast on television. About some things there is very considerable discussion indeed. From a British perspective, the Jamie Bulger case immediately comes to mind as a prime example of the ability of television to inspire and maintain debate. (Jamie Bulger was a little boy who was taken to a shopping centre by his mother; while she was being served in a shop he wandered away with two older boys who beat him to death on a railway siding. Security cameras filmed Jamie walking away with his killers.) Even though Jamie Bulger's death in a suburb of Liverpool was spatially distant from many of the people who engaged in public discourse about what they saw and heard, it was nevertheless experientially close to them. The death was close not just because it resonated with ordinary and, importantly, very common experiences of parenthood ('Where have they gone now?') but also because of the overwhelming banality of the image of a toddler walking in a shopping centre, holding the hand of another child. Jamie Bulger's death was emotionally immediate irrespective of physical spaces. His murder was most certainly quite appalling; but in some sense it was also very ordinary.

It would be quite wrong to dismiss all of this concern about single incidents like the death of Jamie Bulger as trivial and unimportant when they are considered against the background of ethnic cleansing, genocide and mass rape in other parts of the world. Concern about Jamie Bulger (for instance) itself represents a valuable and important form of emotional, and especially moral, engagement in and with the world. All of the talk which incidents like this occasion represents a variation of the sociable conversation which is, according to Simmel, one of the most important means by and through which we respect each other as individuals. For Simmel, the sociable conversation is valuable almost precisely because of its frequent triviality when compared with what else is going on. Simmel believes that the sociable conversation has itself as its own purpose. This means that the content of the conversation is of secondary sociological importance since 'In purely sociable conversation, the topic is merely the indispensable medium through which the lively exchange of speech itself unfolds its attractions' (Simmel 1950: 52).

In order to distinguish the specifically sociable conversation from any other kind of dialogue Simmel says that 'of two externally similar conversations, only that is (properly speaking) sociable, in which the topic, in spite of all its value and attraction, finds its right place, and purpose only in the fictional play of the conversation itself that sets its own norms and has its own peculiar significance' (Simmel 1950: 52–3). Simmel is sure that 'as soon as the discussion becomes objective, as soon as it makes the ascertainment of a truth its purpose (it may very well be its content), it ceases to be sociable'; instead it becomes 'untrue to its own nature – as much as if it degenerated into a serious quarrel' (Simmel 1950: 52). And such a quarrel is an outrage to sociability since 'sociability presents perhaps the only case in which talk is its own legitimate purpose'. Simmel continues: 'Talk presupposes two parties; it is two-way. In fact, among all sociological phenomena whatever, with the possible exception of looking at one another, talk is the purest and most sublimated form of two-way-ness' (Simmel 1950: 53). Simmel himself was quite prepared to blur the epistemological status of sociability and the sociable conversation. On the one hand, he was using sociability as a formal category of sociological analysis. But on the other hand, he was also happy to establish sociability as an ethic and he saw the commitment of the individual to the conversation as something amounting to a moral duty. He tends to lapse into an account of sociability which sees it as a human right and a moral obligation to maintain. Simmel was prepared to contend that 'each individual should offer the maximum of sociable values (of joy, relief, liveliness, etc.) that is compatible with the maximum of values he himself receives' (Simmel 1950: 47).

At a first glance there is a sharp contradiction between the ongoing liveliness of the sociable conversation and the deep reserve of the inhabitant of the metropolis (or, as I would also have it, the deep reserve of the television consumer). The sociable conversation seems to demand everything which the reserved individual tries to avoid at nearly every possible opportunity. Of course, the easiest way around this problem is to stress the conventional wisdom and point out that Simmel was an extraordinarily unsystematic thinker and that contradictions are therefore only to be expected. But that is no answer at all. Indeed, what is noticeable is the extent to which the discussion of the sociable conversation is actually completely reconcilable with the account of the reserved attitude.

The reserved individual does not want to engage in relationships any more than she or he absolutely has to; the reserved individual tries to pull away from any contact which is too close. And in a strange paradox this is an attitude which is wholly appropriate for the demands of the sociable conversation. Simmel points out that the conversation depends on the personalities of the participants: 'But precisely because everything depends on their personalities, the participants are not permitted to stress them too conspicuously' (Simmel 1950: 45). Indeed, the purposeless talk which practically constitutes and maintains sociability is only effective to the extent that '[i]t keeps the conversation away from individual intimacy and from all purely personal elements that cannot be adapted to sociable requirements' (Simmel 1950: 53). For Simmel then, we can be sociable and reserved at one and the same time precisely because sociability requires that we do not give too much of ourselves away; precisely because sociability demands that we engage with the other on the basis of an assumption of a kind of formal equality: 'Wealth, social position, erudition, fame, exceptional capabilities and merits, may not play any part in sociability. At most they may perform the role of mere nuances of that immaterial character with which reality alone, in general, is allowed to enter the social work of art called sociability' (Simmel 1950: 46). Or again: 'Sociability is the game in which one does "as if" all were equal, and at the same time, as if one honoured each of them in particular. And to "do as if" is no more a lie than play or art are lies because of their deviation from reality' (Simmel 1950: 49). Moreover, Simmel's sociable conversation is also able to take account of our tendency to be or become quite blasé: what seems to be implicit to Simmel's argument is an assumption that the sociable yet reserved individuals will not become blasé about their conversations because the content of the talk is so liable to change at a moment's notice; the conversation is liable to such a rapid change that we are slightly less likely to become bored by it. As Simmel says: 'The ability to change topics easily and quickly is . . . part of the nature of social conversation.' He continues: 'For since the topic is merely a means, it exhibits all the fortuitousness and exchangeability that characterize all means as compared with fixed ends' (Simmel 1950: 53). But pictures of horror, of war and violence, cannot be consumed and publicly discussed quite so easily. They do not seem to be so readily and easily amenable to the demands of the sociable conversation. Even though the pictures of the insults and injuries suffered by relatively distant others have been domesticated through the traditionalization of the media, the images are nevertheless prone to create a shiver for the individual. The point is that amongst other things we are all subjects of a social and cultural tradition which emphasizes concepts such as sympathy and concern for suffering (drawing on themes from Arendt, that tradition can be identified with the social question; Arendt 1973). We watch and consume certain pictures or reports and perhaps feel that we ought to be moved by them; but in so far as we are also possessed of a quite blasé attitude in the face of the fleeting and transitory, we are not moved. In fact, we are more likely to want to see more and more pictures of horror simply in order to discover quite how deeply and irredeemably blasé we might have become. In other words, we are likely to respond to televised horror in a way which makes us somewhat ashamed of ourselves. And in the face of that inward shame, reserve becomes our hope and our defender. Instead of having publicly to show that we either do not care about, or do not cry at, or actually slightly enjoy, the spectacle of suffering, we emotionally withdraw ourselves from others. We come to feel a certain contempt for those who do 'wear their heart on their sleeve'.

In these terms, television pictures of horror have a most peculiar status. If they have a profound emotional impact upon the individual, then she or he is unlikely to want, or even be able, to talk about that impact in public relationships. If they have a public dimension they lose any immediate personal value in themselves and, instead, become contingent problems to be addressed in the service of the sociable conversation. It would seem to be the case that television can allow for personal existential concern or public engagement. But television cannot possibly allow for both at the same time, and so it implies either concern without action or discussion without engagement.[1]

NOTE

1 I would like to thank Gill Bendelow and Simon Williams for their helpful and pertinent comments on an earlier version of this chapter. However, I remain wholly responsible for this work. The chapter draws on material discussed at greater length in my book *Moral Culture* (London: Sage, 1997).

BIBLIOGRAPHY

Arendt, H. (1973) *On Revolution*. Harmondsworth, Mx: Penguin.

Bauman, Z. (1993) *Postmodern Ethics*. Oxford: Blackwell.

Benjamin, W. (1970) 'The work of art in the age of mechanical reproduction', in his *Illuminations*, ed. Hannah Arendt. London: Jonathan Cape.

Giddens, A. (1991) *Modernity and Self-Identity: Self and Society in the Late Modern Age*. Cambridge: Polity Press.

Giddens, A. (1994) 'Living in a post-traditional society', in Ulrich Beck, Anthony Giddens and Scott Lash (eds) *Reflexive Modernization: Politics, Tradition and Aesthetics in the Modern Social Order*. Stanford, CA: Stanford University Press.

Kallscheuer, O. (1995) '"And who is my neighbor"?: moral sentiments, proximity, humanity', *Social Research* 62: 99–127.

Mestrovic, S. G. (1994) *The Balkanization of the West: The Confluence of Postmodernism and Postcommunism*. London: Routledge.

Riesman, D., with Glazer, N. and Denny, R. (1950) *The Lonely Crowd: A Study of the Changing American Character*. New Haven, CT: Yale University Press.

Robins, K. (1993) 'The war, the screen, the crazy dog and poor mankind', *Media, Culture and Society* 15: 321–7.

Robins, K. (1994) 'Forces of consumption: from the symbolic to the psychotic', *Media, Culture and Society* 16: 449–68.

Simmel, G. (1950) *The Sociology of Georg Simmel*, trans. and ed. Kurt H. Wolff. New York: Free Press.

Simmel, G. (1990) *The Philosophy of Money*, 2nd edn, trans. Tom Bottomore and David Frisby. London: Routledge.

Weber, A. (1947) *Farewell to European History, or The Conquest of Nihilism*, trans. R. F. C. Hull. London: Kegan Paul.

6 In search of the inner child

Co-dependency and gender in a cyberspace community

Norman K. Denzin

The internet is where my problems blossomed, and maybe with other avenues, it can be where I find some healing.
> (New male reader/member, alt.recovery.codependency newsgroup [a.r.c.], 5 September 1996)

On my first visit to this newsgroup [a.r.c.], it was so wonderful to read about the work of your recovery and the joy of it. As I am just at the beginning of the self discovery and the hard work, I really thank you for sharing that.
> (New female reader/member, a.r.c. newsgroup, 1 September 1996)

INTRODUCTION

In this chapter I examine the gendered, emotional talk, the 'narratives of self' that are posted in an Internet news-discussion group called 'alt.recovery. codependency' (a.r.c.). Alt.recovery.codependency is an on-line newsgroup which draws on the tenets of the Adult Children of Alcoholics (ACOA) and the Co-Dependency (CODA) movements.[1] Alt.recovery.codependency is one of 'more than 5,000 discussion groups, or newsgroups, housed on the Internet' (Hahn and Stout 1994; Walstrom 1996). These newsgroups form 'what is commonly called the Usenet' (Parks and Floyd 1996: 80). The Internet users who participate in these discussion groups post messages which are disseminated 'to all Internet sites carrying the newsgroup. Others may respond to a particular message, thereby creating a "thread" or connected series of messages, or they may read without responding (called "lurking")' (Parks and Floyd 1996: 80; also quoted in Walstrom 1996: 1).

My intentions are to show how a new information technology (IT), Usenet, has created a site for the production of new emotional self-stories, stories that might not otherwise be told. These narratives are grounded in the everyday lives and biographies of the women and men who write them, yet they circulate in the anonymous, privatized territories of cyberspace. The life on the screen (Turkle 1995) that occurs for this newsgroup involves struggles over identity, meaning and the self. A politics of gendered identity is enacted in this site, a politics which intersects with technology and machines (the personal computer), and with embodied, biographical identities (Bardini and Horvath 1995: 44).

This intersection socially creates a gendered computer user who learns how to talk and write within the preferred languages and representational formats of this group. These interactions are shaped by the prevailing cultures of family, therapy, illness (addiction) and recovery that circulate in the international cyberspace recovery movement (Kaminer 1992; Rice 1996). The increasing medicalization of illness in American culture (Conrad and Schneider 1992: 106–7) has spread the disease model to the alcoholic and non-alcoholic family, giving rise to the concept of the dysfunctional family suffering from the disease of co-dependency (see below).

The discourses in a.r.c. join the three dominant discourses from this larger medical meaning system, the discourses on addiction, therapy and family (Denzin 1993: viii). Paraphrasing Rice (1996: 210), everyone now has a disease of their own, the disease of co-dependency which requires a liberation psychotherapy for its treatment. Alt.recovery.codependency is one place where this therapy occurs; virtual reality (VR) thus serves to help repair the ruptures that occur in the real world (RW). This is talking therapy turned into the exchange of written words whose meanings are constantly being deferred as they are debated and discussed.

I will offer intensive readings of two complex threads: the first from a series of exchanges in late 1994, one month after the group went on-line; the second from 2–5 September 1996.[2] I compare and contrast these two threads (Thread One, 'Choices, Holidays and Gifts', and Thread Two, 'Help Me Understand Something') in terms of the above processes; asking always, what are the consequences of this new form of story-telling for the emotional lives of women and men in this historical moment?

LIFE ON THE NET

Internet life in moderated and non-moderated newsgroups is cyclical, and this in a double sense (see below).[3] First, as in a conversation, exchanges follow the comment–response cycle, woven into a thread. One person makes a statement, another person comments, and a third person comments, perhaps on the second person's remarks, and so on. Second, over any given time, a small number of topics, formed into threads, constitute the life on the screen of this particular newsgroup. (Moderated newsgroups clear out their files on a regular schedule, usually every two to three weeks.) A reader's entry into a group is thus shaped by what is on the screen at any given time. The appeal of the group to a reader may differ markedly over any extended time-period, and the public face of the group may be drastically different from time one to time two.

This is what I discovered in the two threads analysed below. Each thread gives a different picture of a.r.c. In Thread One women control the discourse. In Thread Two a male, acting as a moderator, attempts to control the discourse. Thread Two supports the argument (Kramarae 1995: 54; Balsamo 1994: 142) that men tend to control talk on the net, while Thread One leads to the opposite conclusion.

The method of instances

But it is premature and perhaps incorrect to phrase the problem this way. The initial empirical concern is not with *who controls* the discourse over any period of time. Rather, the question involves *how control* is exercised in any given sequence. Once this 'how' question is provisionally answered, the second question, involving *how power* is socially distributed in terms of race, class, or gender, becomes relevant. Following Psathas (1995: 50), the initial (and primary) focus is on the use of the 'method of instances' which is used in conversation analysis. This method takes each instance of a phenomenon as an occurrence which evidences the operation of a set of cultural understandings currently available for use by cultural members. The analyst's task is to understand how this instance works; whether it occurs again is irrelevant, and the question of sampling from a population is also not an issue, for it is never possible to say in advance what an instance is a sample of (Psathas 1995: 50). Collections of instances 'cannot be assembled in advance of an analysis of at least one, because it cannot be known in advance what features delineate each case as a "next one like the last"' (Psathas 1995: 50). Thus large samples of Internet talk are of little use until the analyst has exhausted the method of instances. There is little concern for empirical generalization. The goal is to achieve an adequate analysis of a particular instance or sequence (Psathas 1995: 50) (hence my intensive focus on two threads).

The real and the virtual

Not surprisingly, interactions in a.r.c. erode the boundaries 'between the real and the virtual . . . the unitary and the multiple self' (Turkle 1995: 10). The user who enters this virtual world finds a nascent culture of simulation and meaning which partially overlaps with and maps the real gendered worlds of CODA and ACOA which have been, until recently, dominated by women.[4] In (and around) a.r.c. the writer can interact in 'The 12 Steps Cyberspace Cafe' (a place for hope, help and healing), and confront cyberspace psychotherapists, fellow-travellers, and persons with less than honourable intentions (see Turkle 1995: 10).[5] An on-line community is discovered, a community with its norms, its rules (netiquette), its own emotional vocabulary and its use of emoticons (Turkle 1995: 112), a set of frequently asked questions (FAQs – what is co-dependency? what is recovery?), guidelines for posting, acceptable subjects, regular users, leaders, oldtimers, and a constant circulation of newcomers.

In any Usenet community self and personality are communicated in written form. That is, a gendered computer user writes speech, attempting a form of inscription which may or may not be compatible with their voice and 'their off-screen personae' (see Derrida 1976: 9). The written text that defines the posted message can interfere 'with the transfer of the users' personalities and unique qualities. The result is the creation of [on-screen] "personae"' (Turkle 1995: 118). These on-screen self-images may bear little relationship to the person's interactional self in everyday, non-screen life. On-screen personae are given meaning through the written inter-actions that occur between users. A public, on-screen self is shaped through the use of emoticons and the group's preferred language and style of verbal-written presentation.

Screen interactions are easily transformed into printed texts, actual tran-scriptions of on-screen talk. Thus any reader with a printer can make a per-fect copy of an on-screen text. This gives readers an access to the spoken (now printed) word that they would not otherwise have and allows them to study carefully the printed words of the speaker. Unlike the give-and-take of ordinary conversation where persons may debate what was spoken, or what was meant by what was spoken, on-screen speakers have the original text as a point of reference. Thus screen talk is deliberative, stilted, formal, clearly marked in sentences, with commas, exclamation and question marks, and so on. At the same time, on-screen talk can be directed to a large number of readers, and the identity of the speaker can be masked.

Persons establish their presence in the newsgroup through their regular participation in the conversational topics of the group, which take several forms, each a variant on the adjacency pair (Psathas 1995: 16),[6] including: greetings, questions–answers, responses–replies, closings, complaints–apologies and justifications (Psathas 1995: 16–17). Internet conversational life consists almost entirely of cycles of responses to statements, in the form of adjacency pairs, or to those extended sequences which involve 'tell-ing stories' (Psathas 1995: 21).[7] Both conversational forms lead to the crea-tion of threads. In threads, the cycle of responses to a statement is given in skirmishes, banter, criticism, support, counter-stories, and inflammatory comments (for 'flames', see Aycock and Buchignani 1995: 227; Dery 1994: 4–5). In these ways personality, self and reputation are established (see Turkle 1995: 128–30; Baym 1995b: 49).

ADULT CHILDREN OF ALCOHOLICS AND THEIR OFFSPRING

The major figures in the ACOA and CODA movements, which have been intensively studied by David Rudy (1991) and John Steadman Rice (1996), include R. S. Ackerman, Claudia Black, Janet Woitiz, Sharon Wegscheider, John Bradshaw and Melody Beattie. There are currently over 1,000 ACOA and CODA groups in the USA. Over 100 volumes on the topics have been published, and more than 40 national conferences have been held. At least two national magazines are devoted to the movements and their members (*Changes, Focus*). Over one million copies of Janet Woitiz's *Adult Children of Alcoholics* (1983) have been sold. (At the 1992 democractic presidential convention Bill Clinton publicly announced his status as an adult child of an alcoholic parent.)

The literatures of these two movements argue that adult children of alcoholic parents are co-dependants and, like their alcoholic parents, have the *disease of co-dependency*; that is, 'they let another person's behavior affect them, and they are obsessed with controlling that person's behavior' (a.r.c. 1996: 4). A reader browsing the a.r.c. web page (1996) will find under the heading 'What Is Codependency?' a list of characteristics attributed to co-dependants, including the following: co-dependants are attracted to alcoholics and to drug addicts, they feel a constant need to be in a relationship with someone, they can't end relationships, and they are people-pleasers (a.r.c. 1996: 4). Co-dependency, as indicated above, is a gendered, relational production. It describes, at one level, the interaction patterns that build up between men and women in intimate and non-intimate relationships. The fact that more women than men appear to get this disease speaks to this culture's tendency to feminize illness and to make women-as-victims responsible for their own situations. This is but one more instance of the 'gendered triumph of the therapeutic' in American culture (Mitchell-Norberg *et al.* 1995: 122).

The ACOA and CODA movements are connected to the languages and literatures of the Twelve-Step groups (AA and Al-Anon, and Alateen).[8] In addition, they accept the disease concept of alcoholism. A.r.c. (1996: 15) states: 'we come to see parental alcoholism . . . for what it is: a disease that infected you as a child and continues to affect you as an adult'. This disease concept is generalized to the lived experiences of non-alcoholics. 'As an addict, I probably have multiple addictions . . . work, money, control, food, sexual, approval' (a.r.c. 1996: 15).

The disease of co-dependency is a process addiction: an addiction to a way of life. This should be distinguished from a chemical or ingestive addiction, which is an addiction to a substance. Process addictions now appear alongside substance addictions. (In this literature an addiction is anything persons feel they have to lie about.) Process addictions put people out of touch with their feelings. They mask a dependence on any mood-altering experience that has life-damaging consequences. Co-dependants are dependent on others for their own happiness; they let another person's behaviour affect who they are. Such individuals are obsessed with controlling another person's behaviour. This disease that co-dependants have is chronic, progressive (CODAs want and need to be around sick people), habitual and self-destructive. It is characterized by a variety of disorders, including alcoholism, drug addiction, the eating disorders, obsessive gambling and sexual compulsions.

CODAs seek out and have relationships with alcoholics, drug addicts, the mentally ill, chronically ill individuals, and irresponsible people. CODAs have low self-worth, repress their emotions, are obsessive, controlling, filled with denial, are poor communicators, don't trust others, are filled with anger, often have problems with their sexual identities, and are failures in intimate relationships. CODAs and ACOAs play out the identities of family mascot, hero, scapegoat and lost child.

These texts teach that what happened to you as a child is happening to you now, for your childhood in a dysfunctional family has not equipped you to build healthy, normal, warm, intimate relationships with others, including your children. ACOAs and CODAs come from dysfunctional families, where they never learned true love, or how to express their emotions. They learned shame and guilt, feeling that their failures caused the failures in their alcoholic parents. Lacking a 'carefree childhood', ACOAs and CODAs became young adults at an early age. They never learned how to be normal. They thought (and think) that a chaotic life is normal, while believing in 'Brady Bunch' images of the ideal American family.

Trapped in a cycle, CODAs and ACOAs now reproduce their distorted, dysfunctional childhoods in their adult relationships. Such individuals have a shame-based, co-dependent inner self. The problems experienced today are directly related to an alcoholic childhood. This means that persons must learn how to redefine their past, so that they can get free from it. This is called 'Inner Child' work, the discovery 'of the child within. . . . [W]e each have a young child within us with all the feelings, fears, complexities, simplicities, and needs we had when we were that age' (a.r.c. 1996: 6–7).

Co-dependency theorists make co-dependency an addictive process that requires therapy and treatment. This process addiction, they argue, should become a personality disorder listed in the APA's *Diagnostic and Statistical Manual*, 3rd edn. Co-dependency should be treated as an emotional disease. Treatment and recovery include the use of psychotherapy, Twelve-Step groups, goal-setting, and recovery of the inner, childlike self that was lost in childhood. A new form of family therapy is required, one that uncovers the repressive rules which structure childhood in this culture. This therapy teaches self-love.

HISTORY

Alt.recovery.codependency started in early 1994. The reason for its existence was given thus: 'to create a supportive, loving and safe environment for those of us who consider ourselves to be codependent and wish to interact with others in similar situations' (a.r.c. 1996: 3). In this space, the individual begins to experience recovery. This occurs through a process wherein the individual shares his or her 'experience, strength and hope with others' (ibid.). Through this sharing, the person is able to aid in his or her own recovery and 'to help others make progress on their journey to recovery' (ibid.). Recovery now becomes a process of letting go of a painful past that is damaging the person's life today: 'recovery . . . loosely describes the methods we utilize in order to . . . let go of the pain in our past and present so that we may fully live our lives today' (ibid.: 5). There are different paths to recovery: physicians, friends in recovery, therapists, Inner Child work, Twelve-Step groups.

A.r.c. has few rules concerning postings; any subject relating to co-dependency is relevant, including topics which 'deal with our relationships with other people . . . spouses, children, family of origin, friends, employers, co-workers, most importantly ourselves' (ibid.: 7). There are, however, five general guidelines defining the netiquette of a.r.c.: do not reproduce entire copyrighted documents; avoid posting private e-mail correspondence; if dissatisfied with a particular person take what you like from their posting and leave the rest, or add them to your kill file; if persons respond to your posting on group mail, inform them privately that you do not like this; avoid sending notes that are void of substance (ibid.: 8). Persons are invited to just jump in and post, and those who want to maintain anonymity can use first only or false names, or an anon.id. Posting can occur by using an anonymous server (anon.penet.fi and anon.twwells.com). Lurking is encouraged (ibid.: 9).

Discourse centres on the Inner Child work, discovering the child within us. According to Melody Beattie, a leader of the co-dependency movement, many of us ignore this inner child, and this causes us trouble. The gendered talk that occurs in this newsgroup does not connect to an oral tradition of group storytelling, as is the case for Alcoholics Anonymous (Denzin 1993: 246). There are, however, a number of canonical texts that are referenced, including the AA *Alcoholics Anonymous,* and the works of Bradshaw and Beattie. A monthly list of co-dependency videos is posted, as is an updated list of co-dependency sayings and slogans ('You have a right to choose relationships', '"To let go" does not mean to stop caring').

The emotionality, cross-talk and advice that are avoided in other on-line and real-life recovery groups are valued in this newsgroup. Here, an IT opens up a new space for women (and men) to talk with one another. Their talk is personal and emotional, filled with evocative symbols connected to mothers, families, holidays and children. The women who have found their way into alt.recovery.codependency know what to do with this site. They are talking about things the men in their lives will not listen to, using this new IT to create new identities and lives for themselves. On other sites (and here too) men are still debating the rules of discourse.

THREAD ONE: 'CHOICES, HOLIDAYS AND GIFTS'

Consider the following anonymous postings between persons using the names Jacki, Liz, Diane and Nicki.[9] The postings occurred between the dates 9 and 16 December 1994 under the headings of 'Choices' and 'Holidays and Gifts'.

Choices

The first exchange is between Jacki and Liz. It discusses the pain that is involved in working on the inner child. On 9 December Liz wrote to Jacki, connecting to Jacki's discussion of her past, finding a link to her own childhood:

> Your post reminded me of how I struggled also with the idea of my childhood having effects that lasted past the time of childhood. . . . It was/can still be hard to allow myself to accept that it affected my experiences outside the family home as I was growing up.

Jacki agrees:

> It's funny, cuz all my life and still to this day when I look back on the time when my parents were still married I think of my family as a normal middle-class family with no problems. I still look back through that glass ball and think how can that be, I can't seem to make the connection of the abuse with what I perceived as a normal family. . . . After my parents divorced the abuse was more apparent. It came in the form of neglect and abandonment and that is something I've been able to at least see and try to work on . . . I'm glad my post helped you, I'll look forward to hearing more from you. Hugs and smiles from Jacki

Jacki and Liz converse within a shared space organized around the pain of letting go of childhood experiences and expectations. Both women see connections between their lives as children and experiences outside the family home. Each is doing a version of Inner Child work, and Jacki's hugs and smiles anchor this exchange in a warm, supportive emotional give-and-take. This is recovery talk of the sort endorsed in the a.r.c. statement of purpose.

Holidays and Gifts

The next thread brings mothers into the inner child situation. Each writer is a mother struggling with the childhood loss of her own mother. Diane moves the discussion in this thread to the topic of dead mothers and Christmas:

> My mom died when I was 12 and I was extremely devastated. After 24 years, I still am. . . . Every Christmas since I've had my children, I geared everything towards them and my husband. I even had a stocking

hanging, right along with mine for my husband. Every year I would make sure all stockings were filled . . . I thought maybe my husband would put something in mine. No way . . . Christmas morning would find me with nothing in mom's stocking. . . . Talk about hurt feelings. I finally got wise and stopped filling his . . . but my inner child cries because others are getting things and I'm not.

Nicki thanks Diane for her posting:

Thank you for your follow-up to my post. It is so *easy* for me to feel like the only one going through this particular kind of Christmas pain. I know that it isn't. I have known so few other women who lost their mother in childhood that it just seems that way sometimes. We are the same age, so I can relate to how immediate your mom's absence can seem after many years.

Nicki then discusses the problem of gifts in Christmas stockings:

Someone earlier in this thread mentioned the same phenomenon. I no longer have the post, but if I may risk a paraphrase, the person said she came to realize that it actually upset one of her children that Santa seemed to forget Mom at Christmas. And she began buying things for herself and putting them under the tree because it was important to model to her children that *she* was important too. I thought that was a beautiful idea. All the best to you, and happy birthday! Nicki

Diane and Nicki, like Jacki and Liz, engage in emotional work based on shared histories. Nicki can relate to Diane's empty stocking on Christmas morning. Diane's inner child wants presents. Like a dutiful mother, she learns that she has to buy them for herself. No one else remembers her, even her dead mother can't help. But Nicki is here on-line to help, reporting on other people in Diane's situation who are doing the same thing. Each woman relates to the other's loss and pain, especially the Christmas pain when each mother relives the loss of her own mother.

Within the therapeutic ideology of a.r.c., when Diane buys gifts for herself, she addresses the needs of her inner child. Thus one part of her recovery dates from that moment when she finally got wise and started getting things for herself. Nicki is firm on this: recovery involves putting self first, seeing personal needs and addressing them without guilt or shame. This is what Diane is able to do, and her behaviour undoubtedly served as a model for others who were silently lurking behind this exchange.

These conversations can be interpreted, in part, through the method of instances, which focuses on how meaning and control are interactionally produced. These on-line exchanges involve women talking to women. No men are involved. Each woman knows how to talk the talk of a.r.c. Each writer uses the right language, and each contributes to a gendered discourse centring on family, illness and recovery. No one gets emotionally out of control. There is no flaming and no individual acts as a spokesperson for the entire a.r.c. newsgroup. These exchanges appear to work because each person shares, and appears to be sincerely interested in the other writer's situation. There is an implied merger of on- and off-screen selves, talk between persons who genuinely care about one another. Power is not an issue; rather each woman attempts to share an experience, to create a space which the other can enter. This is not the case in the next thread.

THREAD TWO: 'HELP ME UNDERSTAND SOMETHING'

On Monday 2 September 1996 Lucia, who listed herself as an MSW (medical social worker), wrote:

> Here's the situation: about a couple of weeks ago, my brother asked to cut all ties with us. He's lived on the opposite coast for two years now. He requested our communication to be limited to 1) emergencies, and 2) items he wanted brought from home before he moves to his new apartment. One of those items puzzled me. I would never have gotten suspicious if it wasn't for the fact that I was in the D & A [drugs and addiction] treatment field. Anyway, I asked him, with the preface that if it weren't for my job I would never have thought twice. Knowing my parents, I told him if there was something he wanted to say, I'd be the best person to tell. (This was based on experience.) Well, I got a response earlier last week. He did answer my question. He also reminded me of the boundaries he set up, and reamed me for crossing them. Finally, he told me that I should 'focus on my own addictive behaviors and patterns' instead of someone else's (in terms of my job, this can sound pretty funny). Now here's the kicker – My brother told me he is in the CODA fellowship. I can understand if some distance may be required. He's had that for two years. What I don't understand is if CODA condones a person 'burning his bridges' as he is doing to my family. I know our parents have a lot to do with his behavior, but if anything, he can learn to transcend that without cutting us off completely. Also, I want to know if CODA condones the type of dialogue my brother wrote in this letter. I took this situation to my supervisor, a recovering drug addict, who said this is typical of an addict in denial. Is this type of behavior approved for recovering codependents? Lucia.

This posting was given the label 'Help Me Understand Something'. The next day Richard wrote, commenting on various sentences in Lucia's posting. To the first three sentences, he stated, 'Why would you be suspicious of a plain, simple request like that? Are you your brother's keeper?' To the sentences 'Anyway, I asked him . . . I'd be the best person to tell . . .' Richard observes:

Then again, you may not. He has apparently decided you were not the best one. Likely he is pursuing his recovery, preparing to say what he wishes to his parents when he is ready.

Richard proceeds to further dissect Lucia's posting:

To Lucia's 'and reamed me . . .' Richard retorts: 'Excellent! Saves me the chore of doing again.'

To: 'sounds pretty funny . . .' he comments: 'Not funny . . . but WEIRD.'

To: 'if CODA condones . . .' he states: 'Not at all. You're not helping one bit by taking this stance.'

To: 'without cutting us off . . .' Richard observes: 'Not at all. You're not helping one bit by taking this stance.'

To: 'I know our parents . . .' Richard complains: 'So you're correcting his behavior for the good of the family?'

To: 'If CODA condones . . . to my supervisor . . .' Richard asks: 'Have you discussed your reactions with your supervisor? That would be the appropriate response. It seems quite inappropriate for you to drag a family matter – essentially a family viewpoint, and a highly dysfunctional one at that – to your supervisor for reinforcement. Your brother's behavior is typical of a codep in recovery. YOURS is typical of a dysfunctional family member struggling to scapegoat the recovering member who has broken ties with an obviously toxic family environment.'

To: 'behavior approved for recovering codependents?' Richard answers: 'Lady, we don't approve shit! Each person follows the 12-Steps as best they can for their personal recovery. Your attempt to recruit support in turning a recovering person back into a sick family is in itself insane.'

To Lucia as an 'MSW' Richard takes exception: 'The attempt to introduce yourself with the presentation of credentials is inappropriate to the NG [newsgroup]. We do not welcome professional healers and helpers here. The approach and reasonings used above confirm this as a wide tradition. We, I personally, are unimpressed with your credentials. Further, I am negatively impressed with the illness presented in your post. It is truly frightening that you are in the professional recovery field. Richard'

Thus does Richard directly attack Lucia. Sharing little of his personal experience with her, he positions himself as a spokesperson for the newsgroup. His responses border on flaming ('Saves me the chore of doing [reaming] again'; 'Lady, we don't approve shit!'). Richard reads his way into the unnamed brother's social situation, and then positions Lucia against the brother and the family ('For the good of the family?'). He then suggests that Lucia has a dysfunctional family, and uses the CODA language of toxic environment and scapegoating to explain what she is doing to her brother. Richard then challenges Lucia's credentials, and tells her 'We do not welcome professional healers and helpers here.' This suggests a difference between lay and professional healers. Richard sides with the lay healing traditions, using the phrase 'truly frightening' to describe his reactions to her presence in the professional recovery field.

These are personal attacks. Richard is using his apparently acknowledged position as a frequent reader on this group as a lever for monitoring and censoring Lucia's posting. He treats her as a toxic presence, a presence that needs cleansing. He does not find uniform support for this position. Although the following postings by women seem to endorse some of the same CODA principles that Richard holds, they are not personal attacks on Lucia. They feminize his stance.

Feminizing and resisting Richard

Marny by-passes Richard in her comments on Lucia's posting ('Is this type of behavior approved . . .?') , stating, 'I'm Marny and I'm in the 7th year of recovery, with the help of CODA. . . . Nothing that *I* know of makes anyone say or do anything.'

On 3 September Carmella enters the discourse, essentially agreeing with Richard, again using terms from CODA and ACOA:

> It sounds as if you have taken the position of 'family caretaker' – that you are not respecting your brother's right to pursue his recovery as he sees fit . . . you are making him 'wrong' or scapegoating, as Richard indicated . . . I agree with Richard . . . your brother is not a client and his business is not your supervisor's. . . . To Richard: friend, you pull no punches! Carmella

The next day Dana comments on the fact that Lucia brought her supervisor into this situation. Dana is less critical of Lucia, and is even somewhat supporting:

> Are you prepared to wage a war with your brother over his boundaries? Maybe he is STRUGGLING with not behaving in ways that are not approved by your family. . . . As for the role of CODA in all of this . . . I say that you should give your brother time, and back off a little . . . (my opinion, and you know what they say about opinions . . .). Dana

An anonymous posting sides with Lucia against Richard:

> Although I understand Richard's position, it seems harsh to me . . . Lucia may work in the field . . . but she is hurt and confused and is asking for help. That IS the first step. She knows she needs help . . . I have found the gentleness and acceptance of others as I recover to be more helpful than 'constructive criticism' by others of my old way of thinking. My thinking was no clearer than hers a brief time ago. . . . Harsh analysis of that

thinking would not have benefited me then . . . I hope to never be so complacent and assured of my own recovery that I cannot remember the old me.

This posting is like the exchanges between Liz and Jacki and between Diane and Nicki: it stresses acceptance and gentleness, and love. 'Anonymous' criticizes Richard for being harsh, notes that Lucia is confused and hurt, and underscores the fact that she has asked for help.

Richard will have none of this, and immediately responds to the statement that his position 'seems harsh to me'. To wit: 'Reality is often harsh. Confrontation is harsh. Pain is harsh. I come honestly to these conclusions over years of recovery.' Richard will not accept the proposition that Lucia is hurt and confused. He now engages in a point-by-point refutation of the above post:

> [Hers] is not a request for help. That is manipulation . . . she will get no help from me if she wishes to continue dysfunctional behavior. I may have been direct, even rude, but does anyone dispute the facts I have presented? . . . I agree her thinking is not clear. It is bent in a direction determined by years of steeping in the toxic family of origin. . . . Don't ask me questions you don't really want answers for. I don't have time for it . . . I don't have time for folks that want to wallow in their past. Don't ask me what I think of you, 'cause I might not tell you what you want me to.
> Richard

Richard insists on authorizing one interpretation of Lucia's posting: she is a sick co-dependant, engaged in dysfunctional behaviour. He knows this because of his years of recovery experience. The facts justify his directness. She is using her MSW credentials to manipulate her brother and her family. He doesn't have time for these people, even though he has dominated the postings on her call for help. There may even be a hint of misogyny in his comments.

Nina supports Richard:

> Although many will find Richard's comments to be somewhat harsh, I choose to view them as a reminder that this program is all about self-care and Lucia's brother is struggling to give himself the space and time to practice that self-care.

Lucia re-posts to Richard

Lucia corrects misspellings in her original posting and responds directly to Richard's harsh evaluations of her situation. He counters each of her comments, as if they were in Internet Relay Chat:

Richard: Brother's keeper?
Lucia: No. But I was puzzled.

Richard: Not my point. I see a lot of putting your brother in the position of a patient.

Lucia: I figured that out already.

Richard: I believe it's critical to examine your motives.

Lucia: Excellent! Saves me the chore of doing again?

Richard: You're not hearing what I am saying!

Lucia: Mister! I don't want him to come back to a sick family! I'm not asking for reinforcement. I'm trying to figure out where to go from here. I am working on acceptance.

Richard: If I misunderstood your intentions, I apologize. However, your original post was, upon review, an attempt at solicitation for a position already formed. This is not what we call recovery. Perhaps you do not understand our traditions (traditions are posted as ACOA Bill of Rights). It is truly frightening that you are in the professional field of recovery.

Lucia: It is truly frightening that you read a sincere request with suspicion.

Richard: Call 'em like you see 'em. I did.

This reader can almost visualize Lucia and Richard in the same room, perhaps at an ACOA or CODA meeting, shouting at each other. The emotionality is electric. Lucia gets in Richard's face and refuses to back down: 'Mister! . . . I'm not asking for reinforcement.' In defending her position, which has surely moved and changed since the original posting, Lucia reveals an attempt to help her brother get distance from her sick family. (This understanding was not evident in the original call for help.) Yet Richard will not give her the benefit of this change, insisting that she is still sick, thereby emphasizing his version of what recovery is all about. She retorts, suggesting that his inability to read a sincere request for help without suspicion is 'truly frightening'.

This is more than an IRC give-and-take. A woman with professional credentials is challenging a man, a professed lay expert who is attempting to control the grounds, terms and language of recovery. Richard is acting as if he were the gatekeeper to the recovery process, as that process is structured by ACOA and CODA. Lucia proposes an alternative reading of this language, an alternative which Richard rejects. A gendered conflict occurs, a battle over recovery identities is fought. Lucia will not accept the labels Richard wants to apply to her, and she will not grant Richard the power he claims. She will not accept his language, or his definitions of this situation. Thus in this instance, in this thread, power and control move back and forth from Richard to Lucia, to Marny, Dana, Nina, to Anonymous, back to Richard and Lucia.

Later that day, Lucia again posts to the entire group, thereby ending the thread. Her posting is titled 'Epilogue':

Thanks to those who have posted, and to those who will post as they see my original post. To those who have, or will, accuse of me being the problem: if you recall, my original post asked for HELP. Accusations do not help anyone. If putdowns are what you consider help, thanks, but no thanks. But don't worry, you have not totally dashed my hopes for learning what I need to do. Based on my survey of responses, turns out yours are in the minority. I guess I can use a little advice I hear often: if it don't apply, let it fly. At this point, I am respecting my brother's wishes. I was going to reply, but after my initial reaction, I decided it would be easier this way. We still have some business to complete, and it would be better to do it quick and without conflict from anyone. I can guarantee we won't get his new address – I'd be surprised if he did . . . I have no idea how I'll respond when he decides to open up lines of communication. That's where I'm at. An extra thanks to those who gave/will give their insights. Lucia

Inscribing Lucia's illness

And so ends, for the time being at least, Lucia's foray into this particular on-line recovery group. Her epilogue divides the persons who responded into two groups, the accusers and the non-accusers. Still, she takes something from the accusers, as seen in her decision not to respond to her brother. But she is firm, putdowns are not help, not what she thinks recovery is all about.

The Richard–Lucia exchange centres on three key terms in the ACOA and CODA discourse systems: illness, therapy and family. Lucia is defined as coming from a sick, dysfunctional family. She is told that proper therapy involves detachment from that family, and working on her own problems. Thus by entering a.r.c.'s virtual reality, Lucia receives advice on how to handle problems in the so-called real world.

This is talking therapy in the form of a written text. The written word becomes an instance of the illness that requires therapy. This illness is relational. It involves Lucia, her brother and her family. At one level the problem centres on her brother's desire to cut all ties with the family. But this is not the problem; the problem lies in her response to his request: that is, should she honour it? The situation thickens when she reports that her brother is a member of CODA. This information locates the brother inside the CODA community of recovering persons. Ironically, this same information places Lucia outside the moral boundaries of CODA. Hence the responses to her can be read as ganging up on her, the accusers versus the non-accusers. She is part of the problem, not part of the solution. Thus the very actions that asked for help, are read as being symptomatic of Lucia's illness. A co-dependant tries to control others and that is what she is attempting to do. The illness, or situation she seeks help from, is turned back against her.

Of course her original posting asked for help. But here is the paradox: she asked for help the wrong way. In so doing she was defined, by some at least, as being the source of her brother's problems. In fact, in her eyes, her brother is the source of the trouble that must be dealt with. Little did she know that her original posting would stir up such an uproar.

That posting was publicly responded to (and apparently printed) by five people: Richard, Marny, Dana, Nina and Anonymous. The printed posting now becomes the basis for future discourse. The meanings of Lucia's key questions can be debated and discussed. Her responses now become reflex-ively embedded in this original text which defines her as a dysfunctional person. Her text thus provides a historical document with which all future exchanges can be compared. Lucia takes on a life of her own in this small community of persons who take up the challenge to respond to her posting. Motives and intentions are imputed to her. This motive talk is ACOA- and CODA-based, it uses the language of dysfunctionality.

In attempting to control this discourse, Richard took on the position of a spokesperson for the group. He turned this into gendered talk, a man telling a woman what to do. He did this by siding with her brother against her. This meant he rejected her definitions of this situation. He applauded the reaming she got, labelled her family as dysfunctional, used profanity, mocked her professional degree, located illness in her post, said she was scapegoating.

Not all responders accorded him this power, and the debates that fol-lowed focused, in part, on this fact. Hence Richard, not Lucia, became, for a moment, the centre of the thread (Richard and Anonymous). He became the problem to be dealt with, and thus did Lucia (and her brother) disappear from sight.

Women by-passing illness

Return to Jacki and Liz, Diane and Nicki. Four women talking about mothers, childhood, Christmas, stockings, Inner Child work, and gifts. Same newsgroup, a.r.c. But the talk is different. No one attempts to control the discourse. Gender in its masculinized versions does not operate. No men are present. Experiences as mothers, wives and daughters are shared, common problems are taken up. Pathologies and illness are not inscribed in the talk. Rather each woman addresses a specific (or general) problem, or issue, which is then loosely interpreted from within the ACOA and CODA frameworks. The talk is taken to be symptomatic of what persons in recovery say to one another, including how they describe themselves and their situations. It is not read as an example of pathology. This is in stark contrast to Richard using Lucia's talk as an instance of her illness. The women, instead, by-pass illness and focus either on solutions to prob-lems, or engage in mutual talk about the problem (e.g. Jacki and Liz and their lost childhoods, Diane and Nicki and Christmas stockings). Discussing problems and sharing solutions to them create a form of recovery talk which is mutually supportive, and non-evaluative. As discussed above, this sharing of experience (strength and hope) is basic to the group's purpose. Such sharing is noticeably absent in the Richard–Lucia exchanges.

These women selectively use the languages of CODA and ACOA, stressing the positive over the negative. That is, they resist the negative terms used by Richard (sick family, insane, dysfunctional family member). They create, instead, a gendered space for recovery where a positive culture of family, therapy and illness is enacted.

INFORMATION TECHNOLOGIES AND RECOVERING SELVES

When the self-help industry went on-line, few could have imagined the uses to which this new information technology would be put. Of course in retrospect it all makes perfect sense, and nothing seems at all odd about an on-line '12-Step Recovery Shopping Network', hanging out at 'The 12 Steps Cyberspace Cafe', belonging to any one of several Usenet recovery groups, from Sex Offenders Anonymous, to Smokers Anonymous, to CODA, ACOA, and that old stand-by AA. Kaminer reminds us (1992: 165) that we cannot imagine America without its self-help groups. And we cannot imagine an America that is not in love with technology. Cyberspace and the recovery movement were meant for each other: cyber-recovery.

Like the new information technologies connected to cyberspace, the CODA and ACOA recovery moments employ liberationist ideologies. They purport to free the self from itself, to move the self into a new moral community. In this new frontier old stereotypes are challenged, and new ways of being are not only imagined, but also realized, if only in VR. In this new space persons are encouraged to roam, and to enter freely into new social relationships.

The cyber-recovery movement uses rationalist ideologies, arguing that it is not rational to remain in unhealthy relationships. These are also emotional ideologies, appealing to cultural stereotypes about ideal family histories and ideal childhood experiences. These discourses are anti-institutional and anti-family, for they critique the major institutions of American society. Cyber-recovery ideology rests on a populist conception of treatment. Under this framework everyone is sick. But on the utopian level, it is argued that changes from within the family can change history. In this, cyber-therapy treats the family as the basic institution in society. Everyone, it is claimed, has been emotionally abused. Only the individual can be the judge of the nature and extent of this abuse. We are, as Bradshaw argues, 'the stories we tell about our childhoods'. These stories mutate and multiply in cyberspace, threads within threads, stories within stories, printed texts of on-line oral tales of the self and its miseries; desktop publishing and computerized recovery.

Based on weak, anecdotal cases, this literature creates spaces which anyone can enter, for who can't remember something unhappy about their childhood? These literatures have, in a sense, created a national epidemic of illness; everyone, if honest, today suffers from a process addiction. This amorphous disease now generates millions, even billions of dollars. What were once bad habits have become signs of illness, and Americans, perhaps, have become obsessed with disease. We want to be in recovery, and ACOA/CODA literatures offer steps for recovery for anyone who can read.

Some might argue that the cyber-recovery movements are reactions to the 'selfish' 1970s, where people attempted to get whatever they could out of life. The cognitive therapies of the 1970s (*I'm O.K., You're O.K.*) and the popular religious therapies of the 1950s (Norman Vincent Peale – *The Power of Positive Thinking*) emphasized the individual's ability and power to heal himself or herself. Faith and rational thinking could produce happiness. Like Mary Baker Eddy's 1920s Christian Science movement, the self-help movements of the 1950s, 1960s and 1970s emphasized faith and will-power.

The new self-help movements are different. They shift attention away from the self and place it on the sick society. They encourage a kind of collective fantasy about recovery and being free of the sick family. Ten years of personal computers on the job, in the home and in school have prepared millions of Americans for the cyber-recovery movement. Any computer-literate child over the age of 6 can participate in this discourse.

Couch (1995) argues that the particular consequences of each IT are contingent on how the IT is contextualized within a social structure. The contextualization process involves forms of relatedness and connectedness that organize the social actions of those who use the IT. Users of an IT can be connected and related in a variety of ways, from exchange to charismatic, intimate, or tyrannical relationships (Couch 1995).

In the world of cyber-recovery this new IT is contextualized in each of the above ways; intimate, tyrannical, egalitarian, exchange and charismatic relationships connect users to one another.[10] The discourses that are produced connect to the wider meaning systems that circulate in the real worlds of CODA and ACOA. But this meaning system is fitted to on-line authority relationships that differentially privilege age, gender and recovery experience. The IT is filtered through these defining social relationships. These Virtual Reality relationships frequently tilt in the direction of men telling women how to recover from their experiences in dysfunctional families. In this way virtual reality (VR) reproduces the real world (RW).

WHOSE CHILDHOOD IS IT ANYWAY?

Without cultural narratives about children, without children's literature, there would be no ACOA or CODA movements. These movements require cultural narratives which idealize childhood and family life, and here a subtle reversal in literary production occurs. Under the traditional frame-work, children's narrative, or children's literature (Lukens 1995: xi), is litera-ture written by adults for children. This literature treats children as valued human beings. It places great value on children's emotions, their fears and their intimate, family and peer relationships and friendships. It often locates the child in a world of magical realism where animals and nature talk and express humanlike emotions and feelings. Under the regime of cyber-recovery, adults rewrite children's literature for themselves. A new version of childhood is created, the adult reliving the idealized childhood tradition-ally given to children.

Hence this adult version of children's literature appropriates and repro-duces recurring cultural understandings concerning children, their care-takers and the societies they live in. These understandings include beliefs in the innocent wisdom and kindness of children, their natural curiosity about the animate and inanimate world around them, their love of play, their ability to engage in make-believe and fantasy games, their susceptibil-ity to irrational fears, their need for love, tender care and understanding from the adult world, their need to be protected from a cruel, irrational and harsh world by loving, caring adults. This inner childlike self is one that is joyous, free, innocent, loving, self-confident, and trusting in others. This is the self ACOAs and CODAs are searching for. This is the self that Diane and Nicki are co-constructing as they discuss presents on Christmas morning in Christmas stockings. This is the adult self of a mother modelling childhood behaviour for her children. This mother is showing her children that Santa did not forget Mom on this Christmas Day.

True to the larger cultural narratives that define the recovery movement, this adult literature for the postmodern or contemporary child (who is also an adult) involves stories and narratives about children of divorce, children who have experienced sexual abuse, children of single-parent homes, children raised by their grandparents, children without mothers, children with same-sex parents. Such children never learned how to build healthy, normal, warm, intimate relationships with others. Thus Nicki can tell her children that even though she did not have a mother when she was growing up, they do, and this mother knows how to take care of herself, and them, on this holiday. Together, she and her children will have that childhood she never had.

Recovery from this disease requires that the person find and re-experience the inner child lost to alcoholism, divorce, abuse and other forms of dys-function and neglect. This inner child is the idealized child found in tradi-tional children's literature. Thus do ACOAs and CODAs use children's literature for their self-recovery programmes.

IN CONCLUSION: BACK AT 'THE 12 STEPS CYBERSPACE CAFE'

My reactions to ACOA and CODA parallel those of Kaminer (1992: 163) and Mitchell-Norberg *et al.* (1995: 143–6), who waver between being amused, pleased and disturbed by developments in the self-help recovery movements. Kaminer, Mitchell-Norberg, Warren and Zale take pleasure in seeing people, especially women, getting help, watching them reaching out to one another. But it is disturbing to see only certain versions of recovery being honoured, or endorsed. It is disturbing to see members attack and criticize one another, as was the case when Lucia encountered Richard. It is disturbing to see the accoutrements of recovery marketed on-line in cyberspace. It is disturbing to see men attempting to control this discourse about family, intimacy, self and other.

Usenet technology also presents a problem. The lifetime of any thread on a.r.c. is short, a few weeks, usually a day or two at best. But in that short time the person who asks for help can receive advice from countless, faceless others, others who purport to have help for the person in question. This help comes fast, and it may be critical (Richard and Lucia), or supportive (Liz and Jacki). This is instant, electronic therapy, immediate feedback. In a.r.c. there are no appointments, no weekly sessions with a psychotherapist, no waiting for the next ACOA meeting. The meeting is always there. All you have to do is dial-up and look for help. Of course there is a danger here. A highly susceptible person may get what some would regard as the wrong kind of advice, and even may act on that advice, thereby getting into new kinds of trouble, or creating new kinds of problems for herself or himself.

Karl Marx reminds us that if events of significance occur twice, then the first time is 'as tragedy and the second as farce' (1983 [1888]: 287). Surely ACOAs and CODAs have experienced tragedies of great import. Certainly their attempts at recovery are to be honoured. But on one level the ACOA and CODA movements risk becoming farce. In their attempts to escape a tragic past by enacting a perfect childhood, they idealize what never was; that is, they create an ideal childhood. At the same time some may make a mockery of their present lives, failing to recognize the significance and importance of what they now have. Idealized versions of selfhood, childhood, love and intimacy are just that, ideal versions of what never can be. And here a sense of loss is experienced, for what the person gains may never match what he or she is now willing to give up.

At this level, the conceptions of womanhood, family and gendered relations endorsed by CODA are, as Mitchell-Norberg *et al.* note, unsettling (1995: 145–6). The movement seems to reject the concept of a woman's nurturing identity, while encouraging an independence that protects women from the demands of men and a troubled family past. This may leave women isolated and alone.

In the following posting (25 September 1996) Trish is struggling with just these issues; that is, should she ask her husband to come back home?

> My husband and I separated a couple of months ago. My life has taken a
> steady course downward. Just when I think it can't get any worse it does.
> I have asked my husband to come back. I know now that our problems

came from me. He says that he will have to think about why he is afraid to come back. I really need him. I am trying so hard to put my life back together and I really want him to be there for me. Am I wrong? Trish

Carmella responds:

Trish . . . your husband may be afraid that you are just too needy and expect that having him in your life will 'make it better'. That's a big order. . . . Are you seeing a therapist? Do you have other friends/relatives to whom you can turn for support? . . . If an SO isn't available for us emotionally, friends – sometimes relatives – are. If we need a hug, there are many ways to get one. Being dependent on ONE human being to make our lives better is so disempowering. Peace.

And there is always cybersex.

NOTES

1 The decade of the 1990s has been a time of renewed public interest concerning self-help groups (Kaminer 1992), personal health (Rice 1996), drugs, drinking and the problems of alcohol consumption in American society (Conrad and Schneider 1992: 109). A new temperance movement (Pittman 1991), paralleling the outbreak of a national war on drugs, is one manifestation of this concern. As David Pittman (1991: 775) observes, for the third time in the twentieth century the United States is in the midst of a war on drugs. The first war occurred during those years bounded by Prohibition, 1914–33, the second overlapped with the Vietnam War years, 1965–72, and the third has just begun. Other indicators of this renewed public concern can be seen in the many new recovery groups that have appeared in the last decade, including the Adult Children of Alcoholics (ACOA) and the Co-Dependency (CODA) movements.

2 I was a passive, lurking observer. I never identified myself to the group, nor did I obtain permission to quote from postings, thereby violating many of Schrum's (1995) ethical injunctions for electronic research.

3 In a moderated newsgroup all messages are screened by a moderator for content; only those deemed appropriate for the group are posted (Turkle 1995: 132).

4 Historically these have been female-based movements, ACOA being an offshoot of Al-Anon, the spousal (wife) side of Alcoholics Anonymous (see Asher 1992; Rudy 1991). The participation of males in ACOA and CODA has dramatically increased in the last decade; however, the ratio of females to males is still approximately 2:1 (see Rice 1996: 223). In late 1994 women outnumbered men 7:1 in the on-line a.r.c. conversations. Kaminer (1992: 88–9) argues that CODA is disproportionately female (but see Rice 1996: 44). The welcoming document inviting the reader into a.r.c. is apparently written by a person who uses the name deedee.

5 The user can also go shopping, a recent posting (1 October 1996) announces: 'Shop On The Internet For Your 12-Step Recovery Gift Items. Network 12 Offers Listings of Recovery Stores & Suppliers of Recovery Gift Items Throughout The United States & Canada. Visit Network 12 Recovery Stores & Gift Resources On Line Where A Wide Array of Recovery Gifts Are Available' (http://www.network12.com).

6 Adjacency pairs are at least two turns in length (hello–goodbye), that is, have at least two parts, with at least two speakers, where the sequences are immediate next turns (Psathas 1995: 18). Internet relay chat (IRC), that mode of Internet

talk where people are able to communicate synchronistically on different chan-
nels from disparate locations (Baym 1995a: 151), most closely approximates
these features of the adjacency pair.

7 Stories are narratives, tellings with beginnings, middles and ends. Stories begin
with an initial situation. A sequence of events leads to the disturbance, or reversal, of this situation. The revelation of character and setting is made possible by
this disturbance. A personification of characters (protagonists, antagonists and
witnesses) also occurs. The resolution of this predicament leads to stories
where there is a regression, a progression, or no change in the main character's
situation (Polkinghorne 1988: 15; Polkinghorne 1995).

8 a.r.c. (alt.recovery.codependency 1996: 6) states: 'The three most common
Twelve-Step programs pertinent to those of us dealing with codependency are
Codependents Anonymous (CODA), Al-Anon and Adult Children of Alco-
holics . . . [see] Melody Beattie's *Codependent's Guide to the Twelve Steps*.'

9 I give pseudonyms to all persons quoted in this manuscript.

10 For example, Richard, clearly a charismatic figure, attempts tyranically to manipulate Lucia into accepting his view of her illness. In contrast, an egalitarian
relationship seems to exist between the women who discuss lost childhood and
Christmas.

BIBLIOGRAPHY

alt.recovery.codependency (1996) 'Frequently asked questions and general information about the Usenet newsgroup alt.recovery.codependency.' world wide web
page: http://www.infinet.com/-deedee/arc.html.17 March.

Asher, R. (1992) *Women with Alcoholic Husbands: Ambivalence and the Trap of
Codependency*. Chapel Hill, NC: University of North Carolina Press.

Aycock, A. and Buchignani, N. (1995) 'The e-mail murders: reflections on "dead"
letters', in Steven G. Jones (ed.) *Cybersociety: Computer-Mediated Communication
and Community*. Thousand Oaks, CA: Sage, pp. 184–231.

Balsamo, A. (1994) 'Feminism and the incurably informed', in Mark Dery (ed.)
Flame Wars: The Discourse of Cyberculture. Durham, NC: Duke University
Press, pp. 125–56.

Bardini, T. and Horvath, A. (1995) 'The social construction of the personal computer user', *Journal of Communication* 45: 40–65.

Baym, N. (1995a) 'The emergence of community in computer-mediated communication', in Steven G. Jones (ed.) *Cybersociety: Computer-Mediated Communication
and Community*. Thousand Oaks, CA: Sage, pp. 138–63.

Baym, N. (1995b) 'From practice to culture on Usenet', in Susan Leigh Star (ed.) *The
Cultures of Computing*. Cambridge, MA: Blackwell, pp. 29–52.

Conrad, P. and Schneider, J. (1992) *Deviance and Medicalization: From Badness to
Sickness*, expanded edn. Philadelphia, PA: Temple University Press.

Couch, C. (1995) 'Oh, what webs those phantoms spin', *Symbolic Interaction* 18:
229–45.

Denzin, N. K. (1993) *The Alcoholic Society*. New Brunswick, NJ: Transaction Publishers.

Derrida, J. (1976) *Of Grammatology*. Baltimore, MD: Johns Hopkins University
Press.

Dery, M. (1994) 'Flame wars', in Mark Dery (ed.) *Flame Wars: The Discourse of
Cyberculture*. Durham, NC: Duke University Press, pp. 1–10.

Featherstone, M. and Burrows, R. (1995) 'Cultures of technological embodiment: an
introduction', in M. Featherstone and R. Burrows (eds) *Cyberspace/Cyberbodies/
Cyberpunk: Cultures of Technological Embodiment*. London: Sage, pp. 1–20.

Hahn, H. and Stout, R. (1994) *The Internet Complete Reference*. Berkeley, CA: Osborne McGraw-Hill.

Jones, S. (1995) 'Understanding community in the information age', in Steven G. Jones (ed.) *Cybersociety: Computer-Mediated Communication and Community*. Thousand Oaks, CA: Sage, pp. 10–35.

Kaminer, W. (1992) *I'm Dysfunctional, You're Dysfunctional*. New York: Vintage Books.

Kramarae, C. (1995) 'A backstage critique of virtual reality', in Steven G. Jones (ed.) *Cybersociety: Computer-Mediated Communication and Community*. Thousand Oaks, CA: Sage, pp. 36–56.

Lukens, R. (1955) *Critical Handbook of Children's Literature*, 5th edn. New York: HarperCollins.

McLaughlin, M., Osborne, K. and Smith, B. (1995) 'Standards of conduct on Usenet', in Steven G. Jones (ed.) *Cybersociety: Computer-Mediated Communication and Community*. Thousand Oaks, CA: Sage, pp. 90–111.

Marx, K. (1983 [1888]) 'From the Eighteenth Brumaire of Louis Bonaparte', in *The Portable Karl Marx*, ed. E. Kamenka. New York: Penguin, pp. 286–324.

Mitchell-Norberg, J., Warren, C., and Zale, S. (1995) 'Gender and codependents anonymous', in M. Flaherty and C. Ellis (eds) *Social Perspectives on Emotion*, Vol. 3. Greenwich, CT: JAI Press, pp. 121–49.

Parks, M. and Floyd, K. (1996) 'Making friends in cyberspace', *Journal of Communication* 46: 80–97.

Pittman, D. (1991) 'The new temperance movement', in J. Pittman and H. Ruskin White (eds) *Society, Culture, and Drinking Patterns Reexamined*. New Brunswick, NJ: Rutgers Center for Alcohol Studies, pp. 775–90.

Polkinghorne, D. (1988) *Narrative Knowing in the Human Sciences*. Albany, NY: State University of New York Press.

Polkinghorne, D. (1995) 'Narrative configuration in qualitative analysis', in J. Amos Hatch and R. Wisniewski (eds) *Life History and Narrative*. Washington, DC: Falmer Press, pp. 5–23.

Psathas, G. (1995) *Conversation Analysis*. Thousand Oaks, CA: Sage.

Rice, J. (1996) *A Disease of One's Own: Psychotherapy, Addiction, and the Emergence of Co-Dependency*. New Brunswick, NJ: Transaction Publishers.

Rudy, D. (1991) 'The Adult Children of Alcoholics movement: a social constructionist perspective', in D. Pittman and H. Ruskin White (eds) *Society, Culture, and Drinking Patterns Reexamined*. New Brunswick, NJ: Rutgers Center for Alcohol Studies, pp. 716–32.

Schrum, L. (1995) 'Framing the debate: ethical research in the information age', *Qualitative Inquiry* 1: 311–26.

Star, S. (1995) Introduction, in Susan Leigh Star (ed.) *The Cultures of Computing*. Cambridge: MA: Blackwell, pp. 1–28.

Turkle, S. (ed.) (1995) *Life on the Screen: Identity in the Age of the Internet*. New York: Simon & Schuster.

Walstrom, M. (1996) 'Women with eating disorders: an internet study', unpublished dissertation proposal, Speech Communications, University of Illinois, May 1996.

Woitiz, J. (1983) *Adult Children of Alcoholics*. Hollywood, FL: Health Communications.

7 Emotions, cyberspace and the 'virtual' body

A critical appraisal

Simon J. Williams

INTRODUCTION

As we approach the *fin de millénium*, few would disagree with the assertion that we live in an increasingly 'mediated' age; an information-based society where the media, printed and electronic and other forms of communications and computer technology come to play a crucial role in contemporary forms of (emotional) experience and everyday life (Giddens 1991). Some go even further, claiming that the escalating role of the media in society signifies the transition from the modern world of *production* into a postmodern universe of *simulations* involving a radical semiurgy of signs (Baudrillard 1983a, 1983b, 1988).

It is within this context and against this multi-media backdrop, one involving the explosion of information and communications technology and the recent advent of cyberspace and 'virtual' reality, that the following key questions come to the fore. First, what are the implications of these new forms of technology, and the various 'hyperrealities' they spawn, for human emotional experience? More specifically, *if* contemporary forms of experience are increasingly mediated by modern forms of technology, and *if* we are likely to spend more and more of our time in the future interacting with others in the 'non-place' or 'virtual' environments of cyberspace, then what impact will this have on the *nature*, *depth*, *intensity* and *duration* of human emotional experience? This, in turn, relates to a second, deeper and more knotty philosophical problem concerning mind–body dualism and the associated sociological question of the relationship, or lack of one, between emotions, the body and (self-)identity in cyberspace. Finally, in the light of these developments, a third key question relates to the issue of whether or not we need fundamentally to rethink, modify, or extend some of our existing tried and trusted assumptions and concepts within the sociology of emotions.

It is these key questions – questions which highlight the crisis of meaning surrounding the body, self and emotions in late twentieth-century western society – which this chapter seeks to address. Clearly these are complex questions which defy easy answers: for many, only time will tell. In raising them, my intention is not to downplay or downgrade the (emotional) opportunities which these new forms of information technology (IT) afford. Rather, what this chapter amounts to is a challenge to some of the over-inflated claims and disembodied visions that IT spawns.

LIFE IN MEDIASCAPE SOCIETY: THE 'BLUNTING' OR 'INTENSIFICATION' OF EMOTIONAL EXPERIENCE?

As suggested above, according to writers such as Baudrillard (1983a, 1983b, 1988), the media become key 'simulation machines' which endlessly reproduce a glittering profusion of images, signs and codes in the digital postmodern landscape of our times. These images, signs and codes, in turn, come to constitute an autonomous realm of (hyper)reality in which the relationship between representation and reality becomes radically reversed. From this perspective, the advent of this new multi-media reality means that the real becomes 'hyped' as more 'real than real' through an endless chain of self-referential images or 'simulacra'. As a consequence 'fact' becomes 'fiction', and TV, reality. 'The *medium*', in short, to use McLuhan's famous phrase, becomes 'the message'.

More precisely, the 'explosion' of information technology at the turn of the century has, according to Baudrillard, resulted in the 'implosion' of meaning and the blunting of (emotional) response. In this postmodern mediascape, individuals come to feel isolated and privatized, trapped within a universe of simulacra and a 'radical semiurgy' of signs (Kellner 1989). The distinction between the 'spectacle' and the 'real' becomes blurred, and individuals, as passive consumers of endless images, come to prefer the former to the latter. From this Baudrillardian perspective, information and communication technology result in a dulling or numbing of the senses, the *neutralization of meaning*, and a prevention of response on the part of their audiences. In this sense, not only do the media intensify processes of 'massification', 'saturation' and 'information overload', they also promote a 'chilling' effect; one which freezes individuals into functioning like 'terminals' of the very apparatus of communications technology, thus obliterating the distinctions between public and private, interior and exterior.

Within this teeming network of cool, seductive images and fascinating sights and sounds, the era of interiority, subjectivity, meaning, privacy and inner life has, it is claimed, given way to a new era of *obscenity*, fascination, vertigo, instantaneity, *transparency* and over-exposure; a postmodern world *par excellence* (Kellner 1989: 67–72). The domestic scene is exteriorized, made explicit, in a sort of 'obscenity where the most intimate processes of our life become the virtual feeding ground of the media'. Inversely, the entire universe 'comes to unfold arbitrarily on your domestic screen'. In the 'ecstasy of communication', everything is explicit, ecstatic and obscene in its transparency, detail and visibility: 'the obscenity of the visible, the all-too-visible and the more-than-visible' (Baudrillard 1983b: 131).

According to this line of reasoning, an inverse relationship exists between the frequency of media exposure and its impact in terms of the nature, depth and quality of human emotional response it evokes: issues which are nicely captured in the lyrics of a recent U2 track: 'I feel numb, too much is not enough.' At a broader level, this dulling or blunting of emotional response may also resonate with the more general style of emotional management in contemporary society which Stearns (1994) has appositely termed 'American cool'. For Baudrillard, information is 'directly destructive of meaning and signification, or neutralizes it. . . . Information devours its own content . . . leading not at all to the surfeit of innovation, but to the very contrary, to total entrophy' (1983a: 96–100). In this sense:

> There are no longer media in the literal sense of the term – that is to say, a power mediating between one state of the real and another – neither in content nor in form. Strictly speaking this is what implosion signifies: the absorption of one pole into another, the short-circuit between poles of every differential system of meaning, the effacement of terms and of distinct oppositions, and thus that of the medium and the real . . . the medium and the real are now in a single nebulous state whose truth is undecipherable.
>
> (Baudrillard 1983a: 102–3)

The upshot of this, in Baudrillard's terms, is the 'end of the social' (Kellner 1989: 84–9).

To be sure, there are many problems with Baudrillard's position, not least his sign-fetishism, obsessive preoccupation with 'simulacra', and excessive hyping of the 'hyperreal'. In Kellner's (1989) eyes, this justifiably merits the charge that Baudrillard is the 'Walt Disney', *par excellence*, of contemporary metaphysics. None the less, as Tester's chapter in this volume amply illustrates, you do not have to be a Baudrillardian postmodernist to argue that the massifying effects of the media, as key simulation machines, engender in their audience a bored and blasé emotional response. Yet this is surely not the whole story. The unimaginable, inadmissible nightmares of documentary photographic evidence testifying to piles of dead bodies overseen by nonchalant Nazis in the death camps of the Holocaust; the horror of the burning body of the little Vietnamese girl running down the road to escape napalm; and the newsreels showing the charred, blackened bodies of raped and mutilated women in Bosnia: these, and many other similarly chilling 'mediated' images, lie indelibly etched on our minds, calling forth a variety of emotional responses, from rage to sorrow, anger to despair.

As Walter *et al.*'s (1995) analysis of death in the news clearly shows, the media play a crucial role in what they term the 'public invigilation of private emotion' – i.e. the 'simultaneous arousal of, and regulatory keeping watch over, the affective dispositions and responses associated with death' (1995:

586). Events are reported in such a way that clear appeals are made to news-consumers as to the appropriate emotional response in the face of tragedy – from school minibus crashes and the abduction and murder of innocent children, to the carnage in Northern Ireland. Whilst this does not mean that responses can simply be 'read off' from the content of news messages, there are good reasons for thinking that some sort of personal identification with these tragedies does indeed take place. As they state:

> It may well be . . . that the prominence of this kind of death in the news engenders for some certain voyeuristic pleasures, and perhaps facilitates the response of *Schadenfreude* or some such similar macabre enjoyment of the misfortunes of others. . . . If, however, there is encouragement to engage in some sort of identification with characters whose emotional intensity and social vulnerability are being displayed, news audiences are likely to experience not so much personal pleasure as vicarious pain on behalf of those suffering and/or anxiety that this could happen to them or their children.
>
> (Walter *et al.* 1995: 586)

On a lighter note, few can have failed to notice the wave of emotions which televised sporting events evoke in their audiences: what Elias and Dunning (1986) have usefully referred to as the 'quest for excitement' involving a 'controlled decontrolling of emotions' (see also Wouters 1986, and Chapter 13 in this volume, on informalization/changing tension balances in the civilizing process). As the Liverpool manager Bill Shankly once famously put it: 'Football is not a matter of life and death, it's more serious than that!' Certainly the hearts of the nation were in their mouths when England won the World Cup in 1966, just as they were when England narrowly missed the Euro '96 championship final in a failed penalty shoot-out against Germany. In both cases a tidal wave of (nationalistic) emotions duly followed, drowned in a sea of alcohol to help ease the mood.

This, then, suggests something of a mixed picture; one in which emotional identification and disidentification, intensification and diminution appear equally viable responses in the complex mediascape of late twentieth-century western society. It is to a fuller discussion of these issues, together with the associated problems of mind–body dualism they raise, that I now turn in the next section of this chapter.

CYBERSPACE AND THE 'DISEMBODIED' MIND: HIGH-TECH PLATONISM?

Closely connected with these developments is the recent advent of computerized/digitalized 'cyberspace'. As Featherstone and Burrows (1995) note, 'cyberspace' refers to a cluster of different technologies, some familiar, some recently available, some being developed and others still fictional, all of which have the ability, through computerized technology, to 'simulate' environments in which humans can interact. These range from existing international computer networks (i.e. the Internet) which rely upon only a limited range of human senses, to more co-ordinated multi-media systems such as virtual reality (VR): an artificial interactive sensorium of sight, sound and touch involving headphones, head-mounted stereo television goggles ('eyephones') able to simulate three-dimensional space, wired gauntlets ('datagloves') and computerized clothing ('datasuits') (Featherstone and Burrows 1995: 2–3). In Gibsonian terms, cyberspace is

> A consensual hallucination experienced daily by billions of legitimate operators, in every nation, by children being taught mathematical concepts . . . a graphic representation of data abstracted from the bank of every computer in the human system. Unthinkable complexity. Lines of light ranged in the nonspace of the mind, clusters and constellations of data. Like city lights receding.
>
> (Gibson 1984: 51)

At present the technology is crude, but all the indications are that the level of 'realism' will improve dramatically towards the end of the century (Featherstone and Burrows 1995).

To be sure, as a number of writers have suggested, new forms of emotional intimacy, sharing and meaning are beginning to open up as a consequence of these technological developments. The computer network provides opportunities for people to get together with considerable personal intimacy and proximity without the physical limitations of geography, time zones or conspicuous social status. Indeed, for many, particularly the chronically sick and physically disabled, computer networks and electronic bulletin board systems (BBS) may serve as important 'antidotes' to life in an increasingly 'atomistic' and seemingly 'uncaring' society, functioning as new 'social nodes' for the fostering of fluid and multiple 'elective affinities' that everyday (urban) life seldom supports (Heim 1991). As Stone (1991) suggests, a new and largely unexamined 'field' is beginning to open up, one which is incontrovertibly social, in which people continue to meet face to face, but under new definitions of 'meet' and 'face'. Here, ethics, trust and risk continue, but in radically reconfigured ways, which are constantly changing and evolving. Cyberspace, in other words, may lead to the generation of new forms of 'community', social bonds, emotional experiences and intimate relationships – the harbinger of Giddens's (1991) 'pure relationship' perhaps? – many of which are currently woven around the textual narratives of the BBS.

Many of these issues are clearly brought out by Denzin in Chapter 6 of this volume, on the gendered emotional talk and narratives of self which are posted on the Internet news-discussion group 'alt.recovery.co-dependency' (a.r.c.), a 'virtual group' which draws on the tenets of the Adult Children of Alcoholics (ACOA) and the Co-Dependency (CODA) movements. As Denzin argues, the Usenet has created a site for the production of emotional stories which otherwise might not be told, stories which involve struggles over gendered identity, meaning and the (inner) self. In this new digital world of 'electronic emotions', individuals may begin to experience recovery through a form of talking therapy based on written text instead of the spoken word. Seen in these terms, cyberspace has forged new alliances with self-help, recovery and support groups – from sex offenders to those suffering from eating disorders and a variety of other personal and health-related problems: a development succinctly captured by the term 'cyber-recovery'.

For some, however, the lure of computers is more than simply utilitarian or recovery-led, it is *erotic*. On this reading, the desire to enter cyberspace, to cross the human/machine boundary, to 'penetrate the smooth and relatively affectless surface of the electronic screen', can be viewed as a quasi-sexual experience similar to that achieved through orgasm (Springer 1991: 307): what Heim (1991) has termed the 'erotic ontology' of cyberspace. Certainly, as Wiley has recently shown, 'cybersexuality' (i.e. the 'hot' chat between virtual strangers who simultaneously 'log on' to various systems as an auto-erotic representation of sexual experience) is a '"core" feature of the BBS social world' (1995: 146). Cybersexuality is mindful and interactive: a communicated reality that (re)moves the physical world of things to 'somewhere other' (Wiley 1995: 157). Indeed, in the shadow of AIDS and the panic culture of 'body McCarthyism' (Kroker and Kroker 1988), this may be the 'safest' sex of all, devoid of potentially contaminating body fluids – although computers too, of course, now 'catch' viruses through 'unsafe disk swapping' (Lupton 1994; Williams 1995)! As Wiley states:

> 'Reality' warns that the body is vulnerable. Sexual repression (AIDS and safe sex campaigns) and denial of pleasures (sins of smoking, eating meat, drinking coffee or alcohol, war on drugs campaign and so on) run concurrent with the intensification of technological simulations and voyeurism that satiate the carnal appetite *vis-à-vis* imagination and sex without a body.
>
> (Wiley 1995: 159)

On a more troubling note, as a recent article in *Time* (1995) magazine suggests, cyberporn is now 'big business' – an issue which, alongside 'video-nasties', has generated considerable anxiety amongst parents whose children regularly use the Internet. Here we return to the Baudrillardian notion of obscenity, transparency and over-exposure discussed above, in which the divisions between public and private, interior and exterior become wholly blurred and ultimately 'implode' into one another.

As this discussion of 'cybersex' suggests, one of the pleasures (or threats) of cyberspace is that it promises to free us from the confines of our physical bodies and to lodge our 'disembodied minds' in computer-mediated environments and 'virtual' worlds. Previously, *being* a body stood at the forefront of personal identity and individuality. Now, however, cyberspace simply 'brackets' the physical appearance/presence of participants, either by omitting or by 'simulating' corporeal immediacy (Heim 1991). In cyberspace, in other words, our *warrantability* is no longer grounded in our physical bodies; men frequently use 'female' personae whenever they choose and vice versa (Stone 1991). We are, it is claimed, somehow more equal on the 'net' because we can either ignore or 'create' anew the body (i.e. the 'virtual' body) that appears in cyberspace. According to this line of reasoning, bodies and bodily contact become 'optional' and the secondary or stand-in body reveals as much or as little of ourselves and our identities as we wish: a situation variously referred to as 'springtime for schizophrenia' (Stenger 1991) or 'multiple personality as commodity fetish' (Stone 1991). This, in turn, suggests a critical new dimension to Goffman's (1963) distinction between 'actual' and 'virtual' identity; one which even he could not have envisaged.

Within this scheme of imagery we are returned *par excellence* to a high-tech version of the mind–body dualism stretching as far back as Plato who, in a similar manner to the cyberpunk writers of today that downgrade the body as 'meat', castigated the body as the 'prison of the soul'! For us, unlike Plato and his contemporaries, however, the logic runs as follows: why remain dependent upon the organic body when the extended nervous system of the computer network is available? Or perhaps more succinctly: 'Why jack off when you can jack in?' (Foster 1993). This, in turn, suggests that the boundaries between the social and the technological, biological and machine, natural and artificial are beginning to blur, break down, or collapse altogether. In other words, cyberspace is part and parcel of the 'growing imbrication of humans and machines in new social forms or "virtual" systems' (Stone 1991); the ultimate expression of which is the 'cyborg'.

As Haraway (1991) argues, hypothetically and materially, the cyborg is a 'hybrid' of cybernetic device and organism; a 'scientific chimera', but also a social and scientific reality in the contemporary era; a 'myth and a tool', 'representation and an instrument'. More specifically, cyborgs exist when two types of boundaries are simultaneously rendered 'problematic': that between animals (or other organisms) and humans; and that between self-governing machines (automatons) and organisms, especially humans as models of autonomy. The 'cyborg', in short, is a 'leaky' figure born of the 'interface' between 'automaton' and 'autonomy', nature and culture, masculinity and femininity, self and other, rendering these divisions indeterminate and thus offering the potential to escape from their oppressive confines (Haraway 1991).

Whilst this may sound wild and fanciful, it is clear that the 'cyborg' – 'posthuman' or 'transhuman' – is not just a creature born of science fiction, television, or film. Rather, as Gray observes, there are already many 'cyborgs' among us in society. Indeed, the range of intimate human–machine relationships is 'mind-blowing': from Robocop to your grandmother with a pacemaker, and from the fighter-bomber pilot in a state-of-the-art cockpit to those born through the new reproductive technologies and genetic engineering (1995: 2–3). Even if individuals in late modernity are not (yet) full cyborgs, it is clear that machines are intimately interfaced with humans on almost every level of existence from computer technology to the intensive care unit. As Lupton (1994) notes, a symbiotic metaphorical relationship now exists between computers and humans which draws upon the age-old body/machine discourse; one in which computers have been thoroughly 'anthropomorphized' whilst humans have, in turn, been portrayed as 'organic computers' (see also Berman 1989, and Williams 1995).

This, in turn, suggests that bodies, minds and selves, like all other modernist categories and divisions, are 'coming apart' and being critically reconfigured in cyberspace. As consequence, existing sociological concepts such as self-identity, social interaction, and the 'social construction' (Berger and Luckmann 1967) or 'framing' (Goffman 1974) of 'reality' may need fundamentally rethinking (Chayko 1993). It may also necessitate a critical reappraisal of current concepts in the sociology of emotions such as 'emotion work/management', 'surface' versus 'deep' acting, 'feeling rules', the 'commercialization/commodification' of human feeling, and the traditional (gendered) division between the 'public' and the 'private'; one in which physical warrantability becomes irrelevant, spectacle becomes plastic and negotiated, and desire no longer grounds itself in human corporeality (Stone 1991).

Certainly it is possible to raise a number of objections which call into question the all too easy acceptance of a 'disembodied' virtual future. How long and how deep, for example, are personal relationships which develop outside of embodied co-presence (Heim 1991), how much trust and security can we invest in disembodied 'virtual' identities, and will one ever really be able to make love in cyberspace (Stone 1991)? As Stone (1991) rightly argues, the Cartesian separation of mind and body is 'an old trick', and it is easy to be seduced into thinking that in cyberspace we leave our bodies behind. Stripped of its glittery image, the reality of cyberspace, is, however, quite different. For Heidegger, our relationship to technology is not simply abstract and re-presentational, rather it involves a *praxical* element which relates to our embodied being/*dwelling* in-the-world. We can interact *with* technology, *through* technology, or *within* a technological context, but on each occasion our embodied, praxical relationship to that technology and our dwelling in the lifeworld are central (Ihde 1979, 1990).

As Denzin (1984: 128) argues, emotions are embodied experiences; ones which radiate through the lived body as a structure of ongoing experience, including self-feelings which constitute the inner core of human emotionality. For individuals to understand their own lived emotions, they must experience them socially and reflectively. It is here, according to Denzin, at the intersection between emotions as *embodied* experiences, their socially faceted nature, and their links with feelings of selfhood and personal identity, that a sociological perspective and understanding of emotions can most fruitfully be forged.

A crucial issue here concerns the peculiarly 'disembodied' nature of human 'touch' in cyberspace. Certainly, I can be (deeply) touched by the story someone tells or the relationships I develop in cyberspace, just as I may become physically aroused through cybersex. But what we lose in cyberspace is the depth of emotional experience, warmth and understanding which comes from embodied gestures such as being 'touched' by another human being through face-to-face contact and physical co-presence in the real world (RW). The cuddle for a crying child, the arm of support around a friend in need, the gentle physical caress of a passionate lover, these and many other embodied gestures touch us deeply and communicate a shared sense of trust, intimacy and vulnerability which is grounded in the contingencies of our fleshy mortal bodies. Sexual relationships, for example, are built around an immensely complex structure of embodied tensions and contradictions:

> Contradiction between the body and a developing practice is a continuing fact of sexuality itself. In sexual intercourse . . . there is tension and pleasure in working against immediate bodily demand, holding back, creating rhythms. You can communicate pleasure to a partner by working against your own desire in favour of hers or his; you learn the ways of another body which does not contain your own desire or need. In this way the immensely complex practical edifice of a sexual relationship is built as a structure of tensions and contradictions. That is the meaning of union of two people as distinct from the rubbing-together of two bodies.
>
> (Connell 1987: 82)

In these and many other ways, including the problems of fraud, deception and deceit which a lack of physical co-presence can bring, cyberspace rates a poor second to the pleasures and pains, the agonies and the ecstasies, of the real world where physical embodiment is not an 'optional extra'. In the age of the 'technosocial subject', life is still lived through bodies and 'no refigured virtual body, no matter how beautiful, will slow the death of a cyberpunk with AIDS' (Stone 1991: 113).

Not only does cyber imagery imply that the conscious mind steers our organic body – the meaning of the Greek word *kybernetes* (Heim 1991) – thereby reinforcing centuries of dualist thought, it also upholds the gendered forms of embodiment and subjectivity that it seems to unravel (Cherniavsky 1993; Foster 1993; Springer 1991; see also Denzin's chapter in this volume). Indeed, as Doane (1990) suggests, technology is in fact patterned upon the 'fetishization' of the maternal body, thus rendering Haraway's (1991) and Plant's (1995) optimistic vision of a 'post-gender' world populated by 'leaky' cyborg figures little more than a (postmodern) pipe dream.

As Slouka (1995) argues, despite appeals to the power of the 'disembodied' mind, what those with an interest in the promotion of cyberspace do not wish to talk about is the 'flattening' or 'deadening' effect which computer representation can have on the imagination. What this boils down to is the fact that no computer package, however 'real' or sophisticated it might seem, is going to be able to offer the range of potential 'options' available, free of charge, to the individual imagination. To put it quite bluntly, virtual reality, as the term suggests, does not stand a cat in hell's chance of capturing the subtlety and sophistication of life in the real world, nor should it. Take, for example, a walk in the countryside. I can feel the sun on my face, smell the scent of flowers, taste the sweet blackberries that hang so enticingly on the bush, run my hand through the clear water of a stream, observe the wind caressing the wheat in the fields. I am both in and part of nature, reasserting my carnal roots, and what is more it feels good, it feels right, it feels authentic: my imagination is 'free' to run wild in this 'uncolonized' space. What cyberspace can do, however, is 'limit the imagination, force it to walk along certain paths and not others, reduce it, basically – and us along with it – to a function of technology'. In doing so, despite claims to the contrary, cyberspace is in danger of 'homogenizing'/ 'narrowing down' the rich plurality of our experiences, eroding our autonomy, and turning us all into audiences or spectators of our own demise (Slouka 1995: 133–5). Here we return to the Baudrillardian theme identified earlier concerning the dulling or blunting of emotional response.

This, in turn, leads me to the final point I wish to make about the (potential) risks and dangers of the digital age. As I have suggested, cyberspace, itself a sort of digital 'side-show', is in danger of becoming the 'main attraction', substituting representation for reality, fiction for fact, mind for body, and homogeneity for imagination. To be sure, as pure escapism, this might seem an attractive option to some, but ultimately it may distract us from our responsibilities in the real world. Even the cyberspace recovery network substitutes real world (RW) responsibilities for virtual world (VW) interactions: interactions where individuals 'hide' behind their screens, where 'lurking' is encouraged, and where only certain versions of recovery are honoured and endorsed (see Denzin's chapter in this volume). As Slouka (1995: 48) comments, from Guatemala to the Sudan real bodies have suffered; bodies which could not be helped in cyberspace. Cyberspace is also profoundly undemocratic: it sets up a world of haves and have-nots according to computer literacy and terminal access, not to mention the spectre of an emerging virtual class of *digerati* (i.e. a technocratic elite), including the corporate interests of the multimillion-dollar computer industry (Dery 1996).

Only on the basis of our carnal bonds with others in the real world in which we dwell can a truly human ethics of trust, emotional intimacy and responsibility emerge; one grounded in a shared sense of bodily opportunity, contingency and constraint. Fortunately, there are signs of hope in the shape of the real world (RW) 'life-political agenda' which is beginning to emerge in late twentieth-century western society (Giddens 1991, 1994; Beck 1992). These range from the disability movement to groups concerned with the new genetics, holistic health, animal rights and a range of environmental issues. In each case the politics of embodiment, and the existential and ethical dilemmas this poses, are proving central. As such, life-politics provides an important counterweight to the disembodied visions and dys/utopian myths of cyberspace.

CONCLUSIONS

As this chapter suggests, life in a mediated age sets in train a complex series of opportunities and constraints which carry important implications for contemporary forms of emotionally embodied experience. Here the tensions between *re*-presentation and reality, emotional involvement and detachment, together with the associated high-tech problems of dualism in cyberspace, suggest a number of dilemmas for the individual at the turn of the century; dilemmas which defy easy answers or simple (re)solutions. These developments, in turn, suggest the possibility of having critically to rethink existing sociological concepts: from the 'framing' of 'reality' to the dilemmas of the emotionally embodied self, and from the problems of 'emotion work' to the transformation of 'feeling rules' and the vicissitudes of 'surface' and 'deep' acting in cyberspace.

Yet as I have also suggested, whilst new forms of trust, risk and emotional intimacy may indeed be opening up in the 'erotic ontology' of cyberspace, this glittering digital world of images and events is not without its problems. As Dery (1996) comments, the misguided hope that we will be born again as 'bionic angels' is a deadly misreading of the myth of Icarus: it pins our hopes to 'wings of wax and feathers'. Certainly, the disembodied myths and dys/utopian visions of cyberspace, including Baudrillardian sign-fetishism and its obsessive preoccupation with the hyperreal, need to be treated with (extreme) caution. Not only does this deny the very conditions which make us human (i.e. our mortal, flesh-and-blood links with other similarly *embodied* human beings), it also runs the risk, as a kind of 'digital sideshow', of distracting us from our responsibilities in the real world, founded as it is on technocratically elitist, undemocratic principles, where computer illiteracy is a bar, where 'lurking' and 'deception' all too frequently occur and where the problems of gendered identity are upheld rather than unravelled. Indeed, in this technologically uncertain, digital world of (hyperreal) claims and counter-claims, one would do well to remember the old adage: *Plus ça change, plus c'est la même chose!*

BIBLIOGRAPHY

Baudrillard, J. (1983a) *In the Shadow of the Silent Majority*. New York: Semiotext(e).
Baudrillard, J. (1983b) *Simulations*. New York: Semiotext(e).
Baudrillard, J. (1988) *Selected Writings*, ed. M. Poster. Cambridge: Polity Press.
Beck, U. (1992) *Risk Society: Towards a New Modernity*. London: Sage.
Berger, P. and Luckmann, T. (1967) *The Social Construction of Reality*. London: Allen Lane.
Berman, B. (1989) 'The computer metaphor: bureaucratizing the mind', *Science as Culture* 7: 7–42.
Burrows, R. (1995) 'Cyberpunk as social theory', paper presented at the BSA 'Contested Cities' conference, University of Leicester, April 1995.
Chayko, M. (1993) 'What is real in the age of VR?', *Symbolic Interaction* 16(2): 171–81.
Cherniavsky, E. (1993) '(En)gendering cyberspace in Neuromancer: postmodern subjectivity and virtual motherhood', *Genders* 18: 32–46.
Connell, R. (1987) *Gender and Power: Society, the Person and Sexual Politics*. Cambridge: Polity Press.
Denzin, N. K. (1984) *On Understanding Emotions*. San Francisco: Jossey-Bass.
Dery, M. (1996) *Escape Velocity: Cyberculture at the End of the Century*. New York: Grove Press.
Doane, M. A. (1990) 'Technophilia: technology, representation and the feminine', in M. Jacobus *et al.* (eds) *Body/Politics: Women and the Discourse of Science*. London: Routledge.
Elias, N. and Dunning, E. (1986) *The Quest for Excitement: Sport and Leisure in the Civilizing Process*. Oxford: Blackwell.
Featherstone, M. and Burrows, R. (1995) 'Cultures of technological embodiment: an introduction', *Body and Society*, (cyberspace/cyberbodies/cyberpunk) 1(3–4): 1–19.
Foster, T. (1993) 'Meat puppet or robopath? Cyberpunk and the question of embodiment', *Genders* 18: 11–31.
Gibson, W. (1984) *The Neuromancer*. London: HarperCollins.
Giddens, A. (1991) *Modernity and Self-Identity: Self and Society in the Late Modern Age*. Cambridge: Polity Press.
Giddens, A. (1994) *Beyond Left and Right*. Cambridge: Polity Press.
Goffman, E. (1963) *Stigma: Notes on the Management of Spoiled Identity*. Harmondsworth, Mx: Penguin.
Goffman, E. (1967) *Interaction Ritual: Essays on Face-to-Face Behaviour*. New York: Doubleday Anchor Books.
Goffman, E. (1974) *Frame Analysis*. Harmondsworth, Mx: Penguin.
Gray, C. H. (1995) *The Cyborg Handbook*. London: Routledge.
Haraway, D. (1991) *Simians, Cyborgs and Women: The Reinvention of Nature*. London: Routledge.
Heim, M. (1991) 'The erotic ontology of cyberspace', in M. Benedikt (ed.) *Cyberspace: The First Steps*. Cambridge, MA: MIT Press.
Hochschild, A. R. (1979) 'Emotion work, feeling rules and social structure', *American Journal of Sociology* 85(3): 551–75.
Ihde, D. (1979) *Technixs and Praxis*. Dordrecht/Boston, MA/London: Reidel.
Ihde, D. (1990) *Technology and the Lifeworld?: From Garden to Earth*. Bloomington and Indianapolis, IN: Indiana University Press.
Kellner, D. (1989) *Jean Baudrillard: Media and Postmodernity*. Cambridge: Polity Press.
Kroker, A. and Kroker, M. (1988) *Body Invaders: Sexuality and the Postmodern Condition*. Basingstoke, Hants: Macmillan.

Lupton, D. (1994) 'Panic computing: the viral metaphor and computer technology', *Cultural Studies* 8(3): 556–68.

Plant, S. (1995) 'The future looms: weaving, women and cybernetics', *Body and Society* 1(3–4): 45–6.

Slouka, M. (1995) *War of the Worlds: The Assault on Reality*. London: Abacus.

Springer, C. (1991) 'The pleasure of the interface', *Screen* 32(3): 303–23.

Stearns, P. N. (1994) *American Cool*. New York: State University of New York Press.

Stenger, N. (1991) 'Mind is a leaking rainbow', in M. Benedikt (ed.) *Cyberspace: The First Steps*. Cambridge, MA: MIT Press.

Stone, A. R. (1991) 'Will the real body please stand up?', in M. Benedikt (ed.) *Cyberspace: The First Steps*. Cambridge, MA: MIT Press.

Time (1995) 'Porn on the internet', *Time* (3 July): 34–41.

Walter, T., Littlewood, J. and Pickering, M. (1995) 'Death in the news: the public invigilation of private emotion', *Sociology* 29(4): 579–96.

Wiley, J. (1995) 'Nobody is "doing it": cybersexuality as a postmodern narrative', *Body and Society* 1(1): 145–62.

Williams, S. J. (1995) 'Anthropomorphism and the computer virus: the latest chapter in the illness as metaphor story?', *Medical Sociology News* 20(2): 22–6.

Wouters, C. (1986) 'Formalization and informalization: changing tension balances in civilizing processes', *Theory, Culture and Society* 3(2): 1–18.

Part III

Emotions and the body through the life-course

8 Children, emotions and daily life at home and school

Berry Mayall

INTRODUCTION

This chapter makes an exploratory and discursive expedition into oddly unmapped territory. It is concerned with children, childhood, the body and social life, and with how emotions mediate between these. I do not seek to rehearse the literature on the body and the emotions; instead of making a critical analysis of this new field, I start from another new discipline, the sociology of childhood. I explore ways of incorporating children and childhood into sociological discourse on the importance of the emotions in social life.

Essentially I start, as some feminist research has (e.g. Martin 1987), from the proposition that people experience the body as a complex of understandings. Its physical character is continually under inspection and control in the physical and social environments wherein people move; its social character and value are under construction in interactions with others, and especially with those who have some superiority to the individual person or group; and people's estimation of their own bodily and social value is under constant revision in response to these experiences in a range of social environments and with a range of people. The central proposition explored in this chapter, in relation to children, is that emotions mediate between the social order and the body; they construct how we feel about our bodies. Bodily experience is conditioned, or modified, by the social environment – which itself may be more or less modifiable in response to how we feel about our embodied experience. As Scheper-Hughes and Lock (1987) put it, emotions are shaped and given meaning at least in part by social or, as they put it, cultural forces. Emotions then provide a link bridging mind and body, individual, society and the body politic. Among the deliberations of scholars about how we may think about the body and its relationships to the social order, these ideas seem to me to fit most closely with what we know of children's experiences (though these have been little researched), and they provide a framework within which to discuss these experiences further.

Studying the embodied experiences of children is an important but neglected enterprise, and this neglect comprises one branch of the general sociological neglect of children. Yet our understanding of how people live their lives in relation to social structures will be incomplete if we ignore an important social group. For children are not only numerically important – about a fifth of the population – they are now what all of us have been; and what we learned and experienced then remains with us as adults. The universal success rate with which people leave childhood is balanced by the permanence of the social category of children, whose experiences and activities constitute a significant feature of the social order. Sociological study of children and childhood, through studying the specific factors that operate as opportunities and constraints during children's engagement with other social groups, is critical for a proper understanding of social life.

The case of children, bodies and emotions is interesting sociologically not least because, as I shall argue, children's experiential, emotional learning spans the bodily and the cognitive, and this is in part because the work women do in controlling, enabling, civilizing and regulating children's bodies requires them to take account of links between children's bodies and their minds. Shilling's notion of the body as unfinished, a useful concept applying throughout the life-course, has obvious salience in the case of children: 'the shapes, sizes and meanings of the body . . . can be "completed" only through human labour' (Shilling 1993: 124–5).

Those of us who try to explore children's childhoods from a sociological point of view increasingly find it odd, after over ten years of work has taken place to put children on the sociological map, that most sociological work, including that on the body, ignores children, or confines them to half a paragraph. Examples are legion, and one would not wish to point the finger. The situation resembles that identified by feminists in the 1970s – like women, children have been naturalized. Why is this, one may briefly ask? Scholars tend to stick with what is familiar, indeed with what they experience. Men write about men, women researchers have – naturally! – cornered the market in women; some men will not touch women's studies. Within the sociology of the body and emotions it has been argued that feminist insights have been given inadequate attention by male scholars (Howson 1994). Even within this gendered polarization of sociological work, however, one might suppose the boyhoods and girlhoods of those perennially interesting men and women might be of concern. But most of the literature within, for instance, the men's movement ignores even male childhood (but see Mac an Ghaill 1994). Women have had compelling reasons to distance themselves from an interest in children in order to escape from the classification 'women and children' with its implied connotations of the natural, biologically determined asocial life. And though women have been concerned with the construction of gendered identity, this has been mainly from a forward-looking standpoint: how women acquire identity. But leaving aside scholars' tendency to fight for their own interests, we may note that a principal and common feature of the sideglances at childhood that one finds in the literature is an uncritical reliance on the concept of socialization – used in a simplistic sense. Put briefly, many sociologists, in these asides, revert to Parsonian functionalism: childhood and children's actions are uninteresting, because childhood is preparation for adult life, where people interact with the social order – and that is the proper study of the sociologist. Though routes through symbolic interactionism (e.g. Denzin 1977) and through various versions of social constructionism (e.g. Ingleby 1986) have released children from the more top-down versions of socialization theory, it has taken a separate effort to establish children as the subjects of sociological inquiry.

CHILDHOOD FROM A SOCIOLOGICAL STANDPOINT

Some features of current concepts within the sociology of childhood are relevant here (see for discussion Prout and James 1990; Alanen 1992). The pioneering programme Childhood as a Social Phenomenon (1985–92), carried out in sixteen countries, established the idea of children as a social group, one whose interests were not necessarily coterminous with the adult groups with whom they interact – notably parents and teachers (see Qvortrup 1991, 1994). Indeed children may have interests in common as a group, which differ from and may challenge the interests of adult social groups. Furthermore, like any other social group, children's daily lives, self-appraisal, expectations and opportunities are structured in tension with social policies. But the tensions and the effects will be specific to them as a minority group. For instance, their chances of health and education, their freedom of movement, their opportunities for adequate nutrition and exercise will be affected in specific ways, by comparison with adult groups.

Children are also most appropriately to be regarded as social actors, people who are socially inclined from the outset. The sociality of children, their wish and ability to participate in constructing, maintaining and modifying the social order, is a theme eagerly elaborated by those who live with them – their parents (e.g. Mayall 1996: especially Chapter 4). This experiential knowledge, acquired by parents on the job, runs counter to the traditional view, that it is principally through adult effort that children become social beings. Research is exploring these issues with a focus on younger and younger children; Dunn (1988) has described children's social understanding in the second year of life, arguing that emotional and motivational factors drive forward their understanding and participation in family social life.

As a social group, children are the object of intense and prolonged concern by adults, including both parents and agents of the welfare state ('the psy- complex' in Donzelot's (1980) terms). Living with their children teaches parents that children contribute to the emotional, physical and moral order of the home. But these understandings are balanced by the requirement to prepare children, to make them fit to join wider social worlds (e.g. Halldén

1991). This preparatory work – by adults – comprises civilizing, regulating and constructing children's bodies and minds. Adults civilize children into the social and moral mores of the wider social group (see Elias 1978). They regulate children's bodies and minds in the interests of specific agendas (e.g. the school curriculum), and they propose certain bodily shapes and activities to fit socially sanctioned shapes and skills. These three kinds of activity on the body – civilizing, regulating and constructing – constitute interlinked themes in adult behaviour and children's experience.

Some features of the problematic character of child–adult transactions can be understood within these two features of childhood: the time present and time future of children. Adult structures of thought and institutionalized practices – focused essentially on time future – operate powerfully on children as agents in the here and now. Children's agency looks more severely constricted than that of most adult groups, and children themselves identify adult control as a determining factor in their daily lives.

As a context for the following discussion of emotion as a mediating force between social worlds and the body, I discuss two sets of factors that structure children's participation in child–adult transactions.

Generational proximity

By the term 'generational proximity' I suggest the idea of a continuum ranging from conflict to harmony in child–adult relations. At one extreme, the generations may be experienced as separate, firm, congealed, and standing face-to-face or in opposition to each other, to the extent that the child feels controlled, excluded or defined as an object. At the other extreme, children and adults may be engaged in a joint enterprise, in harmony, with similar goals, and with a mutual emotional reinforcement of their satisfaction with the enterprise and the social relationships embedded in it and strengthened through it. (This idea may be compared to that of James and Prout (1995) who identify the family as a social group with stronger or weaker possibilities for distinctive views and behaviour within its social 'hierarchy'.) Looking at generational proximity means being concerned with relationships between adult and child groups, with how close their interests are, and with how far the separation or intersection of the two groups allows children to participate in constructing the social order.

The concept of generational proximity assumes that child–adult relationships are not fixed but are responsive to social factors, such as goals, pressures, preoccupations and so on. This concept must be conceptualized within wider arguments concerning the separation of adult from child worlds. Engelbert (1994) argues that childhood is a period of exclusion from and protection from adult social worlds; and Ennew (1986: 17), discussing the social conditions within which child sexual abuse has become a noted feature of our societies, refers to 'a rigid hierarchy' creating distance between adults and children. However, Büchner *et al.* (1994) argue that more individualized careers, the pace of social change, and children's rights issues are factors leading to more respectful and equal relationships between children and parents. I suggest we should observe a distinction here between social and psychological distance. Arguably, the social worlds of children are sharply differentiated from those of adults, as evidenced by institutions (such as schools), prohibitions (from driving) and child-oriented services (phone-ins, films and TV programmes). Also, arguably, children are consigned to social distance from adults (Elias 1978) until they have acquired certain socially approved controls over their emotions and bodies. However, in terms of psychological proximity or distance, there are wide variations relating to both individual child–adult relationships and social contexts. Between a given child and parent, a joint enterprise or an adult-controlled enterprise provide varying contexts for the psychological proximity between them. Broadly, too, the home encompasses and promotes greater psychological proximity between children and adults than does the school.

Models of childhood, models of adulthood

The second point concerns adult models of what children are, how childhood should be lived, and how, since childhood is a relational concept, adults should behave in relation to children. These understandings structure how homes, schools, health and welfare agencies operate (Alanen 1994). Most crucially, because of the authority and control adults exercise over all aspects of children's lives, adult models not only importantly affect children's experience, knowledge and identity, they are also critical in constructing the personhood of children (Hockey and James 1993: especially Chapter 2). These models present children with a series of institutions they must attend – pre-schools and schools. They encourage the development of certain sorts of bodies, for instance unobtrusive or athletic bodies. The idea that childhood should be a garden of innocence where children are happy, and the Piagetian notion of play as children's proper work, provide a complex of ideas that condition the assignment of children to the company of their toys, and the separation of children's time-use from adults': while adults carry out household maintenance work, children are meant to play. The requirement that children be happy can lead adults to protect them from knowledge that might sadden them, such as the death of a relative, or the cruelty people enact towards each other. As Freund (1988) has suggested, at the extreme, social controls in the form of the 'social organisation of time, space and human motion, have an impact on the vitality and muscular and skeletal structure of the body'. Girls learn not to develop their muscles, if they are to be socially acceptable, and to restrict their bodily movements within smaller spaces than boys do (Young 1980). People, especially in their relationships with their superiors, are required to control and organize their emotions (emotion work) and to use these controls to organize bodily movement in ways approved by their superiors and by more general social legitimation (Hochschild 1979).

These points about social control are of specific relevance to children, because of their social and political dependency. It is one of the purposes of this chapter to consider how, specifically, children experience the diverse workings of adult social control, in tension with the precise character of the generational proximity in a given situation.

HOME AND SCHOOL AS ARENAS FOR CHILDREN'S DAILY LIFE

In terms of time and social importance, the two sites, home and school, are children's main social environments in the UK. The complexity of each arena for children's experience is provided by the precise character of the intersecting factors outlined above. Children's accounts make clear that in general the home offers more opportunity for closeness, for generational proximity. Essentially, the home is the accepted place where attention to the individual can have priority; it is the first and foremost site of holistic health care. Women's health-care work, relating to the physical, emotional and cognitive character of their children (and of their men), is commonly regarded as their central work (Graham 1984). In this context, therefore, children are likely to experience close attention to their emotions, bodies and minds. Furthermore, that emotional and physical factors are interlinked in determining health status is part of the experiential knowledge of mothers, or of those who care for children continuously. The point is made here by a mother recounting an occasion when her 2-year-old son went 'off his food':

> Change in appetite – it happens about once in every three months or so. He often goes through that. He goes off his food sometimes for three days. It was last week. He drinks plenty of milk, so I put a rusk in his bottle, but when I gave him his food he turned up his nose at it. He only ate a biscuit, tinned soup, milk and rusk. He's too lazy to eat. (Interviewer: Why do you think it happened?) He was a bit irritable – it might have been because I began putting him on the pot. And he wasn't sleeping very well. He'd get up four or five times in the night for a couple of nights. He does that quite frequently. He wasn't ill – playing as usual. Perfectly alright.

Her remedy was to focus on his favourite food (milk), to play down the toilet-training and to offer more affection.

As Dunn (1988) suggests, the emotional closeness of child with parent – sharing the same experiences and concerns – mediates children's participation in the social life of the family. These opportunities for closeness are offered in times and places where adult enterprises and priorities do not take precedence. For instance, Newson and Newson found (1970: 257) that children's wishes took lower precedence than adult and household priorities in the morning, when everybody had to be organized for the day; it was in the evening, and especially towards bedtime, that mothers responded to children's needs for comfort and ritual.

At school, clearly, children's experiences reflect a somewhat different set of conditions. Children report sharp social separation between children's and adults' interests as a feature of their experience. In this example, the social order imposes discomfort on the body, and feelings of alienation:

> Miss X – she shouts all the time. One day I was ill, really sick, and sitting down, and she comes up to me and stands next to me, and starts to shout at me: 'Where's your book, why are you sitting next to the window? Only people who are sick can sit by the window.'

Adults, whether teachers or non-teachers, behave in ways that suggest their close identification with the formal remit of the school. Essentially, here the cognitive is distinguished from and takes precedence over the emotional and physical. Whilst teachers at the outset of their careers may want to mother 'their' children (see Burgess and Carter 1992), their work remit demands they maintain physical and emotional distance from the children and treat them equably and even-handedly (King 1989). The demands of the formal agenda and of the social order lead to tension between these demands and teachers' concern for individual children. Some children too may initially hope for replication of a mother's complex set of functions – 'Some of them do tend to call me Mum', said one teacher. As suggested below, the division of labour for the care of children favours the separation of the cognitive, as priority, from the emotional and the bodily, although both children and teachers may overstep these boundaries on occasion.

Adult models of children thus differ: the mother, or caring parent, has learned holistic knowledge of intersections between the physical, emotional and cognitive; whilst the teacher, in line with training and remit, stresses the cognitive child and the child as developmental project. Children's own ability to participate in the construction and reconstruction of the social order will, in response, be broadly different in the two settings; the first conditioned by close relationships and responsive models, the second by more separated child–adult relationships and by more fixed models of how childhood – during the school-day – should be spent.

This very brief outline of these two arenas is proposed as a basis for more detailed consideration of how emotion mediates between these social orders and children's embodied experience. A brief comparison of story-time at home and nursery school illustrates the points made here.

> At home, just before bedtime, two children climb onto their mother's knee. Her arms are round them and she holds in front of the three a book. The children hold their teddies and are drinking their milk. She

reads the story, and the children point out and name details of the pictures.

At nursery school, at the end of the session, a class of children sit on the carpet, arms folded and facing the teacher. One child (on a rota basis) sits on the teacher's knee. Others claim – unsuccessfully – that it is their turn, and instead move closer to her; two children move closer to me, and lean against my knee. The teacher holds the book up so the children can see the pictures. She reads the story and asks the children questions. Two of the children get up and walk away.

In some ways these two events are similar. The adult exercises control; she aims to quieten children down, to prepare them respectively for going to bed and for going home. In both cases, there is a cognitive element: the story gives an opportunity for thinking, discussing and increasing vocabulary and knowledge. In both cases the adult responds to the children's wish to be physically close to her. However, story-time at home provides an archetypal instance of intricately interlinked attention to the cognitive, emotional and bodily. The emotional mediates the control element. Story-time at school subordinates bodily comfort to control, in the interests of the cognitive. The children must sit still, and not touch each other. The teacher cannot satisfy all the children's requests for the emotional comfort offered by close physical proximity – and school encourages children to leave their favourite objects at home. She maintains a cognitive focus: she asks the children questions designed to ensure they have understood the story and to reinforce their knowledge of colours, shapes and sizes. She emphasises the didactic over what the children have to offer.

CHILDREN'S EMBODIED EXPERIENCE AT HOME AND SCHOOL

Here I discuss in more detail some of the issues outlined above. The data derive mainly from two studies. The first is a small-scale study in one primary school – the Greenstreet Study – in which I explored children's daily life at home and school (Mayall 1994, 1996). I was a participant observer with a class of 5–6 year olds and a class of 9–10 year olds over two terms, talked with them in pairs, and held group discussions with the older children. I also interviewed staff and parents, mostly mothers. On the basis of this study, my colleagues and I carried out a larger-scale study, exploring the status of Children's Health in Primary Schools (CHIPS), using a national postal survey (620 schools responded) and case studies in six schools (Mayall *et al.* 1996). We collected data from children (aged 6 and 10), staff and parents.[1] In addition, I have been privileged as a grandmother to sit about in the private world of the home as a participant observer of preschool children's activities.

Participating in constructing the social order

A striking feature of children's own accounts, and of their mothers', is that children both expect and desire to participate in the activities they see adults engaging in at home. The activities they describe include: bringing home the shopping, unpacking it, cleaning the house, setting tables and preparing meals. Children's accounts also forcibly suggest that this participation should be within their own control: they should choose when to participate, and in what activities. They resist adult ordering of their time-use. Through these activities, I suggest, children feel themselves to be actors with a part to play in collaboration with adults in constructing the social order. To the extent that their participation is accepted, the social order endorses children's feeling that through their work they collaborate with the household enterprise. This point was forcibly demonstrated to me by a child's distress:

> A 4-year-old boy stands facing his parents, looking from one to the other. They are having a heated, fast-moving discussion about a crisis in family finances. He stands in tears, flushed, distressed and angry. He shouts at them: 'You're not to argue!' He moves to interpose his body between them. They turn towards him and explain they are not angry with each other, but have a problem to sort out.

What caused the acute distress the boy showed? A conventional explanation might be that he feared the loss of a parent. But his feelings and actions suggest to me that this was a situation where he felt excluded from participation; his knowledge and experience did not stretch to the topics discussed; and his parents excluded him from the discussion. The generations were distanced from each other, through the adults' view that he had no proper contribution to make to an adult problem. His insistence on making a useful contribution to household problems was indicated on another occasion soon after this one: his mother explained they could not afford a trip, and he offered the contents of his money-box as a solution.

By contrast, a mother describes her 2-year-old son's participation in constructing social relationships, through his active use of body and emotion:

> Oh, when he starts laughing and comes in (to bed) and go on you and kissing you and giving you a hug, when you get up in the mornings. He starts smiling alright? [she laughs] and when you smile back at him, he just roll over and come over you, kissing you.
>
> (Mayall and Foster 1989: 23)

At pre-school and primary school the line between adult and child interests is clearly apparent to children. They perceive teachers as those who act to implement the official remit of the school, and are in positions of authority over the children. Teachers themselves emphasize their task of training the children to behave acceptably within the social norms of the school

(Hartley 1987), though these are commonly implicit as well as explicit norms (Waksler 1991).

Faced with this powerful, separate adult social group, children put great value on activity and achievement and on child social groups as sources of reward and enjoyment. Though they cannot, in the main, participate in constructing the social order, some of the time they feel they exercise limited control over both work and play. For instance, when asked to write about the pros and cons of school, John (aged 9) wrote:

> I think I like learning, but I like learning my own way on my own ideas, for that makes me feel I've accomplished double. I think I liked the infants more because I learned general stuff, like reading (which I thoroughly enjoy now). And general numbers which I like fooling around with. So far the infants have put some knowledge into me. The juniors have yet to have its spark.
>
> (Mayall 1994: 68)

It is notable that where children are allowed to participate with staff in improving the social order, for instance tackling bullying, or drawing up information leaflets for newcomers to the school, they respond with enthusiasm (Mayall *et al.* 1996: 211–14). Child–child friendships are a major source of comfort and reward.

> I felt scared [when I first came to school] in case anybody came along and picked me up and threw me against the fence and I just felt so scared . . . I was really shy, so I just went into Class 1 and everybody was horrible to me – said, buzz off, would ya – and I just felt lonely. (Interviewer: Is it better now?) Yes, I've got billions of friends.
>
> (Mayall *et al.* 1996: 181)

This boy describes his initial feelings of rejection and isolation, involving fear of physical abuse, in contrast to his experience now. Feeling accepted as part of a child group is more than a pleasant part of school, it is critical to mediation of the social order. Bodily security itself is ensured through the membership of friendship groups.

Our data indicate that adult and child social worlds are in tension at school, the social order of the school is formally fixed and children have little chance to take part in its modification. These factors may explain in part why people do not recall their school-days as subjectively important: school is not experienced as participative.

Acquiring knowledge

Within the social order of the two arenas children acquire knowledge of how their bodies are valued, by adults, and, in turn, how they feel about their bodies. The bodily character of children is a marker of their status, their positioning within childhood (Hockey and James 1993: Chapter 3), a positioning marked by orderly progress through life at home, to nursery, to infant and junior school. Children's experience at home, especially in their pre-school years, is of parental praise for their embodied beauty, achievements and progress. The praise no doubt derives from many sources: delighted affection, concern that their child is normal, relief that their child is taking on some aspects of self-care, pleasure that domestic life is less dominated by the physical – the mess that babies create and parents clear up. Children thereby learn that their developing control over their bodily movements may justifiably encourage them to feel proud of their bodies. And their bodily control constitutes a contribution to how the day is organized. As they learn, for instance, to go to the toilet on their own, brush their teeth, climb up and down stairs, dress themselves, ride a trike, family activities and routines also change in response:

> Things like dressing, he tries, he pulls things off, he loves to do that. Now I get his jumper off except for one arm and he pulls it off and he feels very pleased with himself. . . . He's learning a little bit about himself as well, because when he . . . wants to urinate he starts to hold himself and he goes 'Oh!'. But he's learning a bit about his own body now as well. (Mother of 21-month-old son.)

> (Mayall and Foster 1989: 24)

These points extend to the more specific work of managing emotions. Learning not to hit people, to take turns, and to defer to adult agendas provides children with knowledge of what constitutes acceptable embodied modes of being within the social order of the family – and as they meet other children and other adults, in wider social spheres too. Dunn (1988) provides many examples; one concerns a girl who accidentally knocks over her baby brother (Dunn 1988: 28). Mother enters room:

> Mother: What happened?
> Girl: I banged him.
> Mother: Well, you'd better kiss him better.

The girl learns that the moral order of the home is to be expressed through embodied emotional activity.

Home therefore encourages children to feel happy in their bodies, to understand which bodily and emotional achievements and actions are valuable, and to understand how these both link in with and contribute to the social order.

The school presents a different set of orientations to children's bodies. High valuation of their bodies is allocated to discrete times and places at school. The infant (5–7 years) and junior (7–11 years) regimes in some schools are interesting in this respect, for, apart from break-times, infant children may play at will in the classroom after finishing short pieces of 'academic' work, and some of this play includes running about, and devising competitions of physical prowess. However, for junior children physical activity is limited to formal physical exercise sessions. During class-time, the body is to be controlled in the interests of cognitive achievement: in literacy, numeracy and so on. The Greenstreet and CHIPS children indicated that whilst the balance between sit-down work and physical activity in the infant years was acceptable, for junior children there was too much class-room work. 'It's sit down, write down, write up', as one boy said. Further-more, achievement was downgraded: when you finished one piece of work, there was always another waiting for you, with adult pressure to move on continuously.

On the other hand, children also learn at school that the construction of their bodies in socially approved directions is not just a matter for them-selves, but is one component of the formal school remit. School offers the chance to delight in the bodily skills and achievements that school proposes, but also the chance of failure to measure up. One of our case-study schools in the CHIPS study engaged the children in specifically health-related activ-ity (see Kirk and Tinning 1994), as this girl reports:

> He makes us run all around the playground . . . down the road. [At first] I nearly fainted . . . it's really hard. But it's worth it. . . . He tells us about healthy diet, and about too much fat in the body, and not having a healthy heart . . . When I first started in this class I used to be really chubby.
>
> (Mayall *et al.* 1996: 192)

In practical terms, larger classes in finite spaces are currently requiring children to regulate their bodies more closely; both children and teachers reported on cramped working conditions. Also, although sport features as a welcome break to classroom learning, essentially children learn that the social order values their cognitive over their physical abilities. They are required to subdue their bodies to school agendas. The school may be thought of by staff as a site of 'socialization', but its teaching relates mainly to the social order of the school. The good schoolchild is not generalizable to other contexts.

Managing one's body at home and at school

I have suggested that generational proximity and adult models of children to some extent structure how children feel about their bodies. A related issue is the adult view of divisions of labour: how far parents, other adults and chil-dren are responsible for keeping children healthy. Responsibility for the health and safety of children at school is a grey area, with competing claims directed towards the local education authority (especially with respect to the building), the governors and the headteacher. In children's experience, adults provide poor opportunities for child health maintenance in many schools. The buildings themselves, the playgrounds and the toilets are commonly described by children and by teachers as inadequate (Mayall *et al.* 1996: 17–25).

Children's own views on the division of responsibility for keeping them healthy are critical to understanding their experience of managing their bodies. Young children's accounts strongly favour their parents as responsible, with increasing mentions, at older ages, of their joint responsibility with their parents. In the CHIPS study, few 6–7 year olds, but many 10–11 year olds, identified themselves only as responsible (17 per cent compared to 44 per cent). As one 9-year-old boy said:

> . . . we're the ones that have to take care of ourselves. Like when we live by ourselves we will.
>
> Boy 2: So we should, like, do that. We're keeping ourselves healthy by doing things ourselves. It's my body, so it's my job.
>
> (Mayall 1996: 94)

Notably, in the CHIPS study, none of the younger and only 15 per cent of the older children identified school or staff as health carers. They favour the home over the school as the place where they can expect to be cared for and enabled, through parental interest, to manage their bodies themselves. At school it may be difficult to get care, and staff may not be interested in enabling them to carry out health maintenance.

These points raise the question of how far children have control over the management of their bodies during their daily lives, and how far adults operate as enablers or regulators of this control. As suggested earlier, whilst parents encourage and express delight in their children's physical achievements, they – that is, mothers – have a socially ascribed responsibility for delivering a child to the public gaze who, in the sense used by Elias (1978), is civilized, that is, has learned societal norms. However, children experience tensions between this civilizing function and the value of the home as a free zone (Halldén 1991), where individual behaviour is acceptable. At home, in privacy, gender stereotypes may be challenged: a boy may cry and a girl be aggressive. Children therefore have to develop interpretive competence (Mackay 1991) in order to judge the parental mode and goal at any one point in time.

At school, children's ability to manage their bodies is severely limited. They are required to subordinate their bodies to the formal regime. Children have to ask permission to go the lavatory, can only exercise and drink at adult-specified times and places. Whilst children may be in tune with their bodily needs, they may not be able to satisfy them, for adult agendas and authority prevent this (see Freund 1982). However, as noted above, children give high praise to the opportunities they do have for bodily exercise, and particularly high praise to those teachers who themselves value exercise and jointly participate in it with the children. Five year olds point forcibly to adult controls over their bodily management; notably by the age of

9 children have carried out the emotion work necessary to accept these controls (and sometimes circumnavigate them). The price some of them pay is boredom.

> School is boring. It lasts 6 whole hours and 30 whole minutes. From ten to nine till 3.30. When I walk in the school gate at ten to nine I feel tired. When I walk out of the gate at 3.30 I feel happy. I think the most important people in school are children. The best part of the day is when we go home.

(Mayall 1994: 71)

From their earliest months, therefore, children learn that the social order promoted and maintained by adults makes complex demands on them, the children. It is within this complex social order that children negotiate, more or less successfully, the management of their bodies, and experience lower or higher adult evaluation of their bodies; and it is in consequence of how these factors operate that their sense of ease with their embodied selves varies.

Dealing with illness

Illness provides specific and dramatic instances in which to consider children's management of their bodies at home and school. Mothers' socially assigned responsibility for the health care of family members extends to children even when they are in the 'care' of others. Social policy assumes that mothers put health care first, so when a child falls ill at school, it is legitimate for staff to summon her. Mothers themselves, in every study I have done, accept this primary responsibility and indeed welcome being summoned. They also voice concern about the health and safety standards of school: especially as regards the playground, the lavatories and the school meals.

Children's accounts of episodes of illness at home endorse the picture of home as a holistic health-care arena: 'It was really good, cos I just lay on the sofa, with the telly on all day, and my Mum gave me ice-cream and I read my book.' At home the care they get comprises attention to their physical and emotional condition, in one package. The message children absorb is that the appropriate care for a physical condition includes emotional support:

> I remember when I was 7, I was really ill. I think I was ill for a week. I had to lie in my Mum's bed all day. It wasn't boring at all really. Mum was with me most of the time. When Mum wasn't with me, my sister or my brother William was there. William did anything for me, so I took advantage of that. I didn't change much except for the fact that I couldn't walk because I was so weak in the legs. I got a lot of attention and presents. This week I was ill was a school week and I liked that fact because instead of working I'm lying in bed watching TV.

The primary school presents children with a complex lay health-care system, which, though it varies between schools, is essentially based on the add-on character of women's work: both teachers and non-teachers add caring to their paid remit. In seeking physical help and sympathy from adults, therefore, children take chances, dependent on adult busyness, mood and diagnosis. In turn, children must manage their bodies, through emotional control; they may have to wait for help, or do without it and carry on. In the CHIPS study, children's accounts of recent episodes of illness suggested that the commonest symptoms were headache, stomach ache and feeling sick. These symptoms would probably be alleviated by time out from work – in a quiet place, lying down and resting – facilities which most schools do not have. Some children reported a caring adult response, but others said that teachers did not listen, or respond, were suspicious of their sickness bid (see Prout 1986), or suggested the child carried on 'till we see how you go'. Reviewing the episode as a whole, children were dissatisfied in 24 per cent of cases, with staff behaviour as a principal reason. Satisfaction was commonly linked to the arrival of a parent (almost always the mother), to take over. Some children did not seek help at school, but saved up their pains until they got home.

The onset of illness provides a clear case where children's ability to manage their body – to respond to its signals – is structured by the interlocking forces outlined earlier. Sharp separation between adult and child groups, in terms of their interests, and the adult view of how childhood should be lived at school, backed by the formal remit of school, constitute a firm framework, within which sickness bids may be questioned. For instance, one child commented:

> Some teachers say, 'You're acting like a baby – go away!' When it turns out to be serious, they say something different.

Recognizing that teachers are stressed, children have to accept that they may get an unsympathetic rebuff when they ask for help in case of sickness or accident.

> They can't be bothered. They hear too much of the same thing, and they're tired.

Children point to a sometimes unmet need for emotional as well as physical care when they feel ill or have an accident:

> They never take you seriously – they just say, 'Go and sit in a corner!' and things like that, and if you've hurt yourself it's not very comforting.

Thus the social order of the school serves to structure the emotional response of staff to children's bodily distress, and the children have to learn to control and manage their bodies through emotion work. Under these circumstances, support from other children is important:

I feel like I could tell my friends (about feeling ill), but sometimes I feel like I can't tell the teacher. It depends what kind of mood she's in, and sometimes I feel I can't tell her at all.

Emotion work at school comprises both teaching one's body to conform to the social norms and providing sympathetic care for other children. The appropriate emotions in the face of illness or an accident may be stoicism and toughness about one's own condition, coupled with ready sympathy for the conditions of other children.

DISCUSSION

This chapter has considered the distinctive social forces in play in the private world of the home and in the public world of school, how these forces serve to shape children's feelings about their embodied identities, and how children learn to manage their bodies through emotional control. I have argued that within the health-care centre of the home, mothers' understanding of interlinkages between the emotional, cognitive and bodily contrasts with school adults' separation out of these components of identity, with emphasis on the cognitive. So children are likely to feel more comfortable in their bodies at home than at school. Furthermore, at home generally, children are encouraged to value their bodily achievements, and to participate through embodied emotion work in constructing the social order of the home. On the other hand, school encourages high valuation of bodily skills at specified times and in specified places, but generally asks children to subordinate bodies to minds.

I suggest we can improve our understanding of children's experiences by considering goals and behaviour under the headings: civilizing, regulating and constructing. Civilizing children is a central remit of the home – encouraging and enabling children to manage their bodies so that they may participate acceptably in the social order of both the home and wider social arenas. Children's contentment with this enterprise may be enhanced where, with shared interests, they participate in a relatively equal relationship with their parents. By contrast, the school encourages children's belief that their bodies must be regulated in the interests of school and societal agendas. Relatively, civilizing is a joint enterprise and regulation is a top-down enterprise.

Yet cross-cutting these themes is a third counterbalancing one: the construction of children's bodies. Children's physical energy is often in conflict with the limited space at home; they have to learn and enact a restricted and controlled body. At school (though only for an hour or two a week) children's bodies are valued as the site for constructing socially valued physical skills, through sports and games. Almost all the CHIPS children reported pleasure in the activities and achievements available, which allowed them to value bodily skills and the construction of culturally acceptable bodies.

Given current traffic policy and public fears about danger from strangers, children have decreasing opportunities (except at expensive leisure centres) for structuring their bodies through physical exercise. School provides the main arena, both in formal sports and through the social experience of the playground, where groups of children themselves construct their vision of the embodied self – a topic explored in detail in the next chapter.

I have suggested that children's construction of embodied identity takes place in child–adult negotiations. The child group is an important site too. Not only is a child's identity constructed through the social group of children (James 1993; Prendergast and Forrest in Chapter 9 of this volume), but children offer comfort and support to each other, and, more generally, they construct the solidarity of the group vis-à-vis the adult groups. For instance, children's recognition of another child's distress, expressed need for help, feelings of alienation or oppression, or of pleasure in achievement, can constitute ratification of that child's evaluation of her embodied experience. The recognition can also confirm the joint interests of children in an adult-ordered world. Children's caring work for and with each other takes place at home (e.g. Dunn 1984, 1988), and children talk about their common front in face of parental control; but perhaps it is especially valuable at school (see Christensen 1993), where adult caring is less reliable.

Implicit in the discussions in this chapter are tensions between children's time and adult time. How children experience their day in the context of these tensions can be considered in relation to the axes of generational proximity and adult models of adulthood and childhood. From their first days, children are encouraged and then required to fit their behaviour to adult time-ordered norms current in the household and more widely. More immediate and local adult agendas also structure children's time use – 'We can't go to the park till I've done the washing up'. At school, adult time-interests structure the school day, week, term and year, indeed time can be seen as organized in terms of adult interests (e.g. Oldman 1994). For children's sense of wellbeing, therefore, it is critical that they feel themselves to be contributors to the adult enterprise, rather than merely subject to it. Thus, the proximity of adult to child interests, and the extent to which adults regard child participation as appropriate, will serve to determine how comfortable children feel in their embodied experience through the day.

The time present and the time future of children is also at issue. Broadly, the remit of the home pays attention to the expressed bodily and emotional needs of people now, as well as to the civilizing, future-oriented remit. The school, broadly, puts greater emphasis on children's time future – school is preparation for adult life – a point children themselves understand. Gym and sports sessions interestingly combine attention to children's time present and their time future. The value school puts on bodily skills during these sessions combines with media-promoted ideals of an active, slim and strong body to structure children's ideas about how they should develop their bodies now and for the future.

The data explored in this chapter suggest that children are positioned at the intersections of important social values: that people should take control over their emotions, and order their bodies to suit social values, but that ensuring children carry out these remits is a central adult responsibility, in two main arenas, the home and the school. For the quality of children's emotional contentment in embodied living, much depends on how far adults accept the child's personhood and contributions to the structuring of the social order.

NOTE AND ACKNOWLEDGEMENTS

1 In chronological order the studies drawn on in this chapter are as follows. Two studies of parental care of under-fives – The Keeping Children Healthy study (1981–4) (Mayall 1986) and Child Health Care study (1984–8) (Mayall and Foster 1989) – were carried out with funding from the Economic and Social Research Council (ref. no. XC00280002, XC00280001 respectively). Two further studies focused on school-aged children, and collected data from children and adults. The Greenstreet study (1991–2) was supported by the Nuffield Foundation and the Institute of Education (Mayall 1994). The CHIPS study (1993–5) was supported by the Economic and Social Research Council (ref. no. ROOO 23 4476) (Mayall *et al.* 1996). To all these funding bodies I am deeply indebted. I am very grateful to all the people who, variously, collaborated with me on these studies: Chris Grossmith, Marie-Claude Foster, Sandy Barker, Gill Bendelow, Pamela Storey and Marijcke Veltman. Very many thanks to those without whom the studies could not have been done: the children, parents, schools and health-service staff. I am very grateful to Leena Alanen, Gill Bendelow and Gunilla Halldén for discussion about the topics of this paper, and to Gill and Simon for comments on an earlier draft.

BIBLIOGRAPHY

Alanen, L. (1992) *Modern Childhood: Exploring the 'Child Question' in Sociology.* Research Report 50. Finland: University of Jyväskyla.
Alanen, L. (1994) 'The family phenomenon: considerations from a children's standpoint', paper presented at the seminar Children and Families: Research and Policy, London, 28–30 April 1994.
Büchner, P., Krüger, H.-H. and du Bois-Reymond, M. (1994) 'Growing up as a "modern" child in western Europe: the impact of modernization and civilization processes on the everyday lives of children', *Sociological Studies of Children* 6: 1–23.
Burgess, H. and Carter, B. (1992) 'Bringing out the best in people: teacher training and the "real" teacher', *British Journal of Sociology of Education* 13 (3): 349–59.
Christensen, P. H. (1993) 'The social construction of help among Danish schoolchildren', *Sociology of Health and Illness* 15 (4): 488–502.
Denzin, N. K. (1977) *Childhood Socialization.* San Francisco, CA: Jossey Bass.
Donzelot, J. (1980) *The Policing of Families: Welfare versus the State.* London: Hutchinson.
Dunn, J. (1984) *Sisters and Brothers.* London: Fontana.

Dunn, J. (1988) *The Beginnings of Social Understanding.* Oxford: Blackwell.

Elias, N. (1978) *The Civilising Process,* Vol. 1, *The History of Manners,* trans. Edmund Jephcott. Oxford: Blackwell.

Engelbert, A. (1994) 'Worlds of childhood: differentiated but different: implications for social policy', in J. Qvortrup, M. Bardy, G. Sgritta and H. Wintersberger (eds) *Childhood Matters: Social Theory, Practice and Politics.* Aldershot: Avebury Press.

Ennew, J. (1986) *The Sexual Exploitation of Children.* Cambridge: Polity Press.

Freund, P. (1982) *The Civilized Body: Social Domination, Control and Health.* Philadelphia, PA: Temple University Press.

Freund, P. (1988) 'Bringing society into the body: understanding socialized human nature', *Theory and Society* 17 (6): 839–64.

Graham, H. (1984) *Women, Health and the Family.* Brighton: Harvester Press.

Halldén, G. (1991) 'The child as project and the child as being: parents' ideas as frames of reference', *Children and Society* 5 (4): 334–46.

Hartley, D. (1987) 'The time of their lives: bureaucracy and the nursery school', in A. Pollard (ed.) *Children and their Primary Schools.* London: Falmer Press.

Hochschild, A. (1979) 'Emotion work, feeling rules and social structure', *American Journal of Sociology* 85 (3): 551–75.

Hockey, J. and James, A. (1993) *Growing Up and Growing Old: Ageing and Dependency in the Life Course.* London: Sage.

Howson, A. (1994) Book review of Shilling, C. *The Body and Social Theory, Sociology of Health and Illness* 16 (3): 403–5.

Ingleby, D. (1986) 'Development in social context', in M. Richards and P. Light (eds) *Children of Social Worlds.* Cambridge: Polity Press.

James, A. (1993) *Childhood Identities: Social Relationships and the Self in Children's Experiences.* Edinburgh: Edinburgh University Press.

James, A. and Prout, A. (1995) 'Hierarchy, boundary and agency: towards a theoretical perspective on childhood', *Sociological Studies of Childhood* 7: 77–99.

King, R.A. (1989) *The Best of Primary Education: A Sociological Study of Junior Middle Schools.* London: Falmer Press.

Kirk, D. and Tinning, R. (1994) 'Embodied self-identity, healthy life-styles and school physical education', *Sociology of Health and Illness* 16 (5): 600–25.

Mac an Ghaill, M. (1994) *The Making of Men: Masculinities, Sexualities and Schooling.* Buckingham: Open University Press.

Mackay, R. W. (1991) 'Conceptions of children and models of socialization', in F. C. Waksler (ed.) *Studying the Social Worlds of Children: Sociological Readings.* London: Falmer Press.

Martin, E. (1987) *The Woman in the Body.* Milton Keynes: Open University Press.

Mayall, B. (1986) *Keeping Children Healthy.* London: Allen and Unwin.

Mayall, B. (1994) *Negotiating Health: Children at Home and Primary School.* London: Cassell.

Mayall, B. (1996) *Children, Health and the Social Order.* Buckingham: Open University Press.

Mayall, B., Bendelow, G., Barker, S., Storey, P. and Veltman, M. (1996) *Children's Health in Primary Schools.* London: Falmer Press.

Mayall, B. and Foster, M.-C. (1989) *Child Health Care: Living with Children, Working for Children.* Oxford: Heinemann Educational Books.

Newson, J. and Newson, E. (1970) *Four Years Old in an Urban Community.* Harmondsworth: Penguin.

Oldman, D. (1994) 'Childhood as a mode of production', in B. Mayall (ed.) *Children's Childhoods: Observed and Experienced.* London: Falmer Press.

Prout, A. (1986) '"Wet children" and "little actresses": going sick in primary school', *Sociology of Health and Illness* 8 (2): 111–36.

Prout, A. and James, A. (1990) 'A new paradigm for the sociology of childhood? Provenance, promise and problems', in A. James and A. Prout (eds) *Constructing and Reconstructing Childhood: Contemporary Issues in the Sociology of Childhood*. London: Falmer Press.

Qvortrup, J. (1991) *Childhood as a Social Phenomenon: An Introduction to a Series of National Reports*. Vienna: European Centre.

Qvortrup, J. (1994) 'Childhood matters: an introduction', in J. Qvortrup, M. Bardy, G. Sgritta and H. Wintersberger (eds) *Childhood Matters: Social Theory, Practice and Politics*. Aldershot: Avebury Press.

Scheper-Hughes, N. and Lock, M. (1987) 'The mindful body: a prolegomenon to future work in medical anthropology', *Medical Anthropology Quarterly* 1 (1): 6–41.

Shilling, C. (1993) *The Body and Social Theory*. London: Sage.

Waksler, F. C. (1991) 'Dancing when the music is over: a study of deviance in a kindergarten classroom', in F. C. Waksler (ed.) *Studying the Social Worlds of Children: Sociological Readings*. London: Falmer Press.

Young, I. M. (1980) 'Throwing like a girl: a phenomenology of feminine body comportment, motility and spatiality', *Human Studies* 3: 137–56.

9 'Shorties, low-lifers, hardnuts and kings'

Boys, emotions and embodiment in school

Shirley Prendergast and Simon Forrest

INTRODUCTION: ONE FRIDAY, TWO STORIES

Friday a.m. Shirley's story: *Andy and the dead cat*

I am walking through the estate, back to school with Simon and a group of 11-year-old first year Cherrington pupils. There is a buzz of conversation about the morning's events. We are returning from a visit to a local primary school to tell the primary pupils what it is like in 'big' school. Each secondary pupil had been briefed to talk to a small group of the primary pupils, and had some activities to do with them. But the visit hasn't gone quite as planned. In at least two boys-only groups the primary boys behaved badly. They mocked and humiliated the two Cherrington group leaders (Andy and Jane) and wouldn't do the activities. They said that Cherrington was useless, it was a dump, nobody would go there. It was violent and full of wallies.

As we walk the girls talk indignantly with Jane. Andy throws his activities folder over a hedge. Walking with the other boys he is silent, flushed and sweating. Suddenly big tears roll down his face. I draw back to talk to him but he brushes me aside and turns away. We look at the front gardens. Andy notices and asks if I like gardens. I do. He says that he helps his father in their garden, and I ask Andy what they grow. He laughs and says that in fact his dad is a builder. Their back garden is 'a rubbish dump where nothing grows'. Also he says, 'Our garden is full of dog shit.'

We get to the long, rough grass in front of school and Andy says, 'Do you like cats, Miss?' He asks me to come and look at something. It is a dead cat, its stomach torn open, with flies buzzing around. He looks at me. 'It's like liver. Lovely, I think I will have it for breakfast.' He shoves the cat with his foot, and runs off smiling.

Friday p.m. Simon's story: *Perky the monkey*

I am sitting alone, writing, in an empty classroom. Everywhere is hot and sleepy and quiet. A small first year boy comes in. He has lank hair and glasses balanced unevenly on his nose. He is very slight. He asks if he can sit beside me. We sit in silence for a while. I ask the boy what he has been doing this afternoon. He has been doing his technology test. He was the last to finish, he says, but it doesn't matter because there are ten minutes before the home-time bell rings. He tells me he likes puppets – you can tell stories with them. He pulls Perky, his monkey puppet, out of his bag. Sitting on the boy's knee, Perky tells his story. He is born without an eye. He has a plaster over it. Then he goes to hospital, wearing a little nappy, like when he was born. Then his eye comes out of the sky and is put in his face. The boy says puppets are quite difficult to find in shops. He really likes animal ones, but you have to look hard for them. Another, even smaller boy comes in and sits beside us. The two boys and Perky talk. The little boy asks the monkey if he is all right. Perky says he is. He is just tired and his eye is ill.

The boys climb out through an open window behind us and talk to me over the frame. We talk to Perky about what he wants to do. He wants to go on holiday. He wants to grow up and be happy. He is quite sad when he has to go back into his bag but he likes coming to school most times. I walk over to the piano in the corner and quietly start to play. Perky says he knows that song but he can't remember the words. He is humming and the smaller boy comes to the window and leans in, listening. Perky asks if I know any more songs. The bell goes and he says he has to go back into the bag now. The boys slip out.

The ubiquitous focus on feelings in western culture reiterates again and again both the splitting of mind and body and the priority of mind: the body is seen to express what the mind directs. Buytendijk (1974) has noted that we commonly describe the shaking of the fist as a way in which someone expresses a feeling, in this case 'anger'. Rather, he argues the shaking of the fist is not an expression of feeling anger, *it is anger itself* that we see. In similar vein Rom Harré says that to study emotions is to study a certain kind of social act: 'There is no such thing as "an emotion". There are only the various ways of acting and feeling emotionally, of displaying one's judgements, attitudes and opinions in an appropriate bodily way' (1991: 143). For both Harré and Buytendijk emotions are neither exclusively of mind or of body, but hover interactively somewhere between. Their enactment and their embodiment are a part both of the definition of an emotion and of the learning that constitutes it. Emotional and embodied learning then are closely intertwined, and occur largely outside of our conscious awareness and control. In the everyday, emotions are most often first encountered in embodied form, widely acknowledged in the idea of 'body-language' as Johnson (1987) Freund (1988, 1990) Lakoff (1987) and others have noted. We can usually tell if someone is happy or dejected, angry or relaxed, whether female or male, young or old, and whether a stranger or someone we know, long before we see their face. At the same time, none of us can say exactly how, across the myriad factors of the lived experience of each minute, day, week or year, a person takes on this embodiment as their own. For this reason Bourdieu (1986) suggests that embodied learning cannot easily be 'forgotten'; it is hard to modify and is among the most powerful forms of learning we ever undergo.

Harré points to the social aspects of emotions and emotional learning. He notes that while the existence of complex emotional lives, 'whether in Oxford or on Ifaluk' (1991: 160), may suggest deeper residual structures, emotion feelings and displays can be understood only as both natural *and* learned. Their meanings are defined by reference to shared language, cultural beliefs and values and the ways in which an individual is positioned in social encounters (Harré 1986). Scott and Morgan go further: 'This is not just a question of bodily understandings being socially shaped. It is also the fact that social orders have always been concerned with bodies and their control and surveillance and that, in certain ways at least, these concerns have increased in modern societies' (1993: 14). To see emotion primarily as a social act in this way calls for an understanding of how individual bodily expressions are learned and defined within a social context, a repertoire of shared emotional meaning. From earliest times a child's sense of self is shaped in relation to the feeling-acts and feeling-words that define how one interacts with the world at the deepest levels. For example, while a child *could* develop an entirely novel and individual way of 'being angry' (perhaps by rubbing the nose as opposed to shaking the fist or stamping the feet), there is little advantage in doing so. Those around the child would have to learn what was signified, while strangers would have no idea at all. As it is, each child increasingly finds and becomes subject to a socially available repertoire of emotion-acts: love, jealousy, anger, fear in all their variety of forms and degrees of expression. Sarbin (1986) calls this socially acknowledged way of doing an emotion the 'dramatistic', in contrast to the 'dramaturgical' where an individual might also adopt and set aside emotion-acts called for in more routine or ritualistic fashion, expressing caring emotions appropriate to a nurse or sad ones as a mourner, for example.

However, studies of children's emotions suggest that Sarbin's categories may not be quite so distinct, describing complex interrelationships between the social expectations of emotions and their expression. For example, although parents may monitor how, when and where their child experiences, witnesses and expresses emotion, this is not entirely within their control. Parents recall how, with the onset of school, their 5-year-old daughter suddenly became frightened of going to the top of the climbing frame or how, at 2, their little boy began to enact the aggressive stance of a man with a sword or a gun. They wonder what this means: what is the relationship between the expression and the experience of emotion in these examples? Gordon (1989) argues that children do not necessarily follow a classic developmental sequence (having emotional feelings or experiences for which they then later discover a social language). Instead they may well learn the available 'dramatistic role' or 'emotion script' before enacting and therefore learning for themselves the feeling it refers to. The little girl might only become frightened of the climbing frame when she sees other girls scared at school; the little boy copies activities that he does not understand because they seem to signify excitement or power. Even for adults these aspects of doing emotion may not be so discrete as we imagine, as Hochschild (1983) describes in exploring the significance of what she calls 'emotion work' in the workplace: in playing out specifically defined emotional roles as a requirement of the workplace we might actually come to live out, literally incorporate, emotions initially assumed (from the dramaturgical to the dramatistic in Sarbin's sense). Similar arguments have been made by Lawlor (1991) in respect of nursing, Game and Pringle (1983) and Game (1986) in relation to secretarial work.

A number of key points about emotional learning emerge from this brief discussion. First, there is the significance of *gendered* emotional learning. The little girl may act frightened because she learns that this is an attribute of being properly female, and the little boy sees that on the whole it is generally men who point guns, and he too wants to be a proper man. The emotions that can be expressed, to what degree and through what forms of embodiment, are fundamentally tied to social perceptions and enactments of gender. Second is the role of *social context*, particularly the workplace and institutional contexts, in shaping gendered learning (Hochschild 1983; Game 1986; Prendergast 1994, 1995). Work is often framed in a fashion that requires emotional skills and self-management which are gender-specified: as a person of that gender does that job he or she is reinforcing and extending what is almost certainly an arbitrary, learned linkage between gender and emotional expertise. Third is the *embodied* nature of emotional learning. Hochschild's point carries such force for this reason. Emotional learning happens because bodies do not just 'act' emotions for the mind. In acting emotions we (as body/mind) are capable of being changed by them. In this fashion consistent acting may operate as a form of embodied learning (as in Bourdieu) becoming real. To return again to the climbing frame: suppose that, in 'acting scared', the girl actually does becomes less physically stable. Then, maybe she loses her balance and falls, becomes really fearful and avoids the climbing frame after that. In contrast, imagine the boy rehearsing standing firmly on his feet, pointing the gun or stick, finding that other children treat him with respect or avoid him for this reason. He comes to embody the control and aggression he admires. In these cases emotion is both enacted and learned, literally *incorporated* into who we are. By the same token, however, since enactment and therefore learning are ongoing there is always the possibility of change.

These themes of the relationships between social context, learning, embodiment, emotions and gender are explored through observational and interview material gathered from boys and girls in three English secondary schools.[1] We focus particularly on boys' experiences in order to look at the ways in which the context of school offers a forum where the emotions of a proper masculine self might be shaped and learned. These are discussed under the following headings: boys' use of space; the shame of smallness and the language of 'hardness'; hierarchies and cycles of embodied masculinity; and the power of groups.

The concluding section of this chapter asks some key questions about the production of masculinity/ies at adolescence: how do embodiment and emotional configurations and transformations overlap for adolescent boys? To what degree is embodiment both a precursor and a mechanism of masculine group processes? How far can it explain, as boys told us so many times, why boys did things in the company of others that they would not dream of doing on their own? It also highlights more general issues concerning the construction of emotions in a social context. As the reader may already have noted, we the researchers are often present in the data presented here, sometimes as joint voices speaking the narrative, sometimes as a personal voice. This does not signal an absence of other data (on the contrary), nor is it an accident. Rather the choice marks and emphasizes some critical points in our own understanding of emotions as it unfolded through this study: the significance of acts and actions as a sequence of events in a context, the issue of who is present and how their presence contributes to the ongoing social construction of emotions in this context, and the power of stories as a way of presenting, shaping and constructing experience. We end by suggesting that powerful forms of emotional learning take place through these embodied, gendered processes that are a taken-for-granted aspect of the everyday.

EMOTION, EMBODIMENT AND SCHOOL

Boys' use of space

(SHIRLEY AND SIMON) *We are looking down on to the corner of the playground, near to one of the teaching blocks at Priory school. It is seething with young people between about 11 and 15 on a thundery, clammy lunchtime. At first we feel dizzy looking – everything appears chaotic, bodies weaving, ducking, running, struggling. Gradually we notice that in the centre of the space boys are using tin cans and screwed-up bags as footballs, leaping, shoving, rarely still. Around the edges, sitting with their backs to the wall, are small groups of girls. They are talking, looking at magazines, swopping notes and giving each other elaborate hairstyles. Stacked everywhere are heavy school bags, coats, jumpers, games equipment, dinner boxes, big bottles of drink.*

We focus our attention on just one corner. A boy crosses rapidly from left to right on a pair of crutches. Two big boys chase a small boy, turn him upside down and carry him round with his legs waving. We glimpse the crutches again, from right to left, but this time it is a different boy, who leapfrogs some concrete bollards with them. The big boys push the small boy head-first into a large bushy shrub and the culprits vanish. The crutches cross a third time, now it is a girl using them. A sudden wind blows a sprinkling of sweet papers and litter across the yard as it thunders and the sky gets dark. All the pupils run towards a covered way, the only shelter on this side of school.

Time and again our fieldwork notes record that while girls almost always could be found clustered in intense oases of laughter and conversation on the margins of things, boys' noise and physicality almost always completely dominated secondary classrooms, playgrounds and open spaces of school. But what was even more interesting was the ways in which boys did this: controlling the active centre of the playground, tripping each other up, pushing each other to the limits of teasing and aggressive behaviour. A girl or a smaller boy who ventured here was likely to risk rough treatment. One boy was put in a bush, another had his jacket sleeves pulled down and tied behind him. Others were yanked along by their jumpers, or their bags were grabbed and thrown from person to person. Alongside on the grass, smaller boys rehearsed these same dramas in safer forms: grabbing each other by the head, wrestling each other to the ground, tumbling in a dishevelled heap of bodies. One day a very big boy approached this group. He stood there for a moment waiting, and then, all at once, the smaller boys rushed at him. He vanished beneath the pile, rose, smilingly brushed them off and walked away.

In saying that space is dominated by boys then, it is more accurate to say that it is dominated by *bigger boys* who set the terms and conditions on which others may join them. This includes not just girls but also smaller boys. Smaller boys, while they wait, practise with each other, and sometimes rehearse with older boys. They also begin to test themselves against girls.

(SHIRLEY) *I never forget, as part of another study, watching a smallish boy of about 12 or 13 walking the length of the school hall. As he did so he touched the bottoms of at least three older and much taller girls as he passed. In each case the girl looked round, brushed her skirt, but could not identify what had happened or who had done it.*

The shame of smallness and the language of hardness

(SHIRLEY AND SIMON) *One day it suddenly struck us that it was only the smaller boys at Priory who wore the red uniform jumpers. All the taller, bigger boys, even in coldest weather, wore shirts with the sleeves rolled up, carefully loosened ties. This happened both between years and also within years. In the very same class the bigger boys would dress in this way, while the smaller boys wore their sweaters.*

There is an interesting reversal here. For girls as the body develops and matures, display becomes more ambiguous. To display the mature female body is to open oneself up to the gaze of boys, and the risk of being labelled, for example, a slag. Boys may always use girls' bodily development against them, particularly since maturity is also marked by the onset of menstruation (Prendergast 1995). In contrast, boys' bodies appear to be most hidden, least displayed when they are immature, most displayed when they are developed and matured.

Between and within boys' groups physical size and 'hardness' often stood as metaphors of superiority and inferiority, reflected in the language they used about each other. *Hardnuts, kings, big and mighty boys, normal boys, superiors* and the *well 'ards* are contrasted to the *low-lifers, bottoms, weeds, wimps, shorties* who are *wasted* and *sad.* Admired groups were *well 'ard,* acted *dead funny* and *mucked about.* These qualities of size and hardness were epitomized in what boys called the 'strut'. A scathing but accurate description of the strut came from a group of girls. Such boys bounced, they noted, bounced as though they had springs in their shoes, a self-conscious looseness of shoulders and arms, a rolling walk with the head thrown back. The strut not only identified a boy as hard but was a form of challenge at any age. You would get beaten up if you did the strut in the wrong place or in the wrong company.

Among boys, then, embodiment predisposes special opportunities, risks, or dangers in comparison to one's peers. Time and again boys reported being bullied because they were small. Big boys, even if they did not use it, carried with them a seemingly automatic potential to dominate by virtue of their size. There was some evidence that, just as the big boy who used his bigness to dominate others physically would acquire status, another, rarer status might also accrue to a big boy who did not, a kind of 'gentle giant' who came into being because of the very physical qualities that he eschewed. Sometimes small boys could acquire in a ritualized way some of the bodily power of big boys by playing with them, but this is a risky undertaking. In playing with them a small boy is always liable to be reminded of his inferiority and weakness by the conversion of playful push to a painful punch. We saw this trade in bodily power between big and small boys played out in a daily ritual in Priory school:

(SIMON) *Every lunchtime a group of small boys played football on the school fields. They, like other groups of boys, had their particular patch, their place in the occupation of the school space. A group of bigger boys often joined in with their game and took pleasure in getting the ball and keeping it from the smaller boys, who were unable to push them off or catch them when they ran away. In the game the big boys slid into tackles on the smaller boys, knocking them over. Some of the small boys slid into the big boys in return. The big boys laughed and got up. But, sometimes the big boys then tackled the smaller boys with real viciousness, intending to hurt them.*

Of course, the big boys were allowing the small boys to knock them over. They shrugged it off, implying that a small boy cannot hurt them, it is a joke, like a man fighting a boy. They always had the power in hand to hurt the small boys. For small boys, taking the risk, knocking over a big boy, is worthwhile because they gain something: a temporary, ritualized equality of bodily power.

Hierarchies and cycles of embodied masculinity

(SHIRLEY) *One lunchtime I was approached by a group of first years aged 11 to 12. They begged me to make a tape recording of them and we went into the room where we worked. There were about 10 boys and girls, the boys amazingly tiny, and in most cases amazingly scruffy and dirty, compared to the girls. I began just by asking them what their first year of school had been like. A flood of stories and experiences followed. Suddenly Will, a small, sturdy boy with a round face and tousled hair, said that he couldn't wait for next year to start. Then, he said, there would be all the new ones to boss around. The boys explained that this year the older boys had bullied them, taking money and sweets, making them do things, pushing them about, sometimes using physical force. There was nothing the first years could do. Will said, 'You have just got to take it. You can't go to teachers or nothing. But next year it's your turn.'*

Will's honesty was an important key to understanding. Straight from being biggest in primary school, the first year of secondary school seemed to mark an almost intolerable return to being smallest and weakest in the masculine hierarchy. An older boy of 13 told us, 'Like when you're at the bottom of the school you feel really small, and you don't like to fight because you feel you can't control things, don't you? But when you're a year higher, you kind of think, yeah, I can have a go at them – like the year lower.' These forms of passing on violence and control started in the first year but spiralled up into other year groups. We heard how bigger boys of 14, 15 and 16 might threaten to beat a boy up unless that boy, in his turn, hit someone else. For example, it was possible to make even a quiet and unassuming boy do something unpleasant or hit someone younger in order to avoid being hit himself. One group explained, with a convoluted chivalry, that while they 'got' boys smaller than they were, if you saw someone smaller than yourself beating up an even smaller boy, then that medium-sized boy would himself 'get it'!

In the toughest schools, or with the toughest groups of boys, the hierarchy reached its peak when male teachers verbally or physically intervened on the same terms. The longer-term cycle of inherited male injustice was described many times over. For example, boys told us how much they hated Mr Pearl's unfairness:

(SHIRLEY AND SIMON) *Sitting in Mr Pearl's class we witnessed a draconian system of classroom control driven by biting sarcasm towards the boys. He spoke in a artificially low whisper, barely audible, which would suddenly shift into a very loud bellow if a boy overstepped the mark. Both the whisper and the bellow seemed arbitrary and frightening. Mr Pearl, as he constantly told the pupils, kept this kind of control over his class to stop bullying. He had been bullied himself as a child and knew what it felt like.*

In another school Tony, a heavy boy of 14, described how a teacher had begun to call him 'Mr Blobby', 'Chubby-Little', names which the class took up. Tony told us humbly that although he *was* fat, he didn't think he was thick. Then, completely without irony, Tony told us that the teacher's name was 'Mr Small'. In the same school a group of boys and girls described how sometimes male teachers would flick a boy's head with the side of their hand, or stand behind misbehaving boys and twist their ears or arms until they cried out. Such measures escalate as the stakes rise. Boys who saw unemployment ahead saw little reason to work hard, if at all, in school. As in Mac an Ghaill's study, one teacher told him that nobody wanted to teach losers, all the effort went into successful kids. 'The losers, specially the boys, are getting harder to control now they have the extra burden of the scrap heap' (1994). In this way the 'solution' imposed by school itself becomes part of the problem. For some boys, the spiralling up and down of physical control, structured by age and by size, from the smallest boy to the toughest male teacher was endemic to school. Hierarchical, endlessly circular, it appears self-perpetuating, a closed system. This hedging of bets, off-loading of violence, acted like a web which caught even those who wished to have no part in it. Interviews with boys were shot through with a passionate and angry sense of injustice and unfairness.

The power of groups

(SHIRLEY AND SIMON) *Initially, with almost no movement at all other than chairs turned to face each other, the pupils readily make three all-boys groups and three all-girls groups. When we ask about forming mixed groups we are met with blank looks and embarrassed denial. Clearly, under normal circumstances pupils would not choose to sit with members of the opposite sex. In almost every classroom the solution comes in the same way: one group of boys offers to swop some members with one particular group of girls. With significant looks and a great display of unwillingness the girls agree. These are the tables where the most mature boys sit, and, often, the girls they swap with are their girlfriends.*

As we have seen, boys in the schools we visited mapped out highly significant comparative reference points across both age and size: not only were you small or large within your peer group, but the relative size and reputation of other age groups was also a factor that boys must bear in mind both in the everyday life of school and as they moved up through the years. Clearly group formations had a particular power and significance for boys. In the classroom we explored some of the ways in which different groups formed and made decisions about gendered issues, recording them on a worksheet. After the pupils entered the classroom and were sitting where they normally did, we asked them to form six groups, two of boys, two of girls and two mixed. They could do this in any way they wished, as described above. It became evident that physical size was an important factor in how groups were formed. This was clearer amongst boys because of the greater differentials in their height, at any age, than those amongst girls. Almost always it looked as though the biggest, most mature boys would sit together, as would the very smallest boys in the class.

In their groups boys found it much harder to concentrate on the task in hand. Often they would muck about throughout the lesson, casting insults and dominating the room. At the end of the lesson we asked the girls and the boys to form two groups, one of all the boys together and one of all the girls together, to report back on the activity they had been doing. Again a highly predictable pattern emerged: almost immediately the girls gathered in one group, talked things through, came to collective agreement and elected a spokesperson. In contrast the different groups of boys found it almost impossible to move physically to one shared space, let alone talk when they did so. Many boys never moved at all. Decisions were generally made by those boys who shouted loudest and most determinedly what should be written up on the blackboard at the front.

As a boy, being inside a group exerts a powerful influence over how you can behave. However, if you are outside of any group, other more terrifying effects can come into play. In each school were isolated pupils, 'loners', the victims of bullying, teased by bigger boys and objects of pity and embarrassment to girls. Without a group they had no way to fight back. The avenues of bullying others, getting a good reputation – being good at sport or having a close group of friends – had all been closed.

(SHIRLEY AND SIMON) *As we go into the class of third years, aged 13 to 14, a boy is standing outside the door. He won't come in. He is pale and his eyes brim with tears. The teacher insists that he enter the classroom. He resists and starts to sob. He says that he has lost his comb and must go and find it. The teacher sits him with a girls' group and leaves the room. John is totally distraught and distracted. He cannot look at anybody. He is shaking and crying. He wrings his hands and keeps repeating that he must find his comb, can he go, he can't stay here. He manages to tell Shirley that the boys in the group opposite always bully him, for years and years, and the girls confirm this. He hates school, he has always been unhappy.*

John and other boys (and sometimes girls) like him had come to experience what looked to us like terror and despair. With the means to become reintegrated and disappear into a group lost, such pupils became more and more visible. In the end they seemed to break down, attracting more and more contempt, electrifying the classroom with their fear. For them all the normal rules of groups and bigness had fallen apart. They were constantly anxious about being teased, hurt, or bullied, and no place in school was safe for them.

DISCUSSION: TO TOUCH WITHOUT BEING TOUCHED . . .

In one of the most acclaimed fresco sequences in the world, in the Arena Chapel in Padua, Giotto (1298) painted the moment when Mary Magdalene finds Christ newly emerged from the tomb. As she (kneeling) reaches up in amazement, pity and love, he turns away, alone, towards his Resurrection: Noli me tangere, 'Do not touch me.'

We want to conclude this chapter by drawing together some themes relating to emotions, masculinity and embodiment as we observed them in boys' lives in school. We have sought to understand these observations in part by reference to what Harré has called a discursive approach to emotions: that emotion feelings and displays can be understood only as both natural *and* inculcated, defined by reference to shared cultural beliefs and values and the ways in which an individual is positioned in social encounters. Harré and others have pointed out how this view of emotion prioritizes both its lived quality and its linguistic framing. Johnson (1987) in particular has drawn attention to the role of embodied metaphors as a way of conceptualizing lived experience. It is perhaps no accident that dominant markers of size appear to have been so massively colonized by boys: as Hockey and James (1993) and Bodily (1994) note, age is a taken-for-granted explanatory factor in which adulthood, to be big, grown up, is 'normality'. Childhood is the ante-chamber through which we approach adulthood, grow up towards it; while old age is a process of decline, drawing us away, back towards a second childhood. To be childlike, childish, implies feebleness, ineffectiveness, linking diminished size to diminished power. For boys height, hardness, superiority of physique, can give access to a relative adulthood, relative power, ahead of others – the girls, the shorties and the low-lifers in their peer group.

Such metaphors are reflexive with what it is to be actively embodied as masculine in a social world. Young has described how boys' personal use of space tends to be more luxuriant than girls'; boys extend themselves into the physical demands of the task in hand. In similar fashion, our data suggest that in adolescence boys also appear to be increasing their control and command over public space. In dominating public spaces in school boys demarcate a kind of theatre in which their corporeality is acted out, and which they fill with their physical presence. In similar fashion Messner (1987), discussing the 'tribalization' characteristics of young men, points to the significance of public performance effected through bodily display in sport. A relatively big space, the classroom or the playground, a sports field or gym, can be commanded by a few if those few use it without inhibition or without regard for others.

While the domination of public space in this fashion may depend upon collective action – in a ball game, for example – at the same time action is also demarcated and ordered *between* boys: some boys and some forms of display predominate. Our observations suggest that it is the larger, active boys who dominate, not just in relation to girls but also in relation to smaller, more passive boys, predicated on embodied hierarchies of size and age. Space is an arena both for the display of masculinity *per se* and for the performance of embodied power relations between boys: for the assertion of certain forms of masculinities over others. As boys command space to enact such dramas, its theatrical centrality is emphasized by what girls do, in more intimate, private, contained fashion, literally sitting at the margins. For most girls, embodiment is not in the large gesture, shouting, leaping, shoving, tumbling, but in the small: an immaculate hairstyle, an uncreased blouse, the carefully arranged legs and flashing smile. Space makes visible emotional constellations and embodiments of gender: as a group, girls take emotion in, mull it over, extract its meaning. As boys say, girls 'talk, talk, talk, never let it go'. In contrast proper boys enact emotion, transform it into a 'laugh', pass it on, give the responsibility to someone else. At this age then, we might say that spatialized forms of gendered embodiment reflexively interact with gendered emotional experience and learning.

Learning to endure

To this we would add another form of gendered emotional learning which we have called 'learning to endure'. Learning to endure takes at least two forms in our observations, but both require that boys cope with, hide, or repress feelings of unfairness or injustice.

First, as we have already suggested, for boys peer groupings are the primary arena within which comparison and relativity of status thrive. Here it is important to distinguish between achieved (learned, gained as result of effort, generally within individual control) as opposed to ascribed status (given, already existing, generally outside of individual control). Bigger boys are in control while smaller boys, judged as less mature, must accept a lower place in the order of things. Thus during the most formative years of embodied learning, that time when adolescent changes are most intense, the most visibly powerful groups are ones that operate largely with ascribed characteristics (embodied ones) that are unfair and arbitrary. This aspect of group functioning is also often evident in both informal and formal sport in school.

Second, enduring ignominy and injustice may be a test of emotional entry both to a group and to a more adult masculinity. As Will illustrated so readily, if a boy endures long enough without breaking down, he too may (if he wishes) eventually come to police the space of masculinity in a similar fashion. Having suffered from the code, boys may go on to ensure that others suffer too. Cycles of endurance thus might be seen as structurally self-perpetuating: our data recorded not only oppressive behaviours from boys to girls and from boys to other boys, but also from adult males – teachers and fathers – to boys. Some groups unite boys who endure being small, and find a collective identity through this, others may link boys who have endured to become hard. While at their best, small groups give boys friendship and protection, as we saw in class activities, boys did not seem to be able to come together as 'boys', free of small group trappings. In our sample, and as Askew and Ross found in their work with teenage boys (1988), membership of a male peer group was key to the experience of school and for many completely absorbed and displaced interest in any other form of friendship or relationship. As Connell (1987, 1995) has so cogently outlined, hegemonic masculinity (which underpins male dominance as a group over women) depends upon the suppression of aspects of masculinity, of other masculinities, that do not meet the ideal. This seemed to be enacted in our data: a seeming impossibility of an overarching sense of maleness, an inclusive category which brings all boys and all groups together at adolescence. Those who break, like John, often become 'loners', not just excluded from groups but, even worse, the target of male group oppression.

The proper masculine surface: out of reach?

While encounters between small and big boys were often dominated by issues of power and control, there was often too a releasing sense of physical pleasure on both sides. The issue of size is, as we have seen, immensely important for boys. In these ritualized encounters big boys can guard themselves, look after themselves, be in control. They cannot be caught or harmed unless they choose; they are often, literally, out of reach. In contrast, smallness, signs of wimpishness, crying, lack of strength and isolation are despised. Wimps seem to be despised above all, as polluting the male ideal, conveying qualities of softness, emotion and embodiment that are dangerously feminine. Like a girl, a soft boy is pervious to emotions: taking them in and letting them show. In contrast, a proper boy is impervious, lets emotions go by enacting them, passing them on, giving them to another.

Perhaps for this reason we might also say that for boys physical touch carries dangers of ambiguity; it risks crossing into other, emotional, territories of feeling. On the one hand touch cannot be affectionate or gentle (you may be named a poof, a pansy), on the other it must not be too aggressive, a challenge or a threat (you may get embroiled in a fight). There is only a narrow zone within which touch is allowable. Boys told us that some of the most violent fights were not the more ritualistic, planned fights, but 'flash fights', where acquaintances and friends had transgressed or misjudged the boundaries of physical distance and acceptability.

Much that has been discussed here revolves around issues of vulnerability and protection. For a boy, to be small is to be vulnerable, as is to let emotions show. Seemingly the safest place is out of reach, out of touch. Giotto portrayed Christ in this fashion, denying touch (particularly perhaps the touch of a woman) at a critical moment of transition from the profane to the sacred world. Although at one level touch is about surface, to be 'touched' is to be reached emotionally, deep in oneself. At that moment the surface of control may break down leaving you vulnerable, allowing access to what is beneath. Consider here some overlapping examples of embodied emotion-acts and words as together, natural and inculcated, they convey the everyday discursive power of 'touch':

- to 'touch', to 'touch your heart' or 'touching' as something able to reach a deep and truthful part of the self, to be moved beyond reason;
- to be 'in touch', 'out of touch', 'touchstone', 'touchdown' as indicating connection with something grounded, the baseline;
- to 'touch a nerve', to be 'touchy' as reaching a sensitive, painful or difficult aspect that is central to self;
- to be 'touched in the head' as being a little mad.

We have seen the ways in which embodied characteristics are built into boys' judgements of what is ideally male. The boy who is a 'wimp', is 'wasted', 'sad', represents not only a despised form of masculine embodiment (unlike the 'hard' boy, the 'hardnut', the 'king') but also a lack of proper masculine emotional tone. In this fashion there is a free flow of exchange between embodied characteristics and emotional metaphor. This might be understood by reference to the use of touch at both a linguistic level (emotion-words) and in bodily display (emotion-acts).

Between boys, to be acceptable and legitimate only some kinds of touch can be given and received. It is acceptable for big boys to pick up a small boy, carry him upside down and throw him in a bush, for small boys to clamber up bigger boys, or tackle them as they did at football. Touch between boys then might be seen as highly rule-bound: accidental, aggressive, rough, joking, ritualized touch, or as part of a game, is allowable, while the proper receiving masculine surface is deflecting, impenetrable. Big boys are impervious to any damaging form of touch in these encounters because they are hard, small boys must accept what is meted out because that is part of being small. Unless they are exceptionally lucky in negotiating this tricky path, the years of adolescence for boys may be about forms of polarized emotional learning that isolate them from both boys and girls. The first year of secondary school might well mark a boundary beyond which boys no longer feel able publicly to express or receive touching feelings: the last time Perky the toy monkey, with the power as if of some ancient myth, could voice the shared vulnerability of little boys.

The necessity of boys' control over proper masculine touch may also be helpful in thinking of how boys negotiate their emergent sexuality at this age, particularly in relation to encounters with girls. If proper boys are 'everything that girls are not' (Jordan 1995) it is conceivable that boys emotionally and physically engage with girls as 'other', ambiguous, potentially overwhelming, out of control. This is specially so if boys have to *demonstrate* bodily competence and separateness from women in order to belong to the world of their friends and adult males, as Hallden (1995) found in her work with Swedish boys. Seidler too (1993) has written about the relationship between fear and vulnerability for men in western culture, and the necessity to hide this fear. He suggests that this fear is about revealing yourself as less, as what men are *not* supposed to be. If this happens, men may feel rejected by both the masculine (they are not proper men) and the feminine (they are not women, nor the proper men they think women want) worlds. We may see this in the data. Andy lost control of his feelings in public. He regained his dignity by proving he was super-hard: not 'touched' by something that might usually arouse our disgust or sympathy – shit and a dead cat. The route out of revealing vulnerability was to demonstrate 'non-fear'. Here again we might speculate as to the implications and meanings of John's distress. Paradoxically, the necessity of demonstrating non-fear may indicate that 'a fear of fear' is endemic to being properly male. In letting go, did John become an object lesson for all boys, raising the terrifying possibility that hegemonic masculinity is a fragile façade, behind which one's feelings can barely be concealed and from which, therefore, any individual boy may be excluded?

Coda: doing emotion work

This chapter, in focusing upon boys' actions, what we saw and what they said, and making connections between the two, acknowledges our presence in the narratives that punctuate the text. The necessity for this acknowledgement is threefold. First, in school, we quickly realized that in looking we came to know things, long before we were able to speak about them (and find them confirmed) with boys themselves. We began to realize the power of understanding that was locked into the everyday: everyday acts of embodiment, of seeing and of knowing. Body-language is amazingly rich, conveying meanings and possibilities unimaginable in advance, impossible to encompass in any questionnaire. Second were the powerful emotions that we ourselves experienced, which came with and from this knowing, and which had to be articulated. Third, arising out of these discussions, was the alarming possibility that our presence was itself an active factor in some of the events that took place, that we might be a part of the context in which, through which and with which boys expressed themselves. All of these things happened to us and were experienced by us as female and male, arising out of our own histories, our own gendered knowledges both of self and other. Andy may have kicked the dead cat in part because he perceived the act as embodying a properly masculine contempt for feeling, in distinction to Shirley's supposedly feminine upholding of emotion. Andy therefore, in shocking Shirley, showed a contempt for women that proved him a proper boy. Similarly complex understandings may be applied to Perky telling his story to Simon. Indeed these incidents might not have happened at all had we not been present as the gendered beings that we were.

This is not to invalidate the research, but rather to suggest that maybe persons, objects, contexts, the sequence and fabric of everyday life are the medium through which emotions come into being, day to day, a kind of emotional bricolage. Popular magazines recognize that an emotion-act takes place in a setting, which is a material time and place: an evening of seduction may require privacy, comfort, certain music or clothes to be successful. As we have described elsewhere, schools provide persons, structures, settings, rules, a context where some emotional configurations may thrive while others may not. We ourselves became a part of this potentiality: interested outsiders, Simon, a large, kindly man, Shirley, a woman a little like your mother, or Shirley and Simon, a woman and a man working together. The power and spontaneity and 'fit' of our encounters in school suggest that the incidents that happened were not artificial, rather they were within boys' emotional capacity and repertoire, given form in those specific circumstances. As Lyon and Barbalet note: 'Emotion activates distinct dispositions, postures and movements which are not only attitudinal but also physical, involving ways in which individual bodies together with others articulate a common purpose, design or order' (1994: 48).

Persistent configurations, particularly embodied acts of the power and persistence that we saw in school, may become more fixed, although not necessarily permanent, constituents of self. Hochschild (1983) says in her description of *feeling rules* that 'in managing feeling we contribute to the creation of it'. The constant reiteration of masculinities as metaphors of size and hardness, together with the lived experience of practices described above, suggests ways in which embodied learning may be shaped not just for boys but for girls too. The sexes shape a world not in isolation but in intimate relation to each other as different: if girls are soft, boys are hard. This is an embodiment of the emotions. Compared with girls, boys speak hard, act hard and, to our detriment and theirs, perhaps in so doing they actually do become hard. These processes constitute a divisive and brutal form of learning to be male.

ACKNOWLEDGEMENTS

The authors would like to acknowledge the following: the help of the young people who took part in the study and the teachers and headteachers who made it possible; the financial support of the Health Promotion Research Trust in doing the study and the support of the FPA (the Family Planning Association) in giving us a place to meet in London. They would also like to acknowledge the support and assistance of Simon Cavicchia from NACTU (the National Aids Counselling and Training Unit), who contributed to the literature review and in planning the early stages of the work. Finally they would like to thank friends and colleagues for their insightful comments when versions of this chapter were given in seminar form. Three seminars were outstandingly helpful: the BSA Sociology of Emotions study group (Institute of Education, London 1995), the Lévi-Strauss Masculinities seminar (Cambridge 1995) and the symposium on Gender, Body and Love (University of Oslo, 1996).

NOTE

1 The project took place over two years, between 1993 and 1995. During that time the authors worked with young people between the ages of 12 and 15 and their teachers in four secondary schools, three of which are discussed here. The study used small-scale qualitative methods, case studies, focus groups, interviews of individuals or pairs, observation and classroom activities (about 100 young people consulted in all), alongside a questionnaire with a larger sample (about 400 questionnaires). Fully informed, advance consent was sought both from young people and from their parents. Further details of the research can be found in Prendergast and Forrest (1997).

BIBLIOGRAPHY

Askew, S. and Ross, C. (1988) *Boys Don't Cry: Boys and Sexism in Education*. Milton Keynes, Bucks: Open University Press.
Bodily, C. L. (1994) 'Ageism and the deployments of age', in T. R. Sarbin and J. I. Kituse (eds) *Constructing the Social*. London: Sage.
Bourdieu, P. (1986) 'The school as a conservative force: scholastic and cultural inequalities', in R. Dale, G. Esland and M. Macdonald (eds) *Schooling and Capitalism*. London: Routledge & Kegan Paul.
Buytendijk, F. J. (1974) *Prolegomena to an Anthropological Physiology*. Pittsburgh, PA: Duquesne University Press.
Connell, R. W. (1987) *Gender and Power*. Cambridge: Polity Press.
Connell, R. W. (1995) *Masculinities*. Cambridge: Polity Press.
Freund, P. (1988) 'Bringing society into the body: understanding socialised human nature', *Theory and Society* 17: 839–64.
Freund, P. (1990) 'The expressive body: a common ground for the sociology of emotions and health and illness', *Sociology of Health and Illness* 12(4): 452–77.
Game, A. (1986) 'Beyond gender at work: secretaries', in N. Grieve and A. Burns (eds) *Australian Women: New Feminist Perspectives*. Melbourne: Oxford University Press.
Game, A. and Pringle, R. (1983) *Gender at Work*. London: Allen & Unwin.
Gordon, S. L. (1989) 'The socialisation of children's emotions: emotional culture, competence and exposure', in C. Saarni and P. L. Harris (eds) *Children's Understanding of Emotion*. Cambridge Studies in Emotional Development. Cambridge: Cambridge University Press.
Hallden, G. (1995) 'Gender and generation: self-identity in boys' narratives', paper presented at the conference Understanding the Social World: Towards an Integrative Approach, University of Huddersfield, July 1995.
Harré, R. (1986) *Social Construction of Emotions*. Oxford: Blackwell.
Harré, R. (1991) *Physical Being*. Oxford: Blackwell.

172   *Shirley Prendergast and Simon Forrest*

Hochschild, A. (1983) *The Managed Heart: The Commercialization of Human Feeling*. Berkeley, CA: University of California Press.
Hockey, J. and James, A. (1993) *Growing Up and Growing Old: Ageing and Dependency in the Life-course*. London: Sage.
Johnson, M. (1987) *The Body in the Mind*. Chicago: University of Chicago Press.
Jordan, J. (1995) 'Fighting boys and fantasy play: the construction of masculinity in the early years of school', *Gender and Education* 7(1): 69–86.
Lakoff, G. (1987) *Women, Fire and Dangerous Things*. Chicago: University of Chicago Press.
Lawlor, J. (1991) *Behind the Screens: Nursing, Somology and the Problems of the Body*. Edinburgh: Churchill Livingstone.
Lyon, M. L. and Barbalet, J. (1994) 'Society's body: emotion and the "somatisation" of social theory', in T. J. Csordas (ed.) *The Body as Existential Ground of Culture*. Cambridge: Cambridge University Press.
Mac an Ghaill, M. (1994) *The Making of Men: Masculinities, Sexualities and Schooling*. Buckingham, Bucks: Open University Press.
Messner, M. (1987) 'The meaning of success: the athletic experience and the development of male identity', in H. Brod (ed.) *The Making of Masculinities: The New Men's Studies*. Boston, MA: Allen & Unwin.
Prendergast, S. (1994) *'This Is the Time to Grow Up': Girls' Experience of Menstruation in School*, 2nd edn. London: FPA.
Prendergast, S. (1995) 'Learning the body in the mind', in J. Holland and M. Blair (eds) *Debates and Issues in Feminist Research and Pedagogy*. Milton Keynes, Bucks: Open University Press.
Prendergast, S. and Forrest, S. (1997) 'Gendered groups and the negotiation of heterosexuality in school', in L. Segal (ed.) *New Sexual Agendas*. London: Macmillan.
Saarni, C. and Harris, P. L. (eds) (1989) *Children's Understanding of Emotion*. Cambridge Studies in Emotional Development. Cambridge: Cambridge University Press.
Sarbin, T. R. (1986) *Narrative Psychology: The Storied Nature of Human Conduct*. New York: Praeger.
Scott, S. and Morgan, D. (1993) *Body Matters: Essays on the Sociology of the Body*. London: Falmer Press.
Seidler, V. J. (1993) *Unreasonable Men: Masculinity and Social Theory*. Male Orders Series. London: Routledge.
Young, I. M. (1989) 'Throwing like a girl: a phenomenology of feminine body comportment, mobility and spatiality', in I. M. Young (ed.) *Throwing Like a Girl and Other Essays in Feminist Philosophy and Theory*. Bloomington, IN: Indiana University Press.

10 Ageing and the emotions

Mike Hepworth

INTRODUCTION: EMOTIONS, SUBJECTIVE AND SOCIAL

This chapter is about the emotions associated with old age in western culture. Its particular purpose is to review dualistic aspects of the emotions of ageing as they have emerged within the context of the 'ages' and 'stages' model of the life-course.

Given the pervasive influence of dualism over perceptions of the relationship between body, self and society in western culture (Bendelow and Williams 1995; Camille 1994; Elliot 1991; Harré 1991; Shahar 1994), it is not surprising to detect two perspectives on human emotions, the subjective (inner) and the social (outer). On the subjective level emotions are conceptualized as an integral feature of the intensely personal structure of inner meaning and as such at the heart of each individual's sense of self. Consciousness of 'I', as in the well-known observation 'I don't *feel* old', is clearly a state of subjective awareness although it also has a point of reference – 'old' – in the world external to the private self. Emotions therefore always have a 'referential content' (Scarry 1985: 5). A connection is established between subjective experience and the outside world, and the direction during the interplay between the inner and the outer worlds is signposted in terms of culturally prescribed images of the appropriate emotions associated with ageing and old age (Featherstone and Hepworth 1993; Hepworth 1993, 1995).

Subjective emotions are therefore exposed to the social world in terms of culturally determined reference points and modes of expression. To make sense to outside observers each privately experienced emotion must be communicated via a shared language or other forms of accessible non-verbal symbols (Jackson 1993). In the popular cliché 'I don't feel old', the personal emotions of ageing are compressed into a kind of social shorthand which the speaker assumes will make immediate sense to others. Similar considerations apply to the emotionality of words such as 'care' or 'caring', and one that has almost become synonymous with old age: 'burden' (Bytheway 1995; Warnes 1993). Yet for all the necessary closeness of these lines of communication, the nature of the fit between the inner emotional experiences of

a particular individual and the social cliché 'I don't feel old' is fundamentally problematic. One significant difficulty is that the phrase itself
tells us a great deal about the language commonly used in everyday life to
make meaningful references to the socially acceptable emotions of ageing
but very little about the subjective nuances of the experience. The choice
of words certainly reveals that the speaker understands what is required
from a competent social actor – the words that outsiders will understand
– but does not necessarily provide a great deal of insight into the personal
feelings of an individual about old age. An important element is therefore
missing from the equation. This dualistic quality of the emotions of
ageing results in two significant outcomes. First, limitations in the range
of social imagery available may impede the expression of subjective feelings
or, secondly, private individuals may wish to conceal their personal feelings
from public view and concentrate their energies on producing passable performances of the emotions they have come to believe to be socially acceptable. These two issues are, of course, closely interrelated.

A poignant example of the first issue occurs in Barbara Rosenblum's
reflections on her own imminent death from cancer when she asks, 'What
words and images are the best combination to represent a dying being?'
(1990: 242). The problem she is describing is the lack of fit between the existing social vocabulary of emotions and the turbulence and instability of her
personal feelings:

> my emotions change rapidly; they rise and fall, become transformed, go
> in circles and come out in squares. I go from sorrow to joy to anxiety to
> calm all in five minutes. The rapid oscillation of my interior emotional life
> does not easily yield to expression and representation.
>
> (1990: 242)

Barbara Rosenblum's struggle to describe the elusive fluidity of her actual
emotional experience and the lack of fit with a relatively static social
vocabulary is a pertinent example of what Norman Denzin has described
as 'the many faces of emotionality' (1992: 17). In her sociological account
of quite a different social situation, that of the erotic dancer, Carol
Rambo Ronai provides a neat confirmation when she writes:

> I supposedly have a self that is a whole, neatly divided up into parts or
> facets that act to fulfil the tasks of particular roles. But, in reality, each
> facet exists only because my culture demands I frame each separately
> from the others regardless of the clashes and overlaps that result from
> the demands of the roles. The self exists as a process in a constant
> state of transformation and flux; it is the dialogue between the facets.
>
> (1992: 107)

The live experience of self and emotions as fluid processes rather than a
static collection of clearly compartmentalized roles raises important questions concerning the precise nature of the specificity of any of the emotions

associated with ageing. In particular the idea of self as process requires us to look more closely into the culturally prescribed assumption that the emotions in later life are *necessarily* distinctive in some way from those experienced during other periods of life. In what sense can emotions be age-specific, and how do we know? In what ways is anger expressed at the age of 70 different from anger at 20 and what are the sources of any possible difference? Are there in fact any emotions at either subjective or social levels which can be *unambiguously* identified with old age? In a review of a BBC television programme, *Grey Sex*, where a number of older men and women described in vivid detail their continuing interest in sexuality, one critic observed:

> The problem with this programme was that what the old folk had to say about sex was not much different from what young folk or middle-aged folk would have said about it. . . . Old people have sex for the same reasons and in exactly the same way as young people.
>
> (Gill 1996: 2)

In other words, there is apparently no age-specific language for signposting the pleasures of genital sexuality. But there is persistent evidence of a tension between socially prescribed emotions of ageing and private subjective feelings. The paradox of the emotions of ageing can be located in the essential dualism of the western culture of old age: on the one hand, public prescription of feelings it is considered appropriate to display in old age, and on the other, a widespread recognition of a lack of fit between these prescriptions and subjective experience. Thus in a characteristic poem written during his own middle age, 'I look into my glass', Thomas Hardy laments the fact that the ageing of his body has not resulted in a corresponding withering of his emotions. There is the familiar lack of fit between the evidence in his mirror of his changing physical 'frame' and his painful awareness of the still youthful 'throbbings' of his heart (Hardy 1960 [1898]: 33). Both the television critic A. A. Gill and the poet Hardy are in critical opposition to the popular belief that the emotions, like the body, undergo some form of distinctive transformation as one grows older. Hardy, in common with many others who have drawn attention to the masklike nature of physical ageing (Featherstone and Hepworth 1989; Hepworth 1993), is reflecting upon the social unacceptability of the persistence of certain deeply felt emotions into later life and thus making a vital contribution to our awareness of the limitations of age stereotypes. His short poem also implies that the concealment of the subjective emotions behind a mask of physical ageing may itself become the focus of considerable emotional labour.

AGES AND STAGES

The essential cultural underpinnings of the dualistic properties of emotions in later life can be traced to the traditional western model of human ageing as a predictable progression through a number of 'stages'. In, for example, a discussion of the continuity of the tradition linking Shakespeare's 'seven ages of man' with present-day assumptions concerning the life-course, Marjorie Garber (1981) has noted the pervasive influence of an image which includes at each socially prescribed 'age' typifications of activities, physical appearance, speech forms and, we can add, emotions. But although it is widely accepted that the concept of human ageing as sequence of transitions from one stage to another provides a structure of timing, expectations, practices and institutional arrangements, there is also broad agreement concerning its essentially processual nature as lived experience. The fact that 'the stage model is still used extensively today and . . . has considerable power in structuring our lives and the way we think' (Bytheway 1995: 19) exists uneasily alongside an acknowledgement of marked individual and group variations, especially in 'modern people for whom change, movement, and variability have in and of themselves come to be a dominant motif in the very design of life' (Davis 1979: 53).

Indeed, in the late 1960s when Glaser and Strauss constructed their influential sociological model of the life-course as a series of passages from one status or 'resting place' (1971: 2) to another they also went to some lengths to emphasize that the boundaries between different statuses were by no means as unambiguous as might be expected. As they observed, passages should be conceived as dynamic processes rather than invariable structures. To be sure, there was evidence of a number of closely 'scheduled' passages in life, governed by 'fairly clear rules concerning when the change of status should be made, by whom and by whose agency', but the tendency to assume that as a general rule 'status passages were fairly regularised, scheduled and prescribed' (1971: 3) had deflected attention away from their variability. Systematic structural analysis did not therefore include the 'total truth' (1971: 7); status passages had 'multiple properties' (1971: 8), being 'in constant motion' and with 'a constant problem involving control' (1971: 73). Further indications of the experimental and creative nature of the subjective experience of passage could be found in the fact that there were many status passages 'of whose existence passagees are unaware', so that passagees are faced with the problem of discovering the meaning for themselves as they go along (1971: 83). As an example of this more open-ended process of transition they made a very brief reference to the menopause, and it is worth adding that until the emergence of a feminist-inspired literature it is certainly the case that the menopause was often described as a 'silent crisis': a source of private emotional difficulties amongst women who for the most part were denied access to a shareable public language. Significantly enough, parallel processes of cultural signposting can be observed in relation to the public recognition of the 'male menopause' (Featherstone and Hepworth 1985a, 1985b), a highly ambiguous terminology with strong emotional overtones.

There is then widespread agreement amongst sociologists of ageing that the model of the life-course as a series of neat stages is too closely framed to contain entirely the turbulent reality of living. In her study of clubs for older people in south-east England, Dorothy Jerrome has observed an 'absence of clearly defined roles and statuses in old age' and a resulting 'sense of both freedom and confusion' (1992: 5). In this ambiguous situation of freedom and uncertainty, each individual is required to negotiate the transition from middle to old age, a process she precisely describes as 'age brinkmanship' (1992: 5). Age brinkmanship inevitably implicates the emotions because it involves feelings about the appropriate effort that should be made to resist or overcome bodily discomfort in the interests of sustaining claims to a fully acceptable moral self. Each individual is faced with the task of publicly negotiating the level of physical impairment that must be endured before withdrawal from everyday social life is regarded as socially acceptable.

It is evident from this brief discussion of the tensions between subjectively experienced emotions and socially acceptable forms of emotional expression that the ages and stages model raises as many questions about as it provides answers to the problem of the emotions of ageing. In his analysis of emotional development throughout the life-course James R. Averill (1986) has recorded some of the key difficulties. Defining emotions as 'a set of interrelated reactions, instrumental responses, subjective experiences', he argues in a fashion similar to that of the sociologist Norbert Elias (1987) that the way these components are 'organised into coherent syndromes is determined primarily by social and not biological evolution'. Because emotions are essentially learned ways of responding to social situations, they are not fixed once and for all during a period of 'primary socialization' in childhood but are open to transformation as an individual grows older and accumulates a widening range of experiences. But this process of transformation is not over-determined. Whilst there is evidence that individuals internalize the social rules relating specific feelings to defined situations, the social rules as such 'tend to be open-ended, allowing a great deal of improvisation' (Averill 1986: 100). There is therefore the constant potential for variable interpretations of the personal meanings of the rules and appropriate modes of expression. In addition, the lifelong process of adult emotional development tends to be 'slow, piecemeal and cumulative; indeed, for the most part, emotional development is not even particularly emotional' (1986: 112). As an example Averill chooses anger: rules that guide judgement about anger are not themselves peculiar to anger, and words spoken in anger are not necessarily different from those which are used in quite different contexts to express quite different feelings. Immediately, of course, this prompts the question: what is therefore specific about anger in old age?

The difficulties surrounding the identification of the specific emotions of ageing are also referenced in Fred Davis's sociological analysis of nostalgia

(1979). The emotion of nostalgia (broadly defined as an extreme form of 'homesickness') is frequently associated in the popular imagination with old age. Older people are seen as more likely to be emotionally attached to the past than younger people and expected to express a range of feelings including grief and even anger over its passing. The assumption is often made, especially by younger people, that old people have a preference for talk about the past (Coupland *et al.* 1991). Yet the origins of this belief can be traced not to some generic property of old age as such but to the historically determined structuring of the life-course as a series of age-related stages. Noting that 'too little is known about the memory experiences of the elderly' (1979: 70), he asks where the images of old people as essentially nostalgic come from and questions the social functions of the image of the 'immersion of the old in nostalgia' (1979: 67).

For Davis the answer can be found in the concept of the life-cycle itself. The mistaken idea that older people are characteristically 'immersed' in the emotion of nostalgia comes conveniently to hand to endorse a pre-existing socially constructed distinction between younger and older age groups. In other words, the historical construction 'nostalgia' is cited in support of the belief in the 'otherness' of old people. Old age is different because the old, unlike the young, are nostalgic, and people are, of course, nostalgic because they are old. A similar problem has been discovered underpinning the assumption that confusion is peculiar to later life: whilst the emotional state of confusion is experienced with varying degrees of discomfort and intensity throughout the life-course we also assume it is a distinctive characteristic of old age as such (McIsaac 1996). As in the case of sexuality, an assumption is made that the emotion is a sign of essential difference – i.e. there is a close correspondence between subjective experience and social categorization: old people *are* confused. Davis, in his analysis of nostalgia, locates the social value of the concept of elderly nostalgia in the function it performs as a bridge between the 'intensely private quality of nostalgic experience' and 'its sources in society and its consequences for collective life' (1979: 52). It has, in other words, a greater value for society than it does for the individual. At the same time, the fact that the functions of nostalgia in the lives of older people are not necessarily different from those in the lives of young people does not mean that there are *no* differences between age groups. One is the obvious fact of an extended past to look back upon (although it must be noted that reminiscence research reveals a significant number of older people who have no particular investment in the past and live for the present); and another, closely related, is the comparatively short time left to live. Although it must also be noted that attitudes towards the reality of a short future also vary and younger people may well share with some members of the older generation a belief in the value of immediate pleasures on the grounds of 'one day at a time' and 'life is too short'. Short-run hedonism is not necessarily a distinctive characteristic of the old or the young.

If, as Davis argues, the attribution of distinctive emotions to ages and stages of life is a socially determined method of maintaining boundaries between groups of individuals, it becomes much easier to make sense of the tensions existing between public images and subjective experiences. One aspect of this socially generated process has been highlighted by Simone de Beauvoir in her discussion of the dualistic belief that old age 'sets the individual free from his [*sic*] body' (1977: 351). The idea that sex in old age has distinctive qualities is deeply rooted in the Christian belief in the impropriety of strong sexual feelings in old age. The oppositional moral belief that people should get wiser as they get older is sharply dismissed by de Beauvoir as 'mystical twaddle' (1977: 352). The classical example she offers is the sexless image of 'Darby and Joan':

> The purification of which the moralists speak consists for them essentially in the distinction of sexual desires: they are happy to think that the elderly man escapes from this slavery and thereby achieves serenity. In his well-known poem 'John Anderson my Jo', Burns describes the ideal old couple in whom carnal passion has died quite away. The pair have climbed the hill of life side by side and once they tasted blissful hours; now with trembling steps but still hand in hand they must go together along the road that leads to the end of the journey.
>
> (de Beauvoir 1977: 353)

As exemplified in the mask of ageing, dualistic separations of the self from the body provide a fertile breeding-ground for the cultural elaboration of distinctions between emotions that are prescribed as morally worthy in old age and those that are labelled disreputable. The result is a public dis-embodiment of the idealized aspects of old age, as the sexless image of 'Darby and Joan', perpetuated in numerous 'Darby and Joan' clubs throughout the UK, clearly testifies. In order to attract public respect it becomes necessary for older people at the very least to engage in the emotional labour required to socially activate cultural images of respectable elderly emotions. A creditable performance of the appropriate public role (Hochschild 1983) does not, as we have noted, necessarily require the complete surrender of incongruent private feelings. In this quotation taken from David Guterson's murder story *Snow Falling on Cedars* (1996), Nels Gudmundsson, aged 79, is defending counsel at the trial of the accused man. Confronting the wife of the victim he becomes acutely conscious of his age:

> Nels Gudmundsson stood at a distance from the witness stand when it was his turn to question Susan Marie Heine: he did not want to appear lecherous by placing himself in close proximity to a woman of such tragic, sensual beauty. He was self-conscious about his age and felt that the jurors would see him as disgusting if he did not distance himself from Susan Marie Heine and appear in general detached from the life of his body altogether. . . . The bad part was . . . that a woman like Susan

Marie Heine inspired a deep frustration in him. He felt defeated as he appraised her on the witness stand. It was no longer possible for him to communicate to *any* woman – even those his own age he knew in town – his merit and value as a lover, for he no longer had this sort of worth and had to admit as much to himself – as a lover he was entirely through.

(1996: 263)

If the social performance of the respectable emotions of old age requires a self-conscious distancing from subjective feelings then the older person becomes involved in the emotional labour of disembodiment. Historical evidence of the displacement of embodied emotions can, for example, be found in the persistent underground tradition of the sexual and scatological humour of old age. And it is in this subversive tradition that the strong subterranean theme of the emotions of ageing is most disturbingly in evidence. Indeed, recognition of 'dirty' humour in old age itself requires considerable emotional effort because the sexual and scatological humour of old age shares with other humour of this kind the capacity to attack, contradict, shock and disgust. Legman defines sexual humour as a kind of 'mask' beneath which 'society allows infinite aggression, by everyone and against everyone' (1972: I, 9). Sexual humour provides a revelation of concealed hostility and also functions both at a personal and a social level as a means of coping with anxiety. In sharp contrast to the asexual image of 'Darby and Joan', Legman documents an extensive collection of 'dirty jokes' which make explicit physical reference to their sexual difficulties. Far from being sexually disembodied in underground humour, Darby vociferously counters accusations of sexual impotence with vicious complaints about Joan's waning sexual charms (1972: II, 254). This is a far cry from those benign figures of classical antiquity, Philemon and Baucis, an essentially virtuous and self-effacing couple whom the gods rewarded by transforming them into an oak and a lime tree (Grant 1986).

The subversive properties of images of sexuality in later life have proved to be an invaluable medium for the artist who wishes to challenge and extend public perceptions of the emotions of ageing. One of the central concerns, for example, of the German painter Otto Dix (1891–1969) was to confront the 'taboo placed on death, old age, and decay in the sphere of sexuality, eroticism, life' (Karcher 1992: 110). A vivid example of his vision of the persistence of sexual desire into old age is found in the painting *Old Couple* (1923) where a naked old woman is seated across the knees of an old man whose lustful gaze is transfixed on the breast he is holding. In another version of the same theme a partially clothed old couple are pictured in an explicitly erotic embrace. Not surprisingly Dix's paintings were not universally welcomed by his contemporaries although his reputation now continues to grow and he is increasingly celebrated as a master of the twentieth century.

Recent public acclaim of Dix's artistry reminds us of the inherent instability of the public repertoire of the emotions of ageing and of the flexibility of the rules governing their expression. A social climate is emerging within which the display of explicit images of naked ageing bodies is no longer regarded as a sign of 'decadence' or deviation but is seen as posing a legitimate challenge to conventional attitudes. In, for example, her innovative and emotive photographs of the naked ageing body, Jo Spence expanded public awareness of the possibility of alternative roles to those traditionally prescribed for women (Spence 1995). If, until recent times, embarrassment over the ageing body (clothed or naked) has been seen as one of the more enduring negative emotions associated with later life, there are also clear signs that such feelings are subject to historical variation within western culture and are not fixed in tablets of stone.

Another interesting example of cultural flexibility can be found in changes in the public response to images of *caritas romana* ('Roman charity') in European art. According to this legend, a dutiful daughter visits her ageing father who is a chained prisoner in a deep dungeon. Because he is unable to feed himself, she preserves his life with milk from her own breasts. This story, as Robert Rosenblum (1972) shows, is open to a number of historical interpretations. Originally, on the walls of Pompeii, the story was seen to exemplify 'rare filial virtue' (1972: 43) and this reading persisted through the Middle Ages and up to the seventeenth century; the emotional connotations then began to expand and eventually included 'everything from the sacrificial heroism of the French Revolution to the exploratory sexuality of the Marquis de Sade' (1972: 43). Rosenblum observes that as western psychology becomes more complex so the emotional range of the theme is enlarged to include themes of intimacy and eroticism as, for example, in J. J. Bachelier's *Roman Charity*, shown in the salon of 1765. Bachelier, who was an animal painter,

> invests the father and daughter with an aura of intimacy and eroticism that can almost be confounded with the incestuous theme of Lot and his daughters, so popular in the Rococo period. In Bachelier's painting, the brawny old man, his shackled hands raised almost in prayer, seems to be receiving, as if in a saintly vision, an erotic angel of mercy in the form of a blonde Rococo maiden, his very daughter, who relieves his supine desperation with the succour of her full breasts.

> (1972: 440)

A much more recent literary version occurs in L. P. Hartley's short story 'Roman charity' (1972). Hartley's extra twist to the interpretation of an intergenerational relationship, published interestingly enough when he was aged 72, is described as follows by his biographer, Adrian Wright (1996). When Rudy Campion is imprisoned as a spy he is deserted by his wife and daughter. But subsequently he receives a visit from his daughter who offers him 'Roman charity'. Eventually she helps him to escape and takes him to her home where she offers him a drink from her extensive collection of alcoholic refreshments. His choice is a final drink from her breast. Wright comments on the complexity of the theme:

> It would be simple to dismiss 'Roman Charity' as about the potency of incestuous love; as it happens, the daughter's offer of her milk has as much malevolence as lust . . . there is a design in her bounty that is not made clear. Is her father drinking a mother's milk, or tasting gall? The savagery of that final offer, 'another sort of cocktail', is dreadful. Physical repulsion and attraction are married in a story that is at once unsavoury, repugnant and dimly understood. But it gave Hartley, apparently, no doubts.
>
> (1996: 260)

CREATIVE TENSIONS

Evidence of historical transformations in cultural readings of intergenerational intimacy brings us back to the troubled question of the specificity of the emotions of ageing. In particular it opens up the issue, central to ageing, of the continuously changing nature of the relationship between the body and the self, and the bodies and selves of others. A fundamental assumption in the sociology of the body is 'that physical experience is inseparable from its cognitive and emotional significance' (Bendelow and Williams 1995: 89). 'Emotions', Bendelow and Williams argue, 'like pain, lie at the juncture between mind and body, culture and biology' (1995: 90). And it is often in imaginative fiction that we can discover moving perceptions of this subtle interrelationship. Marian Thurm's novel about the May–December marriage of Henry, aged 69, to Kate, aged 28, is an example of the reconciliation that can emerge out of the progressive physical dependence of one member of the family on another. Henry develops an unidentified wasting disease and it robs him of his power of independent movement and the ability to speak distinctly. But his mind is left unclouded and the effects of physical disability on his relationships are portrayed with a mixture of sympathetic irony and humour. The following passage describes Henry in his bath. He is being looked after by Day, a younger man:

> Henry sits in the bathtub wiggling his toes, obviously enjoying himself. 'You know you're okay if you can still wiggle your toes,' he tells Day. 'When that goes, along with the ability to get it up, you know you're *really* in trouble.' The things Henry tells him! The things they tell each other! This intimacy came quick and easy, fostered by the very nature of what Day does for him; his hands so often against the flesh and bone of Henry's failing body. There's something about giving another human being a bath, Day thinks, that relaxes the barriers between people and encourages them to give away all sorts of secrets. It was during the course of one of the first baths he gave Henry, several

months ago, that Day found himself revealing to him that he was bi-
sexual. Henry did not seem at all surprised or alarmed, did not shrug
off Day's hand or stiffen at his touch. He simply nodded, saying 'Good
for you,' when Day told him he'd tested negative for AIDS antibodies
and intended to keep it that way.

(1990: 107)

It is clear that processes of interaction between the body, self and
society do not come in tidy age-specific packages. The very quality of
multi-dimensionality that Averill (1986) has observed is also evident in the
fictional exchange of confidences between Henry and Day. The experience
of 'becoming old' is not unidirectional, nor distinctive of people who are
old but intergenerational and reflexive: the individual moves, as Barbara
Rosenblum testified, through a spectrum of emotions in which the past,
present and future are in essentially unstable combination. The ageing of
the human body as 'the physical referent of . . . selfhood' (Cohen 1994:
66) is, of course, itself evidence of the inevitability of biological change
but its role in the ageing process is not overdetermined and it is possible
for individuals to dissociate themselves from their bodies and to experience,
at least momentarily, in a disembodied self a kind of dualistic liberation
(Bendelow and Williams 1995; Scarry 1985).

The model, moreover, of life as a fluid non-unilinear 'course' rather than a
'cycle' with fixed generically predetermined stages (Hazan 1988) creates the
space critically to oppose the emotions stereotypically associated with
ageing – typically, pessimism (Bailey 1988) and 'gerontophobia' (Freedman
1978) – with more positive feelings towards later life. In her cultural analysis
of ageing in the United States 1910–35, Margaret Morganroth Gullette
challenges the 'constructed fear of ageing' (1993: 28) inherited 'from the
writings of eminent literary figures such as Oscar Wilde' (*The Picture of
Dorian Gray*, 1891) and Thomas Mann (*Death in Venice*, trans. 1911), and
a host of popular novels supporting the 'tendency to think of ageing-into-
the-midlife as a traverse to loss, disaster, or possibly death' (1993: 27). In
this gloomy scenario, created largely, she argues, out of masculine aversions
to physical ageing, a 'developmental schema' (1993: 31) emerged in which
the emotions designated appropriate to midlife are shame, pain, sorrow
and grief. But there is also evidence in this complex and ambiguous process
of positive 'women's emotions of struggle and achievement' (1993: 46).
Subjective experience, in other words, belied social expectations and was
creatively translated by some brave spirits – especially women in this reading – into public expressions of an alternative range of feelings. The mask of
ageing could, in other words, be cast aside. Midlife can thus be regarded not
as a determined stage with invariable states of feeling deriving principally
from the belief in ageing as an inevitably downward motion, but as a
living process of critical engagement with the past, the present and the
future. If we can think of this creative process in terms of the stories we

tell each other about the body and the self growing older, and if we accept the existence of a reflexive tension between the subjective and the social, it follows that we can look to imaginative literature to enhance our under-standing of the contradictions that characterize these perceptions. During recent years a number of scholars in the new field of 'literary gerontology' have made a significant contribution to the analysis of the role of the crea-tive imagination in making sense of the ageing process. Janice Sokoloff (1987) has drawn our attention to the contribution comparative studies of ageing in fiction can make when she warns that the 'paradigms created by psychologists such as Erik Erikson and Daniel Levinson can become mis-leading when they suggest neat, linear stages of growth in a human life-course' (1987: 129). In a similar vein, Anne Wyatt-Brown has urged the importance of understanding the 'entire life' (1989: 55) of the artist if we are to understand the specific qualities of the literary work of an aged artist. There is a need to cultivate 'tolerance of the ambiguous nature of human life rather than insisting on the simple but distorting categories for which human nature longs' (1989: 56). In its concern with the ambiguous struggle to maintain the self, literary gerontology is ideally placed to address the question of the specificity of the emotions of ageing with which this chap-ter began. Anne Wyatt-Brown shows, for example, that distinctive emotional problems in later life may act as a spur to literary creativity, itself seen as an act of self-discovery. For writers like Anita Brookner, Penelope Mortimer and Barbara Pym

> [i]t seems apparent that for the first time they no longer needed to define who they were; instead they longed to reconcile themselves with their fates. Having abandoned any hope of experiencing a miraculous sea-change, their fiction, as well as their diaries, letters and literary journals, reveals that they were seeking some kind of permission to continue to be the person that they had become in the course of their lives. Luckily they discovered that constructing their narrative gave them some hope for the future and some modicum of the wisdom that Erik Erikson says can be possible in old age.
>
> (1989: 61)

From the perspective of literary gerontology, ageing into old age implies a form of movement which some analysts have described as a 'transformation' (Chinen 1987: 119). In his study of fairy stories where the protagonists are not children but adults in midlife, Chinen has detected the presence of 'a single theme – that of *transformation*'. This process is at once an emo-tional, cognitive and social transformation through which 'Traditional mas-culine and feminine roles are changed into new, more integrated ways of life, and the innocent, optimistic worldview of youth must be enlarged to include the darker side of the human heart' (1987: 119). The darker side of the human heart includes an appreciation of 'the humour of mankind's absurd situation' together with an awareness of 'the darkness and tragedy of the human condition'. The functions of fairy tales of midlife or 'middle tales' include an education of the emotions (1987: 125).

Chinen's literary evidence of the complexity of the emotions of ageing comes as a sharp reminder that it is a mistake to regard all the emotions associated with ageing as distinctively harmonious. Indeed, some (perhaps even all) of the emotional problems of later life have their origins in the unresolved conflicts of much earlier life (Rowe 1994); the phrase 'unfinished business' is, after all, a familiar feature of the contemporary social repertoire of ageing. And literary gerontology also extends the vision of emotional conflict in later life to include emotions which are not, in conventional social stereotypes, regarded as morally acceptable.

Some writers, like Henri de Montherlant, live long enough to make a distinctive contribution to what Josephine V. Arnold, writing on the problem of the ageing pederast, describes as 'literature of the life cycle' (1993: 187). De Montherlant, whom we now know to have been a lifelong pederast, 'ended his own life when age and infirmity made it increasingly difficult to cruise the streets of Paris'. 'For him a life without the love of boys was inconceivable and unendurable' and he was only able to perceive old age as a 'cruel joke' (1993: 190). In Arnold's interpretation the pederast who has a fixation on prepubertal boys must ceaselessly search for new loves because the period immediately preceding puberty is so fleeting. She argues that Montherlant's tragedy was that, unlike his body, the object of his desire never aged. There was a conflict between his physical ageing and the agelessness of his desire which he was unable to resolve. He could not, as in the asexual version of Darby and Joan, age alongside a loved one, or, like the legendary Philemon and Baucis, become transfixed for ever in a pastoral idyll. Nor could he be subjectively reconciled with the respectable mask of ageing that he felt forced to wear.

The increase in life expectancy inevitably means that, like the rest of us, imaginative writers tend to live longer. The literary output of Kingsley Amis who continued writing into old age, and about old age, provides a fascinating example of the complex interaction (although he strenuously denied it) between fiction and life (Jacobs 1995). Literary reflection on ageing into old age is, of course, as old as written culture (Cole and Winkler 1994) but there are contemporary signs of an increasing concern to explore the emotional dynamics of ageing and to enlarge the repertoire of public expressions. When authors of fiction write about the emotions of ageing their personal experiences and creative styles lead them to focus on different aspects of these emotions and it follows that their work is likely to provide us with evidence of the wide range of emotions it is possible to experience in later life. Wyatt-Brown observes that the literary output of Barbara Pym, a person with very conventional social attitudes who was schooled to exercise considerable self-control over her emotions, reflects aspects of her particular personal experience of life's transitions:

Growing older added yet another dimension to Pym's work. Her literary career had been problematical from the start. After Oxford, she returned to her parents for eight years while she attempted to convert her fantasies and hurt feelings into novels. During that troubled time, she often longed to grow old quickly, because she assumed that the elderly were no longer afflicted by their passions. The experience of ageing turned out to be far more trying than she had imagined. Not only were her romantic dreams repeatedly shattered, but her professional life unexpectedly disintegrated. . . . In fact, her illnesses gave her badly needed new insights that eventually revitalised her moribund career. *Quartet in Autumn*, the novel she wrote about the difficulties of ageing, is her masterpiece. It won her an enormous audience both in England and the United States.

(1992: 6)

In his discussion of the age-related emotion of nostalgia the sociologist Fred Davis chose to emphasize the distinction between the social functions of boundaries and their variable subjective meanings. Boundaries, such as those between the ages and stages of life, are socially constructed in order to create and sustain distinctions between social categories. The age-categorization of emotions tells us much more about ageing as collective imagery than it does about the complex subjective experience of growing older, but enough has also been said in the ensuing discussion to show that this does not mean that the boundaries are inflexible, both diachronically and in terms of everyday social interaction. And it is our awareness of this flexibility which makes the emotions of ageing problematic. When in the mid-1980s the historian Steve Humphries talked to sixty old age pensioners about their experiences of sex before marriage during the first half of the present century, he was careful to draw special attention to the emotional quality of the interviews themselves: 'the most moving I have ever done'. They often started awkwardly:

there would be an atmosphere of tension and embarrassment, spiked with difficult silences. But after fifteen or twenty minutes the talk would generally flow much more freely. Long-ago hurts would come back, lost loves were remembered, the joys and injustices of the past were relived, often with laughter, less often with tears. The overwhelming emotion which was conveyed, however, was one of pain, suggesting a violence that was done to young minds and bodies.

(1988: 13)

To return to our original question: in what sense are these emotions distinctive of ageing? The feelings so poignantly recalled by these old men and women have their point of reference in the past: the experiences of 'young minds and bodies'. They are not distinctive of old age as such (that is, the present) but of identifiable historical experiences of sexual repression which, Humphries argues, are now alien to present younger generations.

Nor are they obviously inscribed on the visible bodies of these people: in fact, they were often deeply concealed and in some cases had never been revealed to intimate family relations. Unquestionably they are an integral feature of the deepest emotional sense of self, reminding us yet again of the essential ambiguity of human ageing.

BIBLIOGRAPHY

Arnold, J. V. (1993) 'Montherlant and the problem of the ageing pederast', in A. M. Wyatt-Brown and J. Rossen (eds) *Ageing and Gender in Literature: Studies in Creativity.* Charlottesville, VA, and London: University Press of Virginia.

Averill, J. R. (1986) 'The acquisition of emotions during adulthood', in R. Harré (ed.) *The Social Construction of Emotions.* Oxford and New York: Blackwell.

Bailey, J. (1988) *Pessimism.* London and New York: Routledge.

Bendelow, G. and Williams, S. J. (1995) 'Pain and the mind–body dualism: a sociological approach', *Body and Society* 1(2): 83–103.

Bytheway, B. (1995) *Ageism.* Buckingham and Philadelphia, PA: Open University Press.

Camille, M. (1994) 'The image and the self: unwriting late medieval bodies', in S. Kay and M. Rubin (eds) *Framing Medieval Bodies.* Manchester and New York: Manchester University Press.

Chinen, A. B. (1987) 'Middle tales: fairy tales and transpersonal development at midlife', *Journal of Transpersonal Psychology* 19(2): 99–132.

Cohen, A. P. (1994) *Self Consciousness: An Alternative Anthropology of Identity.* London and New York: Routledge.

Cole, T. R. and Winkler, M. G. (eds) (1994) *The Oxford Book of Ageing: Reflections on the Journey of Life.* Oxford and New York: Oxford University Press.

Coupland, N., Coupland, J. and Giles, H. (1991) *Language, Society and the Elderly: Discourse, Identity and Ageing.* Oxford, UK, and Cambridge, MA: Blackwell.

Davis, F. (1979) *Yearning for Yesterday.* New York: Free Press.

de Beauvoir, S. (1977) *Old Age.* Harmondsworth, Mx: Penguin.

Denzin, N. (1992) 'The many faces of emotionality: reading "Persona"', in C. Ellis and M. G. Flaherty (eds) *Investigating Subjectivity: Research on Lived Experience.* London: Sage.

Elias, N. (1987) 'On human beings and their emotions: a process-sociological essay', *Theory, Culture and Society* 4(2–3): 339–61.

Elliot, D. (1991) 'Dress as mediator between inner and outer self: the pious matron of the high and later middle ages', *Mediaeval Studies* 53: 279–308.

Featherstone, M. and Hepworth, M. (1985a) 'The male menopause: lifestyle and sexuality', *Maturitas* 7: 235–46.

Featherstone, M. and Hepworth, M. (1985b) 'The history of the male menopause 1848–1936', *Maturitas* 7: 249–57.

Featherstone, M. and Hepworth, M. (1989) 'Ageing and old age: reflections on the postmodern life-course', in T. Keil, P. Allat and A. Bryman (eds) *Becoming and Being Old: Sociological Approaches to Later Life.* London: Sage.

Featherstone, M. and Hepworth, M. (1993) 'Images of ageing', in J. Bond, P. Coleman and S. Peace (eds) *Ageing in Society: An Introduction to Social Gerontology*, 2nd edn. London: Sage.

Freedman, R. (1978) 'Sufficiently decayed: gerontophobia in English literature', in S. F. Spicker, K. M. Woodward and D. D. Van Tassel (eds) *Humanistic Perspectives in Gerontology.* Atlantic Highlands, NJ: Humanities Press.

Garber, M. (1981) *Coming of Age in Shakespeare.* London and New York: Methuen.

Gill, A. A. (1996) 'The old grey missile test', *Sunday Times* 11 August: 2–3.

Glaser, B. G. and Strauss, A. L. (1971) *Status Passage*. London: Routledge & Kegan Paul.

Grant, M. (1986) *Myths of the Greeks and Romans*. New York: Mentor.

Gubrium, J. F. (1995) 'Individual agency, the ordinary and postmodern life', inaugural lecture, the Open University Centre for Ageing and Biographical Studies, Milton Keynes: the Open University, School of Health and Social Welfare.

Gullette, M. M. (1993) 'Creativity, ageing, gender: a study of their intersections, 1910–1935', in A. M. Wyatt-Brown and J. Rossen (eds) *Ageing and Gender in Literature: Studies in Creativity*. Charlottesville, VA, and London: University Press of Virginia.

Guterson, D. (1996 [1995]) *Snow Falling on Cedars*. London: Bloomsbury.

Hardy, T. (1960 [1898]) 'I look into my glass', in W. E. Williams (ed.) *Thomas Hardy*. Harmondsworth, Mx: Penguin.

Harré, R. (1991) *Physical Being: A Theory for a Corporeal Psychology*. Oxford, UK, and Cambridge, MA: Blackwell.

Hazan, H. (1988) '"Course" versus "cycle": on the understanding of ageing', *Journal of Ageing Studies* 2(1): 1–11.

Hepworth, M. (1991) 'Positive ageing and the mask of age', *Journal of Educational Gerontology* 6(2): 93–101.

Hepworth, M. (1993) 'Ageing and the emotions', *Journal of Educational Gerontology* 8(2): 75–85.

Hepworth, M. (1995) 'Images of old age', in J. F. Nussbaum and J. Coupland (eds) *Handbook of Communication and Ageing Research*. Mahwah, NJ, and Hove, Sx: Lawrence Erlbaum Associates.

Hochschild, A. R. (1983) *The Managed Heart: The Commercialization of Human Feelings*. Berkeley/Los Angeles, CA, and London: University of California Press.

Humphries, S. (1988) *A Secret World of Sex, Forbidden Fruit: The British Experience 1900–1950*. London: Sidgwick & Jackson.

Jackson, S. (1993) 'Even sociologists fall in love: an exploration in the sociology of emotions', *Sociology* 27(2): 201–20.

Jacobs, E. (1995) *Kingsley Amis: A Biography*. London: Sceptre.

Jerrome, D. (1992) *Good Company: An Anthropological Study of Old People in Groups*. Edinburgh: Edinburgh University Press.

Karcher, E. (1992) *Otto Dix*. Cologne: Benedikt Taschen.

Legman, G. (1972) *Rationale of the Dirty Joke*, Vols 1 and 2. London: Panther.

McIsaac, S. (1996) 'Communicating with the "confused": educational implications of the interactionist perspective', *Education and Ageing* 11(1): 44–58.

Rambo Ronai, C. (1992) 'The reflexive self through narrative: a night in the life of an exotic dancer', in C. Ellis and M. G. Flaharty (eds) *Investigating Subjectivity: Research on Lived Experience*. London: Sage.

Rosenblum, B. (1990) 'I have begun the process of dying', in J. Spence and P. Holland (eds) *Family Snaps: The Meaning of Domestic Photography*. London: Virago.

Rosenblum, R. (1972) 'Caritas romana after 1760: some romantic lactations', in T. B. Hess and L. Nochlin (eds) *Woman as Sex Object: Studies in Erotic Art, 1730–1970*. London: Allen Lane.

Rowe, D. (1994) *Time on Our Side: Growing in Wisdom, Not Growing Old*. London: HarperCollins.

Scarry, E. (1985) *The Body in Pain: The Making and Unmaking of the World*. New York and Oxford: Oxford University Press.

Shahar, S. (1994) 'The old body in medieval culture', in S. Kay and M. Rubin (eds) *Framing Medieval Bodies*. Manchester and New York: Manchester University Press.

Sokoloff, J. (1987) *The Margin That Remains: A Study of Ageing in Literature*. New York: Peter Lang.

Spence, J. (1995) *Cultural Sniping: The Art of Transgression*. London and New York: Routledge.

Thurm, M. (1990) *Henry in Love*. London: Bantam.

Warnes, A. M. (1993) 'Being old, old people and the burdens of burden', *Ageing and Society* 13: 297–338.

Wright, A. (1996) *Foreign Country: The Life of L. P. Hartley*, London: André Deutsch.

Wyatt-Brown, A. M. (1989) 'The narrative imperative: fiction and the ageing writer', *Journal of Ageing Studies* 31: 55–65.

Wyatt-Brown, A. M. (1992) *Barbara Pym: A Critical Biography*. Columbia, MO, and London: University of Missouri Press.

Wyatt-Brown, A. M. and Rossen, J. (eds) *Ageing and Gender in Literature: Studies in Creativity*. Charlottesville, VA, and London: University Press of Virginia.

Part IV

Sexuality, intimacy and personal relations

11 Masculinity, violence and emotional life

Victor Jeleniewski Seidler

INTRODUCTION

If men are working with violent and abusive fellow men in the projects that have developed to work with masculine violence, largely as a response to the women's movement, they are centrally concerned with changing men's behaviour and giving protection to women and children. It was feminism, particularly radical feminism, which challenged traditional forms of social theory to make male violence a central concern in the analysis of the workings of patriarchal societies. Functionalist theories that had dominated social theory in the 1950s and 1960s failed to appreciate the importance of violence in sustaining male dominance and women's subordination and oppression. Sexuality was deemed to be a matter of private life and individual choice. It was subjective and personal and so was marginalized within classical forms of social theory that could recognize oppression and injustice as 'real' only when they took place within the public realm of politics. This was true in different ways of Marx, Weber and Durkheim.

Feminism served to challenge an Enlightenment vision of modernity and the dominant rationalist forms of social theory. It insisted on challenging the prevailing distinctions between public and private, personal and political, to show that women's oppression was no less 'real' when women were marginalized and excluded from the public realm. It maintained that power was exercised not only in the public realm of politics but equally in the private realm of sexuality and relationships. It challenged the dominant forms of social theory to rethink the gendered nature of power and its links with sexuality and violence. In questioning the terms of modernity it was crucial to question the relationship between a dominant, white, Christian, heterosexual masculinity and a notion of reason, radically separated from nature. It was a dominant masculinity which could alone take its reason for granted, and as I have argued in *Unreasonable Men: Masculinity and Social Theory* (1994) it was through a disembodied Cartesian conception of reason that the social world was to be known. So it was that a dominant reason was to generate knowledge which was impartial, objective and universal. This was to secure the scientific status for our knowledge of the social world.

A dominant conception of masculinity was able to refigure what it meant to be 'human' within an Enlightenment framework. Within modernity it is a dominant masculinity which can alone take its 'humanity' for granted. For to be human is to be rational and reason comes to be defined as an independent and autonomous faculty which is set *against* our 'animal' natures. It is the categorical split between reason and nature which establishes the terms of modernity. It is a 'fragmentation' that has already been structured into the Cartesian self. So it is that 'identities' are already set within masculinist terms, for it is a matter of a mind that is already separated from bodies that are deemed to be part of a disenchanted nature, as Max Weber has it, and thoughts that are radically separated from emotions. Thoughts are placed in the mind while emotions are separated off and located spatially in the body. Since a dominant masculinity can alone take its reason for granted, it is women, Jews, people of colour, who are all conceived to be 'closer to nature'. They cannot take their humanity for granted but constantly have to prove their reason and rationality.

This helps to construct a dominant white heterosexual masculinity. At some level it means that identities are already gendered and racialized. For the notion of the European self is already constructed in opposition to nature, to animality and the 'uncivilized'. Modernity is set within European terms and appropriates the notion of civilization as an exclusive possession of the west. It is Europe that can claim science, reason and progress as its own. Thereby it sets the terms by which 'others' have to prove themselves. They have to prove that they have been able to resist the temptations of their 'animal' natures. In Kant's terms they have to prove that they are moral beings through being able to 'rise above' their animal natures. Morality is being refigured as a matter of reason alone. In this context it is a dominant masculinity which can assume a moral superiority, for men can alone act out of a sense of duty and obligation. Men can legislate what is good for others, for they can know what is right for others better than 'others' can know for themselves. In contrast women, Jews, people of colour and children are all deemed to be influenced by their instinctual natures.

MASCULINITY AND CONTROL

A dominant masculinity is tied to a particular notion of control. For it is a matter of mind over matter and so of proving masculinity through proving self-control. For within modernity masculinity can never be taken for granted but always has to be proved. At any moment I have to be ready to 'take someone out' to prove my male identity. This control is built around the automatic suppression of emotions, feelings and desires, which are collectively defined as 'inclinations' for Kant. This involves a form of self-regulation and self-discipline that Foucault was exploring in his later work which recognized the self as an ethical category. At some level it involves a relationship of violence, for we have to silence the impulses of our natures which are deemed to be a threat to our identities as rational selves. Rather, a dominant masculinity teaches men to identify with their reason and to assume that they can control their lives through reason alone. We learn to fear the revelations of our natures, for they serve to threaten male identities. This is a form of control as domination.

So there is a fear that as men we are not 'man enough' and a sense that men have to be constantly prepared to prove their male identities. As men learn to explore dominant white heterosexual masculinities they can recognize the need for control. Often men need to be in control of themselves but also in control of others. For as men they should know best, or at least think that they should 'know best' because a dominant reason separated from nature is supposedly an exclusive male possession. This creates a fear of emotions which come to be identified with the 'feminine' and are often treated as a sign of weakness. So within a rationalist tradition, men would often choose to live without emotions at all, treating them as 'distractions' that take them away from the path of reason. It is acceptable for women to be emotional, for this only confirms their weakness, and shows that they need men to be independent and self-sufficient, rocks that can be relied upon.

Within modernity, men are defined as independent and self-sufficient. It is 'others' who have emotional needs, but men often learn that they have to be able to deal with themselves on their own. It is a sign of weakness to ask for help or to need support. Again there are important differences of class, 'race' and ethnicity that need to be taken into account. But there is a dominant white masculinity that sets the terms which women also grow up to conform to. It is important *not* to argue that men are rational whilst women are deemed to be emotional. This is a simplistic notion which fails to come to terms with the power of a dominant white heterosexual masculinity within modernity. An Enlightenment vision of modernity was shaped around a secularized Protestantism and the disdain that it inherited for the body and emotional life. The body is linked to sexuality and so with an 'animal' nature. The body as part of a disenchanted nature becomes an object of medical science. So it becomes difficult to 'listen to our bodies' because the body is not part of our identities as rational selves.

Emotions came to be separated from thoughts and so from the mind, to be separated out and situated in a disenchanted body. In Kant's terms, so influential in the thinking of Durkheim and Weber, emotions are subjective and they are forms of unfreedom and determination. To allow ourselves to be influenced by our anger is to allow our behaviour to be determined by an 'external' force. It is to prove that we are not 'in control' of ourselves. So it is that men and women in different ways learn to curb and control their emotions, which cannot be acknowledged as forms of knowledge. This was part of Freud's challenge. He goes some way to reinstating emotions and feelings as sources of knowledge. He wants to heal the split between emotions and thoughts, recognizing how this serves to impersonalize people's experience, so undermining their sense of reality. But this is difficult for Freud to achieve, wedded as he is to a tradition of scientific rationalism that finds it hard to reinstate the body in its relationship with emotions as a source of meaning and value.

MASCULINITY AND VIOLENCE

We often think of violence as the breakdown of reasonable behaviour. But it might be when we think of the relationship of a dominant masculinity to violence that we also have to think of how violence is linked to control. Within modernity men could take their control for granted, for they were to be the source of authority within relationships and the family. Often men needed to be in control as a way of affirming their male identities. They expected to be respected by their partners and children not so much for what they did but for the positions they held. But feminism challenged the terms of these relationships and threatened men in their very sense of male identity. In traditional working-class families, women were supposed to know their place; a man thought little about giving his wife a 'backhander' to keep her where she 'belonged'. If women were supposed to be emotional then it was assumed that they could not be reasoned with. This is what legitimated the physical violence, though it was not named as such. It was a man's duty and responsibility to keep his wife in her place. This is what she supposedly expected from him.

In the middle-class family there was also domestic violence but this was often hidden. There was a code that people would not go outside the family to seek support but that women would have to put up with what was going on so as not to bring shame or disgrace on the family. Often men felt their control was threatened when their partners talked about their relationships with their friends. This was supposed to be a 'private' matter and it should not be discussed outside the four walls of the family house. The way that feminism helped women to seek emotional support from each other in consciousness-raising groups was often deeply threatening to men. They felt that their partners were 'talking behind their backs' and they resented it. Often it was difficult to accept the autonomy and independence of women, for this threatened the control that men had assumed to be their own. Sometimes men would withdraw into a sullen silence but at other times there would be violence at what was deemed to be 'unreasonable behaviour'. If the woman had anything to say she could say it to him. Men thought they were being reasonable in making this offer, not wanting to recognize the power they were exerting in the relationships.

With feminism women were no longer so prepared to put up with their subordinate positions. They expected men to share more in domestic work and childcare and to be more equal as partners. There was a widespread challenge to the double standards that had operated in different social classes. But as women refused their traditional subordination men were challenged in their masculinities. Often it was women who in the 1980s were initiating divorce. There was a growing awareness of the levels of sexual harassment at work and domestic violence in the home. Women were no longer so prepared to stay in relationships if they felt that they were getting very little from them for themselves. Within the new politics of gender relationships there was a different kind of negotiation: women felt that if their claims were not met by changes in men's behaviour, they would make lives for themselves. This was very threatening to men who had often grown up to think that their relationship, once established, could be taken for granted as the background against which they went on to live their individual lives.

As regards male identities it is the public world, particularly the arena of work, that matters, for this is where masculinities are affirmed and sustained. So it is that men often take their relationships for granted, never having learnt that to sustain them takes time and effort. Traditionally, as Baker-Miller (1986) explored, it was women who were relied up to do the emotional work to keep the relationship going. Often men disdained this kind of work while relying upon it. They were often dependent upon their partners to interpret what was going on for themselves emotionally. They often also relied upon their partners to sustain their social relationships. This was part of a gendered division of labour. But often it meant that men did not appreciate the emotional labour that their partners did for them. Often wives felt they were taken for granted, as if they had become part 'of the wallpaper', and in time they resented this.

But men often grow up to think that it is only necessary to give time and attention to a relationship when it is breaking down or when there is some 'problem'. Since they think of themselves as independent and self-sufficient, it can be difficult for them to recognize the emotional needs their partners have. Rather than listen to what they have to say men often assume that it is their task to provide 'solutions', since often this reflects the ways that men learn to deal with their own emotional lives. Men can feel that women are being *irrational* and *ungrateful* in refusing the help they are willing to give. It can be difficult for them to recognize that their partners want something different, sometimes just the chance to be listened to without offering solutions. So it is that men and women can be talking across each other, since they have often learnt to relate to language in different ways. But when it is men's power and control that is being challenged men often resort to an emotional withholding, refusing to share more of what is going on for them until the woman 'sees reason', or else responding violently. Sometimes this reflects a frustration that men are not used to, for they are often so used to getting their way in situations. When their traditional ways of relating do not work men can feel silently desperate and violence can soon follow.

Sometimes men feel regret and remorse after their violence, for this lack of self-control also reflects on their masculinity. It is more likely for men to want to present this in Kantian terms as an episode, as a matter of being taken over for a brief period by force beyond their control. Men can resist acknowledging this anger as 'part of' who they are. Rather they will treat these emotions as external forces which do not reflect upon their status as rational selves. It will be an episode that men often want to excuse themselves for. They might apologize to their partner and promise that it will never happen again. It was a 'moment of weakness' and they will guarantee to sustain more self-control next time. Often things do not turn out this way and the violence can become habitual in the relationship. But men might still refuse to take responsibility for what is happening. They will want to feel that they can handle the situation themselves and they will resist seeking help, for this is a further sign of weakness.

As issues of men's violence towards women became a central concern in the 1970s and 1980s, it was recognized how silent are traditional forms of social theory. Feminisms were helping to rethink the relation between power and emotion, sexuality and violence. There were projects and refuges that were concerned to support women and children as well as the beginning of projects that were concerned to work with violent and abusive men. Women and men who are engaged in working with the everyday realities of sexual abuse, harassment and violence towards women find it understandable when masculinity is defined exclusively as a relationship of power and dominance. It was important to recognize that sexuality cannot be separated from power and that a situation of rape and sexual violence is an issue not of sex but of male power, control and dominance. This could make it difficult to think of masculinity as anything other than a relationship of power. It could not be imagined as also part of the solution.

MEN, SEXUALITY AND POWER

It is crucial to be made aware of the abiding links between sexuality and power and it is important to be able to analyse the workings of power in their diverse ramifications. As we have learnt to recognize that sexuality is never innocent, so it can be misleading to think that sexuality can be reduced to power or that sexuality is always and exclusively an expression of power. If we are to be able to recognize contact, love and intimacy we need to be able to hold this in tension with relations of power. We know how easily declarations of love can operate as forms of control within intimate relationships, as if the declaration is itself supposed to make the issues and conflicts disappear. Love can operate as a form of control. The words can be hollow and empty because they have become a ritualized response. Rather it helps to open up issues about men's particular relationship to language and emotional life.

Working with violent and abusive men can make people aware of how easy it seems to be for men to deny their responsibility for what they do to their partners. This denial is so common that it can seem crucial to centre an analysis of male violence on confronting men with their responsibilities for what they have done. It is argued that men have to be made aware of the consequences of their actions, consequences they so readily deny. So it can seem that there is little point in progressing unless men are made fully aware of the harm and damage that they have done to their partners. But again it is not enough to secure a ritual acknowledgement; there have to be genuine feelings of remorse. It can be difficult to know whether this has been achieved, especially as men are often so out of touch with their emotional lives. It is easy for them to say what they think the counsellor wants to hear. This opens up important questions about how we understand it to be possible for men to change. In many ways the question of how we relate to the emotional lives of men separates out different analyses that have been provided for men and masculinities.

When we think about men and masculinities in the exclusive context of men's violence it can be difficult to explain why most men are not violent most of the time. As we focus upon the important issues of violence it is tempting to think of masculinities in their diverse forms as relationships of power and dominance. If we reduce sexuality to power so masculinities come to be defined exclusively as relationships of power and the issue is how masculinities can be deconstructed, not whether men can change. We lose heart in the possibilities of change and in the process we often lose hope of being able to reach men emotionally. Rather the focus is placed upon confronting men with the consequences of their actions and it is deemed possible to do this through making them accept responsibility for their abusive and violent behaviours. So it is that masculinity can never be part of the solution, for it is little more than an exercise in power and dominance.

Becoming aware of the violent and abusive behaviours that so often flow from male superiority within a patriarchal society, it is easy to lose touch with the diversity of men's histories, experiences and relationships. This is one of the difficulties of the notion of men against sexism, for it does not say enough about what men are for and how men might change in relation to their emotional lives and relationships. In the United States the change in title from the National Organization for Changing Men to the National Organization for Men against Sexism (NOMAS) was in part a rejection of the too easy notion of men changing and the kind of sex-role theories that fostered a liberalism arguing that just as women were oppressed by the restrictions and expectations of their sex roles so men were also confined by their sex roles that pushed them to identify with work in the public sphere.

This liberalism created some space for men to change but it also fostered a false parallelism in the situation of men and women and failed to illuminate gendered relationships of power. But the shift towards men against sexism could produce its own moralism and it tended to reinforce the notion that masculinity could not be redeemed and that men could not change. It set the men who were struggling against sexism apart from other men who supposedly lacked awareness of how their behaviours were oppressive to women. In a strange way it also maintained the focus upon women, on the forms of female subordination about which men had to be convinced, and it took attention away from the critical analysis of men and masculinities. Somehow it did not help men to rework how they had grown up to identify with a particular masculinity and the unease and tensions they might feel in this relationship.

A radical expression of a moralistic form of sexual politics is presented in John Stoltenberg's *Refusing to Be a Man* (1989). It helped to provide a radical feminist analysis of men and masculinities. This has appealed to many men who feel a deep sense of guilt when they become aware of some of the effects of pornography and male violence. There is a sense of self-disgust and self-hatred that was more familiar in the sexual politics of the 1970s. But in its own way it echoes deeply embedded cultural notions within a Protestant tradition, as I have argued in *Recreating Sexual Politics* (Seidler 1991a), where men are 'bad' and 'evil' so that their evil natures can be redeemed only by good deeds. Through their actions men can prove themselves to be other than what they are, but at some level men can feel haunted by the notion that they are 'good for nothing'. These are difficult emotions to come to terms with and men learn to suppress them, which is why, as Weber understood it, there is such pressure upon men to prove themselves through work within the Protestant ethic. For Stoltenberg the struggle against pornography and male violence is so urgent that it should be men's exclusive concern, for men are largely responsible for the industry and for all the sufferings that it brings in its wake. Men have to be made aware of their status as perpetrators. In this scheme it is men in general who are responsible, for there can be no 'innocent' men and no men who do not at least indirectly benefit from the exercise of male superiority and dominance. So it is, as heterosexual men, that 'we are all guilty' and the sooner that we are ready to admit this the better. In this rationalistic vision that sustains a moralistic politics we do not have to investigate men's experience and relationships. Rather we can 'know' of men's responsibilities, for this is a shared consequence of dominant masculinities. We do not have to consider men's emotional lives, which can be taken to be a distraction to do with men's psyches rather than with power and politics. So it is that the exploration of emotional lives gets suppressed within a rationalistic politics.

We need ways of fully endorsing the realities of male violence and abuse without being forced to accept that the only way of taking these concerns seriously is to follow the kind of moral rationalism which Stoltenberg argues for. How can we value our own lives and experiences when we know that there is such suffering which we are helping to sustain? We can feel the same about poverty and starvation, though we might be implicated in different ways. This is also part of a moral rationalism, a tradition that is linked to a dominant masculinity in its relationship to modernity. At some level, it continues to mean that men have 'all the answers' and that through their relationship to reason they can legislate for others.

EXPERIENCE, POWER AND EMOTIONS

Within social theory the disdain for experience as 'personal' and 'subjective' has gone hand in hand with the disdain for emotions as sources of knowledge. We reproduce the distinction between reason and nature in terms of knowledge and experience. With the disenchantment of nature we have the notion that experience is 'given' and 'ahistorical'. In a rationalist tradition experience is to be constituted through mind and in the twentieth century through language and discourse. Feminism helped to challenge the terms of an Enlightenment vision of modernity through its insistence upon the tensions between reason and emotion, knowledge and experience. It recognizes that experience cannot simply be provided through discourse because it is often a dominant, white, heterosexual masculinity which can produce this language in its own image. It is through men's relationship to reason that they can legislate for others. It is their task to provide an 'analysis' of the experience of 'others' just as it is their task to provide 'solutions' to the emotional problems 'others' have. Men learn to handle problems on their own.

Often men learn to be in control of their experience through suppressing emotions and feelings that might question or disturb the images they live out. They learn to eradicate any emotions that might interrupt the ways they present themselves to others. They learn to silence the revelations of their natures. So it is that the disdain for experience that is a mark of much poststructuralist theory reflects a dominant masculinity. We find this reflected in the analyses of masculinities where, for instance, in Connell's *Gender and Power* (1987) and his more recent *Masculinities* (1995) the notion of men's consciousness-raising is categorized as 'therapeutic' so that there is little sense that men might have to 'learn from' or 'come to terms with' their experience in critical ways. The notion that 'the personal is political' gets too easily dismissed when it is invoked by men as a crucial feminist insight they have learnt from. Somehow in the hands of men it is castigated as an attempt to reduce the political to the personal. This notion was already questioned in the Achilles Heel work; see, for instance, *The Achilles Heel Reader* (Seidler 1991) and *Men, Sex and Relationships* (Seidler 1992).

When men seek to theorize the relationship between emotions and power as part of exploring the tension diverse men often feel in relation to dominant masculinities, this is too readily impugned in Protestant terms as a form of 'self-indulgence'. In refusing to explore the contradictions of contemporary masculinities or to show how men have developed into what they are, we are left with a gulf between 'analysis' and 'experience'. It echoes the moralism which asks how it is possible for men to focus their attention on themselves as men in critical relation to masculinities, when men collectively are responsible for so much suffering to women. How can men justify giving any time and attention to themselves when they are surrounded by so many pornographic images that are degrading to women?

I recognize the force of such political moralism because it was very present in the sexual politics of the 1970s and 1980s. But it is part of the problem rather than the solution and it has made it difficult for men to open a conversation between different generations, for younger men often reject this moralism and the exclusive concern of men's relationship with feminism. Many men who have been angry at the gains they see feminism as making and the loss of power they feel in their own lives have turned towards men's rights movements. Others have been drawn to Robert Bly's work (1990) because he seems to offer a way through, whereby men can learn how to explore masculinities and also to feel good about themselves as men, rather than simply feeling guilty. There are difficulties with Bly's work in *Iron John* (1990), particularly in his understanding of men's diverse relationships to feminism. He misleadingly generalizes, identifying as 'feminized' the men he describes, while at the same time making some sharp observations about how some men have lost their 'gender ground'.

It can so easily seem a 'moral outrage' to open a discussion about what is happening for men when men are aware of how women have been made to suffer. But if we are not to be trapped in such political moralism we need to find a new way of theorizing about men and masculinities that does not get locked into this false polarity. Men can recognize the power that they have as men and the harm and suffering this causes. At the same time men can learn to celebrate revisioned masculinities so that they can teach boys and younger men about different ways of being men and learning to take responsibilities for themselves emotionally. It is important to recognize that for boys to learn to relate emotionally does not mean their being 'feminized'; and although *Iron John* attempts to say that in exploring emotions that have been so long suppressed, men will not have to deal with issues of homophobia, we have to reject any such guarantees. As men learn to draw support emotionally from each other as men, it can be quite scary, for we have often not learnt that there are different ways of loving men.

MEN, VIOLENCE AND EMOTIONAL LIFE

A dominant, white, heterosexual masculinity is tied up with relations of violence. As men grow up within cultures of male superiority, so they learn that if reason does not serve to put women in their place, then they are forced to resort to violence. Women as 'irrational' and closer to nature cannot be reasoned with, so there is no alternative to violence. This is part of the duty that men have. In terms of colonialism white men had similar duties in relation to the colonial 'other'. This is the way European masculinities were framed in relation to the 'native' and the 'savage'. So it is that within an Enlightenment vision of modernity, dominant white Christian heterosexual masculinities were already encoded in terms of hierarchy and superiority. 'Others' who were deemed to be 'closer to nature' were more easily influenced by their emotional lives and this was taken to be a sign of weakness and inadequacy. In the face of this men had to be 'strong'.

Men had to prove themselves to be independent and self-sufficient at least in the public sphere where male identities were sustained. This is the way men had to present themselves, at least in relation to other men with whom they were locked into competitive relations. Any sign of weakness could be threatening, for other men could so easily use it to their advantage to put someone down. So men had to be constantly 'on guard' ready to defend themselves against an attack that could come from any direction. Even friends were suspect; they could never be fully trusted because no man could be sure that a friend would not use whatever information he had if he could see an advantage to himself. Men often learned to bond with each other by projecting on to other men who had less power within patriarchy, their fears and uncertainties. This is very clear in the early years of secondary school when, for instance, many boys go through a period of uncertainty in relation to their heterosexual identities. This is when their fears are often projected on to less powerful boys who can be named as 'queers' and 'poofs'. Sometimes boys who are gay can be forced into 'queer bashing' as a form of self-protection.

As a man you have to be ready to defend yourself. Here, there is a powerful link between masculinity and violence, for there is always a question as to whether you are 'man enough'. Boys often feel that they are being constantly tested. They have to prove that they are not 'weak'. There is a particular fear of weakness as a form of humiliation. If boys feel threatened they will sometimes feel they have automatically to attack. This is particularly so in traditional white working-class cultures. It is as if there is little time to reflect and violence can be used against other men as a form of self-defence. Boys have to learn to defend themselves or they have to seek alliances with older brothers or stronger mates who might be ready to come to their defence if they are attacked. There is a hierarchy in the playground as boys learn how to read the dangers.

Often men can feel good about themselves only by putting other men down, for masculinity is a *relational* concept. I can feel good about myself only by knowing that I am doing better than others. Within a Protestant culture, as Weber has it, men grow up with a feeling that they are 'bad' and that their natures are 'evil'. This leads to particular forms of self-regulation that can also be interpreted as violence to the self. For a dominant masculinity learns to prove itself by knowing that it is self-sufficient and does not need the help of others. This is clear in the public school training of colonial masculinities where men were to be trained partly through the suppression of their own emotional needs. For needs were a sign of weakness and it was only the 'natives' that had needs. They 'needed' the colonizer in order to regulate their lives, which would otherwise be ruled by nature. The masculine voice of reason was radically set against nature. It was to be objective and impartial and to provide order where nature could provide only instinctual chaos. This was the civilized voice which 'others' needed if they themselves were to become civilized. So it was that temptations had to be resisted and a 'superior' masculinity had to show that it had no emotional needs itself. The 'natives' continually reaffirmed that they were uncivilized through the emotional needs they had.

Because the colonizer could take his superiority for granted it did not have to be proved. The 'white man's burden' was a duty to bring civilization where there was only nature. So it was that the 'natives' were defined as 'children' who did not know what was good for themselves and who could not legislate for themselves. As wilful children need to be disciplined to 'break their wills' so colonizers had to be ready to use violence 'for their own good' where there was any sign of disobedience on the part of the colonized population. The iron fist has always to be ready. At some level this was the only language that the colonized could understand. It was the duty of a dominant white masculinity to assert authority whenever it was needed. In relation to the family the father was a figure of authority who would only compromise his position of authority if he got too intimate with his children. He had to maintain his distance if he wanted to maintain his authority. So it was also with the colonial administrator.

A dominant white masculinity is identified with a reason set apart from emotions. Emotions have to be suppressed and silenced as boys grow up to identify with their fathers as rational selves. As colonial men identify themselves with culture and civilization so they set themselves against a nature which is identified with 'others'. Claims to male superiority were tied up with notions of white superiority within an Enlightenment vision of modernity. Women, like 'natives', were identified with children. In their different ways they were defined by the reason they lacked. As Kant has it, only through a child's relationship with a father, or a wife's with a husband, could an inner relationship with reason be established. So it was, for instance, that women had to accept the subordination of marriage in order to find freedom and autonomy. It was only through men that they could know reason and so learn to direct their lives through reason.

In a similar way the 'native' who was deemed to be 'uncivilized' needed to accept the subordination to a dominant white European colonizer in order to seek eventual freedom. The legitimation of colonial power was tied up with the legitimation of male superiority. Gender and race were entwined in the formation of a dominant white European masculinity. In the reordering of gender relations there was the violence of the witchburnings as the scientific revolutions of the seventeenth century helped to consolidate a new order of gender relations in which a dominant masculinity could appropriate to itself to science, knowledge, reason and progress. In their different ways these were set against a nature that needed to be dominated and controlled. So it was that culture was set against nature, as reason was set against emotion. A dominant white masculinity had identified reason with culture as the hallmark of modernity. As a new order of heterosexual gender relations was legitimated the violence that had been crucial to their ordering was rendered invisible. The Enlightenment was to be told as a gender-neutral story of a universalized notion of reason emerging out of the darkness of former times. A dominant masculinity had been able to shape modernity in its own image.

The reorganization of colonial relations and the creation of white Christian superiority went hand in hand with slavery. It was a story of violence, murder and brutality. But as it is taught it is part of the history of people of African descent. It is rarely established as part of the history of European Enlightenment and the reordering of relations between culture and nature. As we learn to think in terms of the growing influence of reason and rationality, so slavery becomes 'irrational'. We lose a sense of how it is tied up with the conceptualization of reason in its opposition to emotion in the west. The links between violence and a dominant masculinity get lost, for we lose a sense of how violence was an everyday part of these colonial relations and of how these relations were gendered and sexualized. Susan Brownmiller's *Against Our Will* (1986) served to show how women of African descent were deemed to be the sexual property of their masters.

MEN, MASCULINITIES AND EMOTIONAL LIFE

Within modernity a dominant white heterosexual masculinity is identified with being independent and self-sufficient. As rational selves men are not supposed to have emotional needs. In identifying with culture men deny their own natures, bodies, sexualities and emotional lives. Rather, men learn to control their lives through reason alone. This fosters a form of self-denial, as I have explored it in *Recreating Sexual Politics*. As men learn to suppress their emotions as part of silencing their natures, often they do not experience a conflict. This is what makes the devaluation of experience as a category, when set against reason or discourse, so easy for a tradition of male rationalism. Rather men learn to project, as Freud understood, their unconscious feelings and desires on to 'others' who are made to carry them. This also happens in relationships where one partner, for example, might have to 'carry' the unexpressed anger. It can be the woman who feels she is always getting angry while her partner in a heterosexual relationship feels superior because he does not lose his 'self-control'.

Social theory set within the terms of a dominant masculinity has similarly excluded and marginalized emotions as sources of knowledge. If they are acknowledged at all, it is as a subjective response to an objective situation. So, for instance, in medical practice, if emotions are recognized they will often be left to the nurses to deal with. They will not be able to affect the nature of clinical judgement. As Alderson (1993) has shown, the emotional knowledge that parents have of their children could affect the kind of heart treatment that might be appropriate for the child. But this knowledge is rarely validated, being devalued as 'subjective'. It might come into the picture only when there are discussions about how the child is coming to terms with the operation.

Often men are not skilled at dealing with their emotions, for this is work that they leave to their partners within heterosexual relationships. As they grow up with little contact with their emotional lives, they are often 'out of touch' with themselves emotionally. This links to men's relationships with their bodies as a site of proving their male identities. Sometimes they will not even register their tiredness, thinking of this as a kind of limit they have to prove themselves against. The body as a machine is there to be used and often it is chastised or punished if it lets us down through illness. For within the rationalist terms of modernity the body is not 'part of' who I am as a rational self. The body is there as property which is at the disposal of my will. It is an instrument that I use, and a matter of testing male identity against its limits often arises.

As part of a disenchanted nature the body is reduced to matter and so silenced. The body does not exist as a source of meaning and value, but like nature the only meaning it can have is provided through the use we put it to. As within the prevailing discourses of modernity there is no sense of communicating with nature, so there is little sense of the idea of listening to our bodies. Outside traditions of alternative medicine there is little sense of an emotional body that we can come to respect and learn from. Ecology has helped us question the terms of modernity in its recognition that nature can be a source of meaning and value, so that we have to rethink an appropriate relationship to animals and nature. This fundamentally challenges the split between body and mind, reason and emotion, that has crucially set the terms for modernity.

It is easier to project on to others when we have not learnt how to take responsibility for ourselves emotionally. A dominant masculinity teaches us that we should not have emotional needs. A rationalist culture encourages us to identify with what is 'right' and so automatically to discount emotions, feelings and desires that might lead us in a different direction. Rather, within a masculine culture of self-denial, we often resent those who seem not to be making the same kinds of emotional sacrifices. We resent their pleasure. At some level we learn to live as if we do not need to be nourished as men, for we supposedly do not have needs ourselves. We might keep ourselves busy, scared of having much time and space for ourselves because of the ghosts that might emerge from our unconscious. But this is very different from having a somatic knowledge of what we want or need for ourselves. It is striking at the difficulties men can have in naming what they want. They can be so identified with what is expected of them in their jobs and relationships that it seems as if they do not exist for themselves.

This can make men even more controlling within relationships. They become identified with *being* their reason and so with legislating for others, before, as I explored it in *Rediscovering Masculinity* (Seidler 1989), learning to express more personally for themselves. This can make it difficult for men to negotiate in more equal relationships, for they can be so out of touch with themselves that it is difficult to say what they want. This has important ramifications for how we theorize men's power in relationships. At some level men can have a great deal of power and control whilst at the same time they feel they get very little for themselves. It is also possible for men to be relatively powerless in relation to other men at work and so feel more pressure to throw their weight around at home to affirm their male identities. Men can want to seem 'reasonable' in their negotiations with their partners, whilst at the same time feeling that they 'know best'. This becomes a form of control which can be difficult to deal with when men claim they are getting very little for themselves.

Within a Protestant culture men can feel that it is 'self-indulgent' for them to get their needs met. This creates difficulties in relationships; for example, it can leave women feeling guilty about satisfying their own needs. A man might volunteer to look after the children because he feels that it is 'fair', and that he ought to do it, though at another level he is very tired. It might be better if he attempted some kind of renegotiation by sharing what he feels with his partner, who might be happy to organize a swap. Instead he feels he *ought* to be able to do it, though later he is shocked at the level of his anger at the children, a level quite inappropriate to the situation, which belongs elsewhere. But it might be difficult for him to recognize this because the moralism can stand in the way of his developing more of a relationship to himself emotionally.

The kind of political correctness that too often went along with an anti-sexist politics meant that men were anxious to do the right thing in relation to feminism. It made it difficult for men sometimes to develop a critical relationship with feminism even where this was about the conceptions of men and masculinities. At some level this was a continuation in a political context of the difficulties men had in acknowledging what they wanted and needed for themselves. This involves a critical relationship to men's emotional lives, one they often find difficult to develop because they are so concerned not only to do what is 'right' but also to have the answers. This is why it can be important to question a tradition of moral rationalism that, in Kantian terms, automatically subordinates emotions and feelings when they come into conflict with thoughts. Again this is not a distinction that can be made abstractly; it involves men learning, possibly with the help of psychotherapy, to develop more of a relationship with their emotional lives.

Anger can be an exercise of power, especially when invoked by men as a way of controlling a sadness or fear that is breaking the surface of conscious life. It can be too threatening for men to acknowledge their vulnerability in this way so that automatically, before consciously registering what is going on, they find themselves getting angry as a means of sustaining an acceptable male identity. Anger can be oppressive to women as an exercise of male power and control, but it does not help for men to reject and swallow their anger as an 'unacceptable' and 'negative' emotion. This is a form of self-sacrifice that can only create distance in a relationship because at some level women recognize what is going on, at the same time as it is being denied. This creates a dishonesty in the relationship.

It is more helpful for men to be able to acknowledge the anger they carry, often from the ways they have been treated as boys, when they were often expected to put up with brutalizing behaviours without complaining. Boys learn to prove their male identities by showing that they can endure and put up with whatever the world throws at them. Even white upper-class boys are expected to put up with zinc toilets and cold rooms; to ask for a duvet can be a sign of a weakness identified with femininity. Foucault in his rejection of the notion of repression does not help us to be able to recognize the kind of emotional baggage that boys carry from their childhood. It does not mean that these emotions are waiting in some kind of pristine state to be expressed. But this is not Freud's conception. The relationship between present anger and past humiliations, for instance, is complex. Sometimes it is in the context of men's therapy groups that some of the connections can be explored, for it might not be appropriate to think that these emotional histories can be worked on in the context of an intimate relationship.

Often men find it hard to acknowledge that they need help, for we grow up with a strong belief that we should be able to handle our own emotional lives. Along with this it is threatening to be in a group of men because it is easy to feel they will take advantage of any weakness that a man might show. Men say in interviews that they feel much closer to women and that they talk emotionally with women, in a way that they do not with men. This is sad: there are ways that men can support and help each other because there are often significant resonances in shared histories. But this kind of trust between men can be difficult to develop, though it can be crucial as part of a resistance to a patriarchal heterosexuality in which it is too often assumed that women will have to take the burden of men's emotional lives. It is better if men can learn to take more responsibility for their emotional lives, including their anger and violence.

Somehow we need to develop an analysis of men's power that does not diminish this kind of emotional work as 'therapeutic' in the way Connell (1995) tends to do, setting it in contrast within a structural analysis of masculinities. As so often happens, the move towards a more generalized analysis of gender relations, to be set along class relations and relations of 'race' and ethnicity, will be very tempting for a rationalist tradition. But this is part of the problem, for it threatens to lose the feminist insight that the personal is political. Too often, we invoke psychoanalytic theory as a way of providing a theory of subjectivity that is recognized as an absence within a structural analysis. Again this can be helpful, but we often find our thinking trapped within its terms, unable to break free from its gender and racial assumptions.

Although the move towards a theory of masculinities has been helpful in revealing both their diversity and the relationships of power that separate them, it has made it difficult to open up the tensions between men and masculinities. Again, too often these structured masculinities determine men's emotional lives and relationships. In its own way this makes it difficult for men to change; too often we end up trapped into thinking of masculinities as relationships of power and dominance. We need different ways of thinking about the relation between the institutional and the personal; we want an analysis that is able to illuminate the importance of the emotional lives of men, as part of a more general theoretical shift able to validate emotions and feelings as sources of knowledge.

Within the terms of an enlightenment vision of modernity emotions are gendered as 'feminine' and this is still reflected in the ways boys often think of sadness as an emotion but not so readily of anger. Emotions in these discourses are linked to vulnerability and so to 'weakness' and 'femininity'. This is reflected not only in modern forms of social theory and philosophy, but in interviews with diverse men. Since it is so important for men to sustain control over their experience, they often do not want to listen to what their partners have to say lest it threaten their sense of self. Sometimes they use anger and violence so as not to be able to hear and then go on to deny the violence because they are so identified with their own notions. This denial is fostered within modernity by the idea that men can control their experience through controlling the meanings they assign to it. This is part of an authority that a dominant masculinity often insists on. It can be further sustained within a discourse theory that does not allow for the tension between language and experience but insists that discourse is able to constitute experience and identity.

Sometimes men can live with the rejection of their partners, knowing that what matters is the support of other men within the public realm, for this is where male identities are sustained. Often it is only when a relationship is broken that men realize what they have lost. Some men learn to blame their partners, rather than take responsibility for their own violence. Others begin a process of change and recognize that this involves an exploration of values, beliefs, emotions and feelings. This can be a difficult process because men can be so unused to listening to themselves, fixed as they are on constantly proving themselves within the public sphere of work. The fear of failure still keeps many men away from recognizing their intimate relationships as a source of meaning and value rather than simply a background against which they live their individual lives.

Within a postmodern world, relationships can no longer be taken for granted and women will refuse marriage and commitment if they feel they are not getting something for themselves. Traditional forms of intimate relationships have broken down and there is a demand for men to 'get their act together' both emotionally and physically, for so many more women have changed under the influence of feminism than men. The way that emotions have been discounted as forms of knowledge has served the purpose of male power within patriarchal heterosexual relationships. As men envision different forms of relationships, both straight and gay, so men are having to take greater responsibility for their emotional lives both theoretically and practically. If men are to change their violent behaviours they have to find ways of moving beyond guilt and blame so that they take more responsibility for their violence as well as for exploring different ways of relating and living as men. Part of this process will involve learning how to feel better about themselves as men.

BIBLIOGRAPHY

Alderson, P. (1993) *Children's Consent to Surgery.* Buckingham, Bucks: Open University Press.
Baker-Miller, J. (1986) *Towards a New Psychology of Women.* New York: Beacon.
Bly, R. (1990) *Iron John: A Book about Men.* Shaftesbury, Dorset: Element Books.
Brownmiller, S. (1986) *Against Our Will: Men, Women and Rape.* Harmondsworth, Mx: Penguin.
Connell, R. (1987) *Gender and Power.* Cambridge: Polity Press.
Connell, R. (1995) *Masculinities.* Cambridge: Polity Press.
Seidler, V. J. (1989) *Rediscovering Masculinity: Reason, Language and Sexuality.* London: Routledge.
Seidler, V. J. (1991a) *Recreating Sexual Politics: Men, Feminism and Politics.* London: Routledge.
Seidler, V. J. (1991b) *The Moral Limits of Modernity: Love, Inequality and Oppression.* London: Macmillan.
Seidler, V. J. (ed.) (1991c) *The Achilles Heel Reader: Men, Sexual Politics and Socialism.* London: Routledge.
Seidler, V. J. (1992) *Men, Sex and Relationships.* London: Routledge.
Seidler, V. J. (1994) *Unreasonable Men: Masculinity and Social Theory.* London: Routledge.
Seidler, V. J. (1995) *Recovering the Self: Morality and Social Theory.* London: Routledge.
Stoltenberg, J. (1989) *Refusing to Be a Man: Essays on Sex and Justice.* Portland, OR: Breitenbush.

12 'Stepford wives' and 'hollow men'?

Doing emotion work, doing gender and 'authenticity' in intimate heterosexual relationships

Jean Duncombe and Dennis Marsden

The feelings I don't have, I don't have.
The feelings I don't have, I won't say I have.
The feelings you say you have, you don't have.
The feelings you would like us both to have, we neither of us have.
(From 'To women, as far as I'm concerned', D. H. Lawrence, 1986)

INTRODUCTION

In our earlier work, we have tried to understand how couples manage to stay together in long-term marriages, now that feminism has promoted a greater awareness of women's exploitation in marriage, and when there is a growing emphasis on the alternative pursuit of self-fulfilment in the 'pure couple relationship' (Giddens 1992; Rubin 1991). We have argued that it is mainly women who help to keep such marriages alive by doing 'emotion work' (Hochschild 1983) on *themselves* as well as on their husbands, to sustain the image that 'we're ever so happy, really' (Duncombe and Marsden 1993, 1996a, 1996b).

However, we have grown uncomfortable that our work has sometimes been read as merely reproducing the patronizing gender stereotypes that women become like 'Stepford wives', who lose awareness of their exploitation by doing emotion work on behalf of emotionally 'hollow' men. Indeed, we believe that there is now a need for a broader exploration of the concept of emotion work, which will examine more closely the kinds of emotion work that not only women but also men are said to do, and which will question whether doing emotion work invariably results in a loss of self-awareness and 'authenticity'.

Paradoxically, the need for this exploration arises from the growth in contributions to discussions of emotion work from a variety of theoretical and ideological perspectives. For example, while some women angrily deny that they are programmed to nurture men, Delphy and Leonard (1992) claim that women's emotion work is merely another demonstration of their 'false consciousness' under male hegemony, and hardly worth exploration. Similarly, some male writers on heterosexual masculinity ('masculinity' writers) deplore men's emotional hollowness, but others angrily maintain that men do express emotion and perform emotion work in their personal and organizational relationships, or that they *could* do so in the right context or with help from women, other men or therapists (Cohen 1990; Connell 1987, 1995; Craib 1995; Farrell 1974; Jackson 1990; Metcalf and Humphries 1985; Roper 1994; Seidler 1985).

More generally, it is argued that the categories 'men' and 'women' are essentialist, and should be replaced by a pluralistic model of gender and behaviour (Connell 1995; Morgan 1992). And the concept of emotion work has itself been criticized as a crude over-simplification of mental processes such as 'repression' and 'denial' which continually occur in the unconscious or preconscious areas of the minds of all men and women – and which sociologists should leave to psychoanalysis (Craib 1995).

This chapter is therefore an attempt to clarify some of the confusion now surrounding the term 'emotion work', which has been adopted, adapted or criticized to such an extent that it is in danger of becoming a catch-all cliché. However, we will still use the terms 'men' and 'women'; for we agree with Morgan, who advocates a recognition of pluralities while recognizing that these are 'variations on a deeply entrenched theme', whose abandonment may 'blunt the critical edge of feminism . . . and [bring] a danger of losing a sense of dominance, of patriarchy and control' (Morgan 1992: 46).

We will begin by trying to find empirical examples of the kinds of emotion work that women and men do in marital and couple relationships. We will then use recent theories of gender pluralism and 'doing gender', to discuss the suggestion in Hochschild's work and psychodynamic theory that doing emotion work may lead to a loss of authenticity. And finally, drawing on our own research on couples, we will show how attempts by individual men and women to preserve their sense of authenticity may vary, depending on what we will call their 'core identities'.

WOMEN, MARRIAGE AND EMOTION WORK: SOME EMPIRICAL EXAMPLES

Hochschild (1983) originally described 'emotion work' in terms of the emotional effort made by individuals – both men and women – to 'manage' their feelings to bring them into line with the societal 'feeling rules' which prescribe how they 'ought' to feel in particular social situations. However, she insists that there are gender differences in emotion work which embody the 'psychological effects of [men] having and [women] not having power' (Hochschild 1983: 162–7) – a distinction that remains central to her later discussion of marriage (Hochschild 1990). Gender differences appear in the way that women make 'defensive use of sexual beauty [and] charm and . . . make a resource out of feeling and offer it to men as a gift in return for the more material resources they lack. . . . So for women being becomes a way of doing, acting is the needed skill and emotion work is the tool' (Hochschild 1983: 162–85). Men, on the other hand, are seen as being more rarely called upon to do emotion work, characteristically in the role of looking tough and being in control.

In studies of marriage, what is conventionally described as women's 'nurturing', 'mothering', 'caring' or 'supporting' behaviour with others (Miller 1986) has also been variously described as: doing emotion work or shadow work, providing emotional capital and backstage wealth (Hochschild 1983, 1990); providing emotional resourcing, carrying emotional baggage (Rubin 1984); doing invisible housework (Miller 1986); doing emotional housework and providing emotional servicing (Hite 1988; Cline and Spender 1987). However, beyond these rather general and amorphous phrases specific empirical examples of women's emotion work proved relatively difficult to find.

In their couple relationships, women say they try to make men talk openly about their feelings and confront their problems partly for men's own peace of mind but also to promote the sense of intimacy they themselves value. Hite concluded from her research that there is a kind of '"emotional contract" in which the woman is expected to nurture the man, take care of his emotional needs': as one of her respondents explained, 'I work more at keeping us together, planning things to do, trying to understand and hear how he feels' (Hite 1988: 30, 34). Reviewing the (largely US) literature, Thompson and Walker (1989) found that women monitor couple relationships and work to foster intimacy, by smiling and laughing more often than men and giving their partners hugs or kisses when something nice happens; and they communicate more – and more personally (Tannen 1991). Many women say they repress their own sexual desire to avoid pressuring their partners, and most had 'faked' orgasms for their husbands (Rubin 1991). There are similar findings from the UK concerning wives' sexual behaviour and efforts to promote intimacy, to build up their husbands' image by overvaluing their husbands' careers and small domestic and parenting input, and undervaluing their own activities (Backett 1987; Coward 1992; Mansfield and Collard 1988). Indeed, Cline and Spender claim that women habitually engage in 'reflecting men at twice their natural size' to 'make men feel good', by 'hiding and minimizing [men's] failure, encouraging, boosting, sympathizing and flattering'. Among women's most significant emotional gestures and arduous tasks are 'mandatory' smiling and the faking of orgasms (Cline and Spender 1987: 112–18).

In relation to wider networks of kin and relationships, Rubin found that 'women make lists of birthdays and anniversaries and friends to keep in touch with, even when they're not doing it they're still thinking about it and figuring out how to do it'. And in the context of the family, one of her respondents described how she listened, almost subliminally, to the children quarrelling in another room so she could anticipate any fighting: 'It's like there's a radar inside me that knows what's going on all around me all the time, and you can't just switch it off' (Rubin 1984: 135, 165–7).

Overall, we would suggest that the available empirical evidence indicates that most women's behaviour in relationships *appears* to fit the dominant gender stereotype of the Stepford wife, yet it also illustrates the basic difficulties in researching and describing emotion work, which must often be interpreted from the sometimes self-contradictory things that people say, and from physical gestures (Duncombe and Marsden 1995). Also, writers tend to stress or assume that emotion work is indeed effort or *work* (as Hochschild's phrase was intended to convey), and the question of whether women may sometimes find emotion work tolerable or even rewarding is seldom raised, unless it is dismissed as 'false consciousness'.

MEN'S EMOTION WORK IN MARRIAGE AND COUPLE RELATIONSHIPS

The blandness of descriptions of women's emotion work makes it easy to understand why many men (and some women!) are irritated by the suggestion that only women do emotion work 'in support of' their relationships. In surveys, most men claim to work for their families and not themselves (Cohen 1990; Duck and Gilmour 1981; Weiss 1990), so, surely, the emotional effort they expend on being breadwinners is a similar kind of support?

Also, as we noted earlier, there are claims that men's emotional behaviour in relationships is changing. So what are we to make of the studies of marriage (mostly by women, but also by a few 'masculinity' writers) which consistently describe men as emotionally remote, and the various studies which argue that even fathers who are physically present in the home are often 'functionally absent' (Acock and Demo 1994; Furstenberg and Cherlin 1991)?

In fact, Bob Weiss's description of how men 'compartmentalize' their lives clearly reveals that men *do* perform emotion work, but with a different focus from women. Men worry about work-related problems, but try to keep these from their wives to save them from worrying about issues that men think they cannot understand or alleviate. However, men then expect their wives to do the emotion work in the home by organizing a stress-free and supportive environment – the 'gender division of emotion work' first proposed by Parsons (Parsons and Bales 1956). An example of one man's emotion work in the home is when he tried hard 'to put out of his mind' his resentment at his wife's repeated failure to provide the breakfast orange juice that symbolized for him both her care and what he regarded as their 'compact': 'I work hard . . . and she has the whole day, she is supposed to make sure there is orange juice' (Weiss 1990: 146–7). However, his emotion work was not successful and his resentment resurfaced in other disagreements.

Several 'masculinity' writers have described how the birth of their first child had caused them (as we would say) to put more emotion work into their careers, and to expect more emotional servicing from their wives

(Cohen 1990; Seidler 1985; see also Lewis and O'Brien 1987). Although their wives had desperately needed emotional validation and servicing (emotion work) from them, these men had found they could not respond, or had even failed to perceive their wives' needs. For example, Cohen noticed his wife looked tired and often cried, but 'it never occurred to me she might be unhappy . . . we always made passionate love and that I imagined was a sign that everything really was OK' (Cohen 1990: 49). His wife, however, complained that he 'wasn't there'. And in Weiss's study, some 'workaholic' husbands confessed to spending so much of their emotional energies in thinking about work that they then could not do the emotion work of pushing thoughts of work out of their heads sufficiently to make love to their wives (Weiss 1990).

However, some wives felt that men's 'remoteness' was not merely a 'psychic absence' but resulted from men doing emotion work on themselves to *resist* becoming intimately emotionally involved: 'He tunes out . . . he has this amazing capacity to just stop being there. . . . There's a wall around him that you can't get past' (Rubin 1984: 164–6; see also Brannen and Collard 1982; Mansfield and Collard 1988). As one wife told us, men want only 'the picture', i.e. home, wife and children, in their heads, but not close emotional participation.

A few 'masculinity' writers reveal how they themselves have done emotion work in sexual relationships. For example, Jackson reports his discomfiture when he could not get an erection with a willing partner: after all, 'Real men were always ready for it at any time, weren't they, irrespective of how they were feeling. No matter how loudly I cursed it inside my head, my estranged penis refused to join in' (Jackson 1990: 133). And Jensen too describes how pressures to 'be a man' had betrayed him into situations where he had to fantasize to keep his erection, and he says he envies macho men who 'don't have to invent their roles [i.e. do emotion work on themselves] every minute of the day!' (Jensen 1974: 220). These examples reveal that some men *do* emotion work and even sometimes fake orgasms, but in these instances they do it primarily on themselves, in order to conform to their *own* ideology of masculinity, although in practice this ideology often seems to be supported by (even feminist) women partners (Cohen 1990; Jackson 1990; Duncombe and Marsden 1996b).

To sum up, the sparse research evidence and the few accounts of *personal* experience from 'masculinity' writers conform to the gender stereotype that men are emotionally 'hollow'. Yet although men *appear* emotionally remote when at home, they are doing emotion work – as they see it in support of their relationships – by coping with the stresses of 'being a breadwinner'. And they also do emotion work in relationships to conform to the ideology of 'being a man'. However, we would suggest that since men's emotion work appears to be primarily *on themselves* – 'in their heads' – and is devoted to *suppressing* rather than expressing emotion, it is not surprising that to their wives they appear emotionally remote. We should stress that we are talking only of white Anglo-Saxon men, and not about men's behaviour at work and in predominantly male groups.

LOSS OF AUTHENTICITY: HOCHSCHILD'S MODEL AND PSYCHODYNAMIC THEORY

In the remainder of this chapter, we will explore the suggestion – in both Hochschild's work and psychodynamic theory – that those who do emotion work are in danger of behaving 'inauthentically'. Hochschild suggested in her earlier research that in shallow or 'surface acting', individuals remain conscious of the gap between their 'real' feelings and the ideological feeling rules concerning how they 'ought' to behave, but in 'deep acting' they lose their sense of their real feelings, and consequently they lose their 'authenticity' and begin to 'feel phoney': 'Am I acting now? How do I know?' (1983: 37–55).

Hochschild pointed out several scenarios for how individuals might react to pressures from feeling rules and loss of authenticity, ranging from over-identification with the required role, with the risk of 'emotional burnout', through the recognition that the role requires emotional acting, but feeling guilt and insincerity, to becoming estranged and cynical (Hochschild 1983: 187). We suggest that as a convenient shorthand these processes may be summarized as: 'self-loss' as a result of 'deep acting'; varying attempts to retain authenticity through 'self-distancing' in 'shallow acting'; and ultimately 'self-withdrawal' and a refusal to do any acting at all.

As we noted earlier, Hochschild's model has been criticized from a psychoanalytical perspective for oversimplifying the complex mental processes of denial and repression. And it is true that Hochschild's attempt to establish 'the management of emotion' as a distinct field, separated from discussions of social institutions, and from psychodynamic or biological accounts of emotions and feelings (1983: Appendix A, 201–23), tended to stress the broader emotional contrasts between women's and men's emotional behaviour, but neglected emotional differences among individual women and men. A more fundamental problem is that the concept of 'authenticity' implies 'real feelings' coming from a 'real' self. Psychodynamic theory would tend to question whether the self that we have developed from experiences in early childhood and adolescence is in some privileged way 'authentic' – although individuals may experience their 'core selves' and identities in this way.

Unfortunately, psychodynamic theory itself does not, in our view, offer a reliable guide to authentic feelings and behaviour. Recent feminist psychodynamic theorists and practitioners have modified Freudian theory to focus on women's psychological development in male-dominated society (Chodorow 1978; Gilligan 1982; Miller 1986), and Hochschild herself (1983) has suggested that such theories may help to explain why women reveal greater propensities, capacities and skills in doing emotion work.

For example, Miller (1986), in a very generalized discussion, asserts that women become attuned to recognize the emotions and needs of others, and to believe that these can and should be served. As a result, she claims that in relationships women measure themselves by whether they are 'giving' enough and they 'try to interact . . . in ways which will foster the other person's development', but that this behaviour is virtually *obligatory*; in other words, women continually 'act' on behalf of others but they do not 'act from their true centre' and their behaviour is therefore 'inauthentic; "women" develop a psychic structuring for which the term *ego . . .* may not apply' (Miller 1986: xx, 32–9, 50, 69, 73, 92). In the object relations literature generally, women's 'selves' tend to be depicted as less independent and self-sufficient, and more 'permeable' to others' needs (Chodorow 1978; Gilligan 1982).

In contrast, it is argued that males are encouraged to pursue maturity through independence and separation from the feminine aspects of weakness and vulnerability in their natures; consequently: 'men have egos; women do not' (Cline and Spender 1987: 13). Men's behaviour is therefore more likely to emerge as 'doing', and a man may 'choose' to serve others by doing practical tasks or providing services, but as a 'luxury' he feels he 'can afford *only* after . . . he has become a man *by other standards*' (Miller 1986: 50, 69, 92). However, as 'masculinity' writers have also stressed, to the extent that men suppress the feminine side of their nature, they fail to develop ways of thinking and talking about feelings (Jackson 1990; Mac an Ghaill 1994), so they 'fail to develop an inner life' (Seidler 1985) and they are 'automatons' (Metcalf and Humphries 1985). In short, men's behaviour too is 'inauthentic'.

Yet we remain highly sceptical whether this psychodynamic literature explains differences in individual selves or describes 'authentic' feeling, since its theoretical base appears to be largely underpinned by highly gender-stereotyped and essentialist assumptions, about family processes and human emotions (Duncombe and Marsden 1996c; Segal 1987). For our present purposes, then, psychodynamic models are best regarded as elaborate 'metaphors' which usefully stress that gender-stereotyped emotional differences may be 'deeply rooted' in childhood and adolescence, so that it is difficult for individuals to recognize consciously what they are doing and to change their behaviour by rational reflection.

'DOING GENDER', 'DOING EMOTION WORK' AND AUTHENTICITY

Recently, attempts have been made to escape from such gender stereotyping by combining psychodynamic models with new sociological theories of the cultural and historical variability of gender and personality (Connell 1987, 1995; Ferree 1990; Segal 1987). New theories of 'doing gender' also offer ways of seeing individuals as actors with some degree of self-awareness who may resist societal pressures to engage in gender-stereotyped behaviour. For example, Connell argues that in any society at a particular moment there will be a 'hegemonic' gender ideology, which prescribes socially acceptable sexual orientations and behaviour, although this will be challenged by alternative competing, but subordinate, ideologies. Individuals who try to adopt and live according to such non-hegemonic ideologies, perhaps under the influence of the lifestyles of figures they currently admire or local peer groups, will risk social and perhaps legal sanctions. But in addition, how *easily* an individual can adopt and conform to a particular gender ideology will depend on how well it fits the 'self' and 'identity' that have developed through the processes of socialization, development and attachment during early childhood and adolescence.

Sociologists have also suggested that gender should be seen not as a set of static attributes and behaviour, but in terms of a process – 'doing gender' – where an individual's gender is continually being re-established, sustained, or modified, according to how far his or her everyday actions, and the rationales offered for them, conform to particular gender ideologies (Berk 1985; West and Zimmerman 1987). Some writers have taken the view that 'self-identity' can be continuously 'reflexively' rewritten through an ongoing dialogue with the self, as new experiences and social pressures are encountered (Giddens 1991; Jackson 1990). However, we suggest from our earlier discussion that the processes involved in becoming an emotionally warm and sensitive 'new man' or a ruthless 'career women' are not merely a matter of rewriting self-identity to conform to a rationally chosen gender ideology. 'Doing gender' will involve displaying the emotional skills, capacities and propensities to do emotion work in a manner appropriate to the chosen gender ideology. In this process individuals may experience the strain of the emotion work involved in bridging the gap between the feeling rules of the gender ideology to which they now aspire, and how they 'really' feel as a consequence of the 'core self' or 'core identity' (as we will call it) developed in early childhood and adolescence. We would suggest that it is particularly in such circumstances that individuals may develop a sense that they are not behaving authentically.

HOCHSCHILD'S STUDY OF MARRIAGE

Interestingly, Hochschild (1990) derived a similar model of gender from her empirical exploration of marital conflicts about which partner should do the 'second shift' of unpaid housework and childcare when both were in paid employment. She identified a major division in gender ideology between modern 'egalitarian' sharing as opposed to traditional segregation, which 'seemed to run not only between social classes, but between partners within marriages and between two contending voices inside the conscience of one individual' (1990: 189–90). The most important internal contradiction was between the feeling rules of the 'surface' ideology that a person *said* he or she believed, and (what Hochschild calls) the 'underneath', 'covert', or 'real' feelings rooted in childhood and adolescence. She suggests that apart from the effort of emotion work required to bring 'real' feelings into conformity with the 'surface' ideology, the clash may provoke secondary feelings of guilt and confusion, or even a '"flip-flop" syndrome' of rapid alternation between contradictory ideologies (Hochschild 1990: 189–91). This means that although doing emotion work is still integrally linked with doing gender, individuals' feelings and actions can be only partially inferred or predicted from the gender ideology they *say* they believe.

This model would potentially cover a wide range of different behaviours (some of which are described in Hochschild's very detailed case studies). However, Hochschild argues that in practice, occupational change and feminism have meant that 'by far the most common form of mismatch was that between . . . an egalitarian [woman] and a "transitional" [man]' – that is, a man who pays lip-service to egalitarian ideology but remains traditional 'underneath' (Hochschild 1990: 56, 193–95). Hochschild suggests that to avoid collision with their husbands, wives collude in living 'a [jointly devised] "family myth", even a modest delusional system' that they have a happy sharing couple life, by belittling their own input, reducing their husbands' obligations to tiny symbolic tasks, becoming 'supermoms' who cope with jobs and the second shift, and (guiltily) lowering their standards of childcare and housework. As a result, wives often need to do a great deal of emotion work in order constantly to maintain and refurbish the feeling that the relationship is a good one and, try as they will, resentment and cynicism resurface in different areas of the relationship.

Hochschild argues that women are forced to live the family myth by the continued gender imbalance of power in the marital relationship, and says that whether women's emotion work is seen as 'a matter of denial . . . [or as] intuitive genius', it 'is often all that stands between the stalled revolution (of American feminism) and a wave of broken marriages', so that ultimately 'couples pay a price in authenticity for their marital myths' (Hochschild 1990: 44–6, 210, 261).

While Hochschild's study of marriage represents a valuable development of her earlier model, we note that she continues to describe 'underlying' feelings as 'authentic'. We would suggest that there is further room for probing variations in the nature of the 'authentic' selves that individual men and women have developed as a result of their earlier childhood and adolescence, to see whether we can find variations in individuals' propensities and capacities to do emotion work. Also (because Hochschild does not discuss them in her study of marriage) we suggest that there is room for further discussion of Hochschild's scenarios for individuals' reactions to pressures from feeling rules and degrees of loss of authenticity. Earlier, we summarized these scenarios as ranging from self-loss (with the possibility of 'burnout') through 'self-distancing' to 'self-withdrawal' in order to preserve authenticity, but at the cost of cynicism and guilt.

THE TRADE-OFF BETWEEN EMOTION WORK AND INDIVIDUALS' SENSE OF 'AUTHENTICITY'

In order to explore questions of authenticity, we need to tap into the 'conversations in people's heads', to ask questions in interviews (or to listen like counsellors), to learn how individuals feel about the emotion work they do, both on and for others and on and for themselves. From gender theory and Hochschild's work, we have also suggested that individuals may become more aware they are doing emotion work when they experience a clash between their 'core identity' (from their early experiences) and the feeling rules in their current situation, or when they receive contradictory messages from different ideologies, a situation that Hochschild suggests may lead to oscillation (or 'flip-flop') between different ideologies. However, Vaughan (1987) has suggested an irreversible change over time, where individuals who begin by deep acting to suppress incipient doubts about their partner tend later to distance themselves in shallow acting and to acknowledge their partner's faults, and indeed to claim that 'at some level' they had always known them (Duncombe and Marsden 1996a, 1996b).

The following quotations from our research have been selected to explore these processes of growing self-awareness and changes in doing emotion work, in relation to how authentic individuals feel, and the costs they pay (Duncombe and Marsden 1993, 1996a and 1996b). Although we should, of course, stress that difficulties of interpretation mean that our discussion must remain highly tentative.

Men, emotion work and authenticity

As we noted earlier, many men appear to fit the first of Hochschild's scenarios in the way they 'lose their selves' in conforming to the stereotype of the emotionally remote or 'hollow' man, so that they actually resist or do not find it easy to talk about their intimate emotions. However, careful listening confirmed that many husbands had been made aware of pressures to change their emotional behaviour when confronted by problems in their marriage.

For example, Mr Palmer's authentic behaviour seemed to have been to do little emotion work directly in support of couple and family life, until his wife had reacted by having an affair and refusing to sleep with him any more:

> Life's not been . . . a bed of roses . . . but over the years, I've just had to tell myself I'm really lucky, she's a really great woman, she's a great mum. Sometimes it's terrible about the sex . . . I think she might even still be having an affair. Then I tell myself not to be so stupid. But don't get me wrong, we're really happy, life's been good to us.

Mr Palmer's wife's self-distancing had jolted him into doing emotion work on himself in the interests of maintaining family life and the semblance of a couple relationship, but this was proving difficult, perhaps because it clashed with his core identity as a man. Mr Foster also described how he had been pushed into doing emotion work by his wife's pre-menstrual moodiness, which had meant that in 'self-defence', but also to make life easier for his wife and children, he had sometimes taken over responsibility for meals and seeing to the children:

> At first I thought she was just moody . . . but luckily I eventually came across a problem page article somewhere that opened my eyes, so after that I was ever so careful to keep my eye on the diary. . . . The only thing is . . . I'm not what they call a 'New Man', so it doesn't come naturally . . . when I'm tired I can't be bothered so much, and I have to confess that as time's gone on, I often find being considerate a bit of a drag. I'd rather just go off into reading the paper, or get out of her way with a bit of work from the office. I feel 'safer' . . . more peaceful.

Apparently, Mr Foster had never felt authentic in doing the kind of 'family work' that women habitually perform, so over time too he was tending to retreat into a perhaps more authentic male remoteness. Finally, Mr Graham described how he had easily learned to do emotion work – once the need had been made clear to him by his wife!

> I've noticed I'm a bit like my mother – I seem to worry about other people in the same way, and . . . perhaps that makes me take a bit more notice of what my wife says. . . . When we were first married she used to go on and on about me being basically selfish . . . but now I've taken this on board to such an extent that I regard myself as a prime exhibit of a 'New Man'. You know, she feels confident to ask me when she wants sex, and to say what she'd like, and I don't feel 'threatened' . . . I even get to feel that this New Man has become the 'real me' . . . encouraged. But the depressing thing is that . . . when I'm really stressed out by work, or tired and kind of 'off my guard', then suddenly something will happen and I'll feel, 'Oh, sod it! Caught out again!' It seems like the real me hasn't changed at all.

Unusually for a man, Mr Graham seems to have found it relatively easy to do emotion work on behalf of others, but interestingly even he was occasionally forced to wonder whether his new self was really authentic. More generally, although a number of husbands had managed to learn that shallow acting could make couple life easier, very few seem to have felt authentic, and most had sooner or later stopped doing the emotion work necessary to sustain 'being a couple', although not apparently that required to 'be a man'.

Women, emotion work and authenticity

Most of the long-term married women we interviewed seemed aware that they sometimes engaged in shallow acting, and Mrs Walker's comments clearly illustrated the complex focus and multiple benefits of her emotion work:

> [My husband] can be a very sarcastic man at times, although I do love him . . . so I find myself softening what he says, tidying it up and smiling to make it seem like a joke – which perhaps it is, but people can't tell. Sometimes I get fed up of being on my guard, but it's important to me, to be seen to be living with a decent man. In a funny way, I feel it would rub off on me if everyone thought he was awful.

Mrs Walker did emotion work on others on behalf of her husband, and by improving his image to help him, she too felt rewarded by the way her own social standing was increased along with his. Like other women who had very mixed feelings about their husbands, she confessed that emotion work was sometimes difficult: 'It's just that resentment pops out sometimes . . . but don't think we're not happy together because we are.'

In the longer term, some women said they had tired of what they had come to perceive as the unfairness and inequality of relationships where they did all the emotion work and seemed to get no direct emotional benefits in return. Mrs Nolan said:

> I used to say to my husband when he got home things like 'Go and see Paul, he's had a very bad day at school, I know he's being bullied. Pretend you don't know and get him to talk to you about it, perhaps give him a cuddle and tell him you love him', you know the sort of thing. . . . [And] they thought their dad was excellent and I sort of got off on that . . . I felt like we were a real good family. But as the children have got older, to tell you the truth, I've got fed up of doing it, because I supervise the homework and I'm the one who has to keep on at the kids . . . and he's always Mr Nice Guy. In fact I tell you what I do now . . . I say, 'Take Kate to see that film, it's on and she wants to go', but when Kate comes to me and says, 'Dad's a really great bloke, he even remembered I liked Mel Gibson', I tell her, 'He didn't remember, I told him.' It's awful really, 'cos I see the hurt come across her face. Cruel, eh?

Nevertheless, Mrs Nolan later confessed that she occasionally started to build her husband up again 'because it suddenly seems to me that I'm not being very nice'. Apparently, her self-withdrawal had made her realize the rewards that not only her children but also she herself gained from doing emotion work to build her husband up as a father and family man. And although she had grown cynical about her husband, she occasionally engaged in self-distanced shallow acting in relation to her husband for the benefit of her family life and sense of authenticity as a mother. Some women described their growing cynicism about doing emotion work for their husbands by saying, 'I've realized that I don't love him any more.'

These are all examples of how wives had started out by feeling authentic while doing emotion work, but to differing degrees they distanced themselves or even withdrew into intermittent, selective, calculated, or even cynical shallow acting, where they felt 'more able' to preserve some sense of authenticity.

However, the more interesting situations we encountered seemed to raise questions concerning the first of Hochschild's scenarios – 'self-loss' – which at first glance appear to correspond to the stereotype of the 'Stepford wife'. Although we did not find anyone who matched this stereotype, we were tempted to call some women 'Stepford pretenders', because they appeared so determined in their efforts to deep act away their knowledge of their husbands' manifest faults. For example, Mrs Darnley said:

> I know lots of people don't like [my husband], and I suppose if I thought about it [hesitation] there's lots of things I know I wouldn't like. . . . Sometimes people try to tell me things, and I just don't want to hear . . . I mean I wouldn't like to watch anything about violence or, say, disabled or poverty-stricken people on TV, because I would know it would upset me, so I choose not to think about it. I'm afraid I cope with most unpleasant things in life like that, and my marriage is just one of those things. We're happy as we are. [Pause . . . then a smile] Ah, well, such is life!

Of course, there are pressures on women to deep act away doubts about their partners, but what strikes us most is how Mrs Darnley seemed to cope not only with her marriage but with most other things by actively resisting self-reflection. We would suggest that although Mrs Darnley could not remain totally unaware, her sense of authenticity was as 'someone who does not think about unpleasantness', and this may be one major personality difference among women – and perhaps a trait shared by many men (Weiss 1990).

Finally, in relation to the stereotype of the Stepford wife, the most interesting woman we encountered was Mrs Saint. She appeared to devote her life totally to being helpful and supportive, not only to her children and her husband – whom she loved, though admitting he was rarely there and made no domestic input – but also to many other people and good causes. Mrs Saint appeared fully aware of the toll that all her emotion work on behalf of others took on her own emotional resources, but offered her own explanation for her behaviour:

> Sometimes I'll have spent all day, listening to everybody's problems, an endless stream, and the kids come home and I listen to them and then [my husband] comes home and he's had a bad day and he wants me to pamper him, and I love him, he's a good man. But inside my head I'm

screaming. I'm so tired . . . it's like I need to shut myself away in a room. But it's bound up with my upbringing and the church. I care very deeply for others and . . . I see it as my duty to make the world a better place. It makes me feel better. It's important to me to *know* I'm a good person. But that's how I am, it's my personality. I get really fed up when my feminist friends tell me I'm suffering from some kind of 'false conscious-ness' . . . as if I'm somehow really stupid. They get cross, they say I should think about myself for a change, harden myself up and do things for me rather than other people. But pleasing other people *is* for me.

Mrs Saint raises, in the most acute form, the question we have been address-ing in this chapter, concerning the trade-off between doing emotion work and loss of authenticity. In fact, in every respect – including what Hochs-child calls emotional 'burnout' – she fits the scenario of self-loss through doing emotion work which we have suggested corresponds to the stereotype of the Stepford wife. Yet despite her knowledge that she was exploited and her feminist friends' exhortations to become more authentic by acting for herself, she insisted that she experienced a sense of authenticity from seeing herself as 'someone who gives'.

IN CONCLUSION: THE SEARCH FOR AUTHENTICITY

In conclusion we will briefly return to the following questions posed at the beginning of this chapter. What exactly is the emotion work that women do? Can and do men also do similar emotion work in their intimate couple rela-tionships? Are there variations in how individual men and women do emo-tion work? Must individuals who do emotion work inevitably lose their authenticity? And would that loss be better described in Marxist terms as 'false consciousness', or by psychoanalytical terms such as 'repression and denial'? Clearly, these questions are too many and too difficult to answer in one short chapter – as we now realize more clearly than when we began this exploration! However, we believe that some of the issues can at least be further clarified.

We would suggest that disagreements about gender differences in doing emotion work have proliferated because of the amorphous and bland use of the concept. Evidence from empirical research confirms that in intimate couple relationships, most women and most men do indeed *appear* to conform to the gender stereotypes of 'Stepford wives' and 'hollow men'. However, this is partly a consequence of the difficulties of researching men's emotional behaviour, but also of the way that women's and men's performance of emotion work – on and for others, and on and for them-selves – tends to be done in the context of gender inequalities of power and resources, in response to different ideological feeling rules with different goals, and is undertaken with the broadly different emotional skills, propen-sities and capacities which individuals have developed in early childhood and adolescence. Recent gender theory suggests there might be individual variations among men and women in how they do emotion work, and indeed our research has suggested that such individual variations can be seen. Yet we must conclude with Morgan (1992) that these are still 'variations on a deeply entrenched theme'.

Finally, in relation to loss of authenticity, we have suggested that there has been a tendency to take at face value the implications of the phrase emotion *work* and there has been too little research on how individuals feel about the emotion work they do – particularly whether individuals find emotion work burdensome and alienating, or whether it may sometimes be rewarding. This is perhaps understandable in view of the methodological, ethical, theoretical and philosophical difficulties involved (Duncombe and Marsden 1996a). But we also noted earlier that Marxist feminists have been inclined to discount women's consciousness as 'false', while critics from psychoanalysis and psychotherapy (and indeed also from sociology) have doubted whether sociologists are equipped to research and understand emotions.

These doubts bring us back to individuals like Mrs Saint, who appears to be fully aware of how she behaves and even how she is exploited, but who hotly denies the charge of 'false consciousness'. Psychoanalysts or therapists might want to insist that she is deeply repressing or denying her own 'real' needs, as a result of influences in early childhood and adolescence, and we would agree that, at this level, sociologists cannot offer to explain *why* Mrs Saint is like she is, and how her present self and identity have developed through her earlier experiences.

As sociologists, we can only (as Hochschild originally intended) offer a description of how Mrs Saint behaves under the influences from social feeling rules. But unlike Hochschild we would be more careful to distinguish between 'authenticity' and 'real feelings', and individuals' *sense* of authenticity in relation to the core self and identity that they have developed through their earlier experiences. Reversing Hochschild's comment that for women 'being becomes a way of doing', we would suggest that for Mrs Saint 'doing becomes a way of being': she assesses the authenticity of her behaviour against herself as 'someone who gives'. It seems to us that in the end – lacking any independent guide to truly 'authentic' emotional behaviour – we have to accept that some individuals may derive their *sense* of authenticity from 'core selves' and 'core identities' which various commentators might want to criticize as deeply inauthentic – although at the most fundamental level they can do so only on ideological or essentialist grounds.

BIBLIOGRAPHY

Acock, C. and Demo, D. (1994) *Family Diversity and Well-Being*. London: Sage.
Backett, K. (1987) 'The negotiation of fatherhood', in C. Lewis and M. O'Brien (eds) *Fatherhood Reassessed*. London: Sage, pp. 74–90.

Berk, S. (1985) *The Gender Factory*. New York: Plenum.
Brannen, J. and Collard, J. (1982) *Marriages in Trouble*. London: Tavistock.
Chodorow, N. (1978) *The Reproduction of Mothering*. London: University of California Press.
Cline, S. and Spender, D. (1987) *Reflecting Men*. London: André Deutsch.
Cohen, D. (1990) *Being a Man*. London: Routledge.
Connell, R. W. (1987) *Gender and Power*. Cambridge: Polity Press.
Connell, R. W. (1995) *Masculinities*. Cambridge: Polity Press.
Coward, R. (1992) *Our Treacherous Hearts*. London: Faber.
Craib, I. (1995) 'Some comments on the sociology of the emotions', *Sociology* 29: 151–8.
Delphy, C. and Leonard, D. (1992) *Familiar Exploitation*. Cambridge: Polity Press.
Duck, S. and Gilmour, R. (eds) (1981) *Personal Relationships*, Vol. 2. London: Academic Press.
Duncombe, J. and Marsden, D. (1993) 'Love and intimacy: the gender division of emotion and emotion work', *Sociology* 27: 221–41.
Duncombe, J. and Marsden, D. (1995) 'Can men love?; "reading", "staging" and "resisting" the romance', in L. Pearce and J. Stacey (eds) *Romance Revisited*. London: Lawrence & Wishart, pp. 238–50.
Duncombe, J. and Marsden, D. (1996a) 'Can we research the private sphere?', in L. Morris and E. Stina Lyon (eds) *Gender Relations in Public and Private*. London: Macmillan, pp. 141–55.
Duncombe, J. and Marsden, D. (1996b) 'Whose orgasm is this anyway? "Sex work" in long-term couple relationships', in J. Weeks and J. Holland (eds) *Sexual Cultures*. London: Macmillan, pp. 220–38.
Duncombe, J. and Marsden, D. (1996c) 'Extending the social', *Sociology* 30: 156–8.
Farrell, W. (1974) *The Liberated Man*. New York: Random House.
Ferree, M. (1990) 'Beyond separate spheres: feminism and family research', *Journal of Marriage and the Family* 52: 866–84.
Furstenberg, F. and Cherlin, A. (1991) *Divided Families*. Cambridge, MA: Harvard University Press.
Giddens, A. (1991) *Modernity and Self-Identity*. Cambridge: Polity Press.
Giddens, A. (1992) *The Transformation of Intimacy*. Cambridge: Polity Press.
Gilligan, C. (1982) *In a Different Voice*. Cambridge, MA: Harvard University Press.
Hite, S. (1988) *Women and Love*. London: Viking.
Hochschild, A. R. (1983) *The Managed Heart: The Commercialization of Human Feeling*. Berkeley, CA: University of California Press.
Hochschild, A. R. (1990) *The Second Shift*. London: Piatkus.
Jackson A. (1990) *Unmasking Masculinity*. London: Unwin Hyman.
Jensen, K. (1974) 'Naked change: revising sexuality', in M. King (ed.) *One of the Boys*. New Zealand: Heinemann.
Lawrence, D. H. (1986) *Poems*. Harmondsworth, Mx: Penguin.
Lewis, C. and O'Brien, R. (eds) (1987) *Fatherhood Reassessed*. London: Sage.
Mac an Ghaill, M. (1994) *The Making of Men*. Milton Keynes, Bucks: Open University Press.
Mansfield, P. and Collard, J. (1988) *The Beginning of the Rest of Your Life?* London: Macmillan.
Metcalf, A. and Humphries, M. (1985) *The Sexuality of Men*. London: Pluto Press.
Miller, J. B. (1986) *Towards a New Psychology of Women*. Harmondsworth, Mx: Penguin.
Morgan, D. (1992) *Discovering Men*. London: Routledge.
Parsons, T. and Bales, R. (eds) (1956) *Family, Socialization and Interaction Process*. London: Routledge & Kegan Paul.

Roper, M. (1994) *Masculinity and the British Organization Man since 1946*. Oxford: Oxford University Press.

Rubin, L. (1984) *Intimate Strangers*. New York: Harper & Row.

Rubin, L. (1991) *Erotic Wars*. New York: Harper & Row.

Segal, L. (1987) *Slow Motion*. London: Virago.

Seidler, V. (1985) 'Fear and intimacy', in A. Metcalf and M. Humphries (eds) *The Sexuality of Men*. London: Pluto Press, pp. 150–81.

Tannen, D. 1991: *You Just Don't Understand*. London: Virago.

Thompson, L. and Walker, A. (1989) 'Gender in families: women and men in marriage, work and parenthood', *Journal of Marriage and the Family* 51: 845–71.

Vaughan, D. (1987) *Uncoupling*. London: Methuen.

Weiss, R. (1990) *Staying the Course*. New York: Fawcett Columbine.

West, C. and Zimmerman, D. (1987) 'Doing gender', *Gender and Society* 1: 125–51.

13 Changes in the 'lust balance' of sex and love since the sexual revolution

The example of the Netherlands

Cas Wouters

INTRODUCTION

In Victorian statements such as 'the more spiritual love of a woman will refine and temper the more sensual love of a man' (Calcar 1886: 47), the sensual love and carnal desires of women are hardly acknowledged, if at all. Such statements typify an ideal of love that is as passionate as it is exalted and desexualized (cf. Stearns 1994), with a rather depersonalized sexuality as a drawback and outlet for his 'wild' sensuality behind the scenes of social life. Although in the twentieth century a 'sexualization of love' and an 'erotization of sex' (Seidman 1991)[1] have continued, until the second half of this century the dominant social code regarding the sexuality of women and men continued to represent a lust-dominated sexuality for men and a complementary (romantic) love or relationship-dominated sexuality for women. This 'traditional lust balance' was attacked in the 1950s, when the topic of female sexual pleasure and gratification gained considerable importance in sexual advice literature. Especially from the 1960s on, the sexual longings of all women, including the 'respectable' and the unmarried, could openly be acknowledged and discussed. Then, for the first time, women themselves actively took part in public discussions about their carnal desires and sought a more satisfactory relationship between the longing for sexual gratification and the longing for enduring intimacy (love, friendship) – a more satisfying lust balance. These longings are interconnected, but not unproblematically. Today, some people (mostly men) even view them as contradictory. In any case, changes in individuals' codes and ideals as well as changes in public morality regarding sex and love have coincided with rising tensions between the two types of longing. From the 1960s on, topics and practices such as premarital sex, sexual variations, unmarried cohabitation, fornication, extramarital affairs, jealousy, homosexuality, pornography, teenage sex, abortion, exchange of partners, paedophilia, incest and so on, all part of a wider process of informalization, implied repeated confrontations with the traditional lust balance. As studies into the connection and the tension between love and sex are rare, while historical studies into this area are even harder to find,[2] what follows is an 'essay'. It is an attempt at sketching a coherent picture of these social and psychic changes within and between the sexes, and to unfold a perspective that is inherent in the concept of the lust balance. This concept is taken from Norbert Elias, who used it in a wider sense, indicating the whole 'lust economy' (1994: 456–519). Here, the concept is used to focus on the relationship between sex and love, a 'balance' that is perceived to be polymorphous and multidimensional (just as in Elias's concepts of a power balance and a tension balance): the attempt to find a satisfying balance between the longing for sex and the longing for love may be complicated by many other longings; for instance, by the longing to raise one's social status or by the longing for children.

Empirical evidence is drawn from a study of changes in the popular Dutch feminist monthly magazine *Opzij*[3] (Aside/Out of the Way!), established in 1973, and from sexual advice books. In addition, reference is made to data resulting from sociological and sexological research, as well as from the experience of these decades. Some of these data refer to changes in actual behaviour but most of them refer to changes in codes and ideals of behaviour and feeling. This selection of empirical evidence also implies a stronger focus on women, the women's movement and the emancipation of women, and, by implication, on female sexuality. The reaction of men, their accommodation and the restraining of their sexuality will receive less attention, partly because for men there is no source of evidence comparable with *Opzij* that could be studied as diachronically and systematically: accommodation processes are rather 'quiet' on the whole.

Central to this study is what might be called the lust-balance question: *when and within what kind of relationship(s) are (what kind of) eroticism and sexuality allowed and desired?* This question is first raised in puberty or adolescence when bodily and erotic impulses and emotions that were banned from interaction from early childhood onwards (except in cases of incest) are again explored and experimented with:

> Sexual education predominantly consists of 'beware and watch out'. The original need for bodily contact or touching, which has a very spontaneous frankness in children, also becomes prey to this restriction in the course of growing up. Sexuality *and* corporality are thus separated from other forms of contact. Whenever two people enter an affair, the taboo on touching and bodily contact has to be gradually dismantled. For most people, this is a process of trial and error.
>
> (Zeegers 1994: 139)

In this century, especially since the 1960s, it seems that a similar process of trial and error has been going on collectively, bringing about a collective emancipation of sexuality, that is, a collective diminution in fear of sexuality and its expression within increasingly less rigidly curtailed relationships. Sexual impulses and emotions were allowed (once again) into the centre of the personality – consciousness – and thus taken into account, whether acted upon or not. Both women and men became involved in a collective learning process – experimenting in mainstreams and undercurrents – in which they have tried to find new ideals and ways of gratifying their longing for both sex and love. The questions and answers with which they were confronted will have shifted and varied along with changes in the spectrum of prevailing interpretations of what constitutes a satisfying lust balance. This chapter aims at a description and interpretation of this collective learning process.

CHANGES IN THE LUST BALANCE

The sexual revolution

The sexual revolution was a breakthrough in the emancipation of female sexuality even though many women throughout these years continued to think of sex in terms of duty (Frenken 1976), sometimes worsened by the new 'duty' to achieve orgasm. Due to the 'pill' and an increase in mutually expected self-restraint (mutual consent) in interactions, the dangers and fears connected with sex diminished to such a degree that there was an acceleration in the emancipation of sexual emotions and impulses. Women's sexual desires were taken more seriously: men became 'more strongly directed at clitoral stimulation' and their aversion to oral sex diminished considerably – from more than 50 per cent reported in the early 1970s to about 20 per cent ten years later (Vennix and Bullinga 1991: 57). This means that increasing numbers of men learned to enjoy the woman's enjoyment and that many women have opened up to sexual fantasies and titillations. In a relatively short period of time, the relatively autonomous strength of carnal desire became acknowledged and respected.[4] For both genders, sex for the sake of sex changed from a degrading spectre into a tolerable and thus acceptable alternative, allowing more women and men to experiment with sex cheerfully and outside the boundaries of love and law. Until around 1970, the slogan of the advice literature that accompanied this process was that 'men should restrain themselves somewhat more and women should be a bit more daring' (Röling 1990: 90), a slogan that was obviously attuned to men who came too quickly and women who did not come at all. From then on, interest and attention shifted from joint pleasures towards discovering one's own sexual desires and delights. In close connection with this, the ideal of love shifted further away from the Victorian ideal of a highly elevated marital happiness towards individual happiness and greater scope for both partners to develop themselves (Blom 1993; Mahlmann 1991; Swidler 1980). In the early 1970s, the growing emphasis on individual development also came to be expressed collectively in the deliberately created 'apartheid' of discussion groups, refuge homes, pubs, bookshops, etc., 'for women only', expressing an outlook of 'emancipation-via-segregation' (cf. van Stolk 1991).

Sex-for-the-sake-of-sex was first and to a greater extent accepted among homosexual men, and the far-reaching liberation of sexuality among them was a topic that was also frequently discussed outside their circles, with both an envious and a frightened tone. The comparison with homosexuals also had another function, put into words by Joke Kool-Smit (commonly credited with having triggered the second feminist wave in the Netherlands):

> feminists and homosexuals are each other's natural allies for they are facing a 'common struggle' [she explains] not only because both groups are discriminated against, but from a much deeper similarity between the liberation of women and of homosexuals. Both demand the right not to behave like a woman or a man ought to, they do not accommodate to their sex role of strong man and soft woman.
>
> *(Opzij* 11 (1973): 26)

The struggle for liberation from the straitjacket of sex roles obviously had priority, but as far as sexual liberation was concerned, Kool-Smit referred to lesbian women as a model:

> lesbian feminists could be an example for other women with regard to their relationships and in finding a distinct identity. For in these relation-ships where men are absent, emotional warmth need not come from one side/partner only, and erotics can at last be separated from dominance.
>
> *(Opzij* 11 (1973): 26)[5]

In their quest for a more satisfying lust balance, the two sexes tended to go in opposite directions, led by their gender-specific definitions of lust: men towards lust-dominated sexuality, towards sex for the sake of sex as (imagined) in the world of homosexual men, and women towards a love- and relationship-dominated sexuality in which physical love and psychical love are integrated and set apart from domination as (imagined) in the world of homosexual women. As many women and men will have experi-enced, the relationship between carnal desires and the longing for enduring intimacy is an uneasy one and the continuation and maintenance of a (love) relationship had on the whole become more demanding. The feelings of insecurity, shame, guilt, fear and jealousy, as well as the conflicts, divorces and other problems related to their drifting lust balance, were all perceived and discussed, for instance, in the encounter and sensitivity movement, but hardly, if at all, by the women's movement. At the time, the spirit of libera-tion from the straitjacket of older generations and their morality, and the fervour of the movement did not allow much attention to be given to the *demands* of the liberation.

From 'sexual liberation' to 'sexual oppression'

In several respects the sexual revolution ended towards the end of the 1970s, as the voices against sexual violence became louder and louder. At that time, as the study of *Opzij* shows, in addition to sexual assault and rape, sex with children – incest in particular – and pornography also came to be included in the category of sexual violence. In the early 1980s, sexual harassment was added. As the women's movement turned against sexual violence, attention shifted from differences between the generations to differences between the sexes. Opposition to the sexual practices and morality of older generations diminished, while opposition to those of the dominant sex gained momentum (van Daalen and van Stolk 1991). 'Greater sexual openness and more acceptance of sexuality had brought sexual abuse into sight' (Schnabel 1990: 16), and this was another reason for the shift of emphasis from sexual liberation to sexual oppression. In the media, the misery surrounding sex came under the floodlights. In the women's movement, heterosexuality was sometimes branded as 'having sex with your oppressor', a sentiment also expressed in the lesbian slogan 'more sun, fewer men'. Hardly anything but 'soft sex' – sex that is not aimed at intercourse – still attracted positive attention, and the phrase '*potteus bewustzijn*' (lesbian consciousness) became popular as a kind of yardstick for feminism.[6] Retrospectives on the 'years of sexual liberation' were also increasingly set in a negative tone.

The change of perspective and feeling from liberation to oppression, occurring from the end of the 1970s into the first half of the 1980s, did not imply an increase in attention to the demands of liberation, that is, increased demands on self-regulation, such as the capacity to negotiate a more ideal lust balance. Whereas before the fervour of the struggle against the old morality had prevented this, now moral indignation about oppression functioned as such a barrier. This indignation also produced a blinkered view of the (gender-specific) difficulties connected with the emancipation of sexual impulses and emotions. Directing public attention to the difficulties of women in particular was met with moral indignation by feminists; it was branded as 'individualizing', that is, as reducing structured male oppression to individual problems of women. While the perspective did shift collectively from the other (older) generation to the other sex (men), it remained almost exclusively directed *outwards*: the origin as well as the solution of all difficulties was to be found in oppression by men.

Banning the psychical demands of emancipation from public discussions and from sight did not, of course, facilitate the quest for a new lust balance, as may be concluded from two extreme ways in which it was sought. One extreme consisted of a romanticization of old we-and-I feelings – of traditional female solidarity and identity – and an attack on pornography as a form of sexual violence. Here, the implicit lust balance strongly emphasizes love and soft sex, coupled to tenderness and affection. This view was the dominant one, and also advocated by the intellectual avant-garde of the women's movement. Only one author deviated strongly from the general trend by expressing regret that a monthly like *Playgirl*, in comparison with magazines for homosexuals, contained so few pictures evoking a visual pleasure that presupposed 'a pleasure in sex without the ballast of love' (Ang 1983: 433; Wouters 1984). Other contrasting voices did not go nearly as far and, taken together, in the early 1980s their force seems to have shrunk to a marginal whisper. In that margin, the other extreme was to be found. It consisted of a tipping of the lust balance to its opposite side. According to tradition, a woman should have sexual desires and fantasies only *within* a romantic relationship, which was meant to last a lifetime. In a lust balance that is tipped the other way, a woman's sexuality could be aroused only *outside* such a relationship, in almost anonymous, instant sex. All public discussion focused on the first of these two extremes, while the second remained virtually in the shadows. A closer inspection of both extremes follows in the next two sections.

The anti-pornography movement

During the first half of the 1980s, protests against pornography were numerous and sizeable, sometimes even violent. In 1980, a massive anti-pornography demonstration was held in Utrecht. Slogans such as 'pornography is hatred of women' and 'pornography is sexual violence' became well known. In 1984, a Dutch ministerial report on sexual violence was strongly against pornography and against 'the process of pornographization in the media, in the advertising industry and in mass-produced literature' (*Nota* 1984: 47). To the extent that this stance was explained, reference was made to a romantic ideal of love, thus preventing any public recognition of the appreciation of sex, and certainly not of sex for the sake of sex.

Although pornography certainly contains many examples of images that are degrading to women, the rejection of the whole genre was nevertheless remarkable. For one thing, the numerous protests against pornography usually suggested that only men were susceptible to this kind of titillation of the senses, and that therefore only men were responsible for the process of 'erotization', referred to as 'pornographization' in the ministerial report. In view of data derived from experimental research, available at the time, this is quite unlikely: images and fantasies of fortuitous sexual conquests by sexually active and dominant women could certainly titillate the female senses. This kind of research suggests that it is plausible to assume that both women and men are more strongly sexually aroused by fantasies and images of sexual chance meetings than by those of marital or bought sexual intercourse (Fisher and Byrne 1978), that fantasies about 'casual' and 'committed' sex make no difference in women's sexual arousal (Mosher and White 1980) and that women, just like men, are more strongly sexually excited by fantasies and images of sex that is initiated and dominated by someone of their own gender (Heiman 1977; Garcia *et al.* 1984; at a later date also: Dekker 1987: 37; Laan 1994). Furthermore, it also suggests that the difference between the sexes in experiencing pornography was relatively small, provoking more arousal and fewer conflicts and guilt feelings if women had been able to explore their sexuality more freely, just like men, and had developed a more liberal, 'modern' sexual morality (Sigusch and Schmidt 1970; Straver 1980: 55). An interesting (later) finding in this context is that on the whole, genital arousal – vasocongestion – occurs 'even when the erotic stimulus is evaluated negatively or gives rise to negative emotions and when little or no sexual arousal is reported' and that 'the gap between genital and subjective sexual arousal is smaller for women who masturbate frequently (10 to 20 times per month) than for women who masturbate less often or not at all' (Laan 1994: 78, 164, 169). This finding suggests the interpretation that women who masturbate often are better informed about their carnal desires and/or indulge more (easily) in them. In addition to frequency of masturbation, frequency of coitus also yielded higher correlations between genital and subjective sexual arousal (Dekker 1987).

Women's public opinion on pornography was also remarkable in comparison with that towards prostitution and 'pornoviolence' – imagined violence as the simple, ultimate solution to the problem of status competition (Wolfe 1976: 162). There have been hardly any protests by women against 'pornoviolence'. In the second half of the 1970s, next to pornography, prostitution also became a significant issue. At first the women's movement was ambivalent about prostitution, but in the 1980s the voices defending prostitutes increasingly drowned out the sounds of protest against them. Prostitutes even succeeded in winning the support of the mainstream women's movement. Yet in fact, on even more adequate grounds than those which apply to pornography, prostitution can be seen as a perverted expression of a sexual morality directed only towards male pleasure and to keeping women in the position of subordinates and servants. As far as 'consumption' is concerned they relate to each other as imagination (pornography) to action (prostitution), while the conditions and relationships of 'production' seem also to be in favour of pornography: the dangers for women are most probably larger in prostitution than on 'the set' or in a studio, and they are absent in the representation of sexual fantasies in books or paintings. In sum, the differences in moral indignation between pornography and prostitution are not likely to be explained by a difference in the dangers of production or consumption. Nor can this difference be explained by a reference to the prostitutes' organization *De Rode Draad* (The Red Thread), which was established only in 1985.

Except as a symptom of women's solidarity, the comparatively small extent of moral indignation at prostitution may be largely understood from women's sensitivity to the argument that there is little difference between the selling of sex in prostitution and in marriage – 'for the sake of peace, or as an expression of gratitude for a night out or a new dress' (*Opzij* 7–8 (1979): 41). In this 'sex-is-work' view, prostitutes may seem to have the upper hand by staying more independent and obtaining higher financial rewards. In this view, lust has no place and sex brings more displeasure than pleasure: women appear predominantly as sexual objects, not as sexual subjects. As such, it mirrors another view that was still widely held in the 1970s, the belief that men are entitled to have sex with their wives. In 1975, a detective of the Amsterdam vice squad was still shameless enough to say: 'I'm almost 60 years old now and I've raped my wife quite often. Yes, if she didn't want to [do it with me]' (*Opzij* 3–4 (1975): 38). In addition to this sex-is-work view, the image of the 'prankster' emerged: 'naughty' women who (more often than not) enjoy the sex they are paid for – an example of women turning traditional double morality upside down.

The protests against pornography also evoke surprise because they go against the flow of the twentieth-century process of informalization (increasing behavioural and feeling alternatives) and its inherent 'erotization of everyday life' (Wouters 1990, 1992). Together, all these arguments seem to permit the conclusion that the anti-pornography movement to a large degree was an 'emancipation cramp'. It was predominantly an expression of the problems connected with the emancipation of sexuality: the attack on male pornography was a sort of 'best defence', concealing as well as expressing a 'fear of freedom' (in Erich Fromm's famous phrase), a fear of experiencing and presenting oneself as a sexual subject.

What is the price of sex?

In the margin of the public debate, some of the difficulties attached to the emancipation of sexual feelings sometimes surfaced more or less casually, one of them being the risk of tipping over to the other extreme of the traditional lust balance. At this other extreme, sex was isolated by excluding sexual intimacy from most other forms of intimacy, as these had come to be experienced as obstacles to sexual pleasure. Sexual desires went to a 'sex without the ballast of love', while the forces which formerly forbade this – the social code and individual conscience – still had to be avoided with such energy and determination that their absence, so to speak, loomed large. This was expressed by a woman who said:

> For years and years I did not want any emotional commitment with men. . . . What I did do regularly at the time, though, was pick up a one-night stand. In fact, that suited me well. . . . Because I was not emotionally committed to those men, I was able to take care of my sexual needs very well. . . . It also gave me a feeling of power. I did just as I pleased, took the initiative myself and was very active.
>
> (Groenendijk 1983: 368)

A statement like this shows more than a shift of accent in the traditional mixture of love ('emotional commitment') and carnal desire. Here, the price of sex, to put it dramatically, is nothing less than love. The formulation – particularly the word 'because' – indicates that the lusts of the flesh can be given a free rein only if the longing for love is curbed radically, as radically

as lust was curbed before. The coexistence of an abhorrence of subordination to men with a longing for a loving relationship will have made
many women suspicious of their relational longing. They feared that if
they gave in to this craving for love, they would lose 'the feeling of
power' since they would (as usual) almost automatically flow into the
devouring dependence of a self-sacrificing love (cf. Dowling 1981). Therefore, what at first sight appears to be a fear of intimacy is in fact another
expression of the 'fear of freedom'.

As an undercurrent, this lust balance formed the negative of that propa-
gated by mainstream feminism, i.e. the anti-porno movement. It is an open
question as to how many women who in public turned against pornography
and, by implication, against male sexual fantasies, to some extent combined
this attitude in private with an escape from emotional commitment into
volatile sexual affairs. What may be concluded, however, if only from the
coexistence of these two extremes, is that in this period there must have
been a tug-of-war between and within women: *between* women who ventured into giving free rein to sex for the sake of sex, and women who rejected
this; and *within* women to the extent that women encountered both sides in
themselves, and met them with ambivalence. The question of how many and
how intensely women experienced this tug-of-war or ambivalence cannot be
answered. From a longer-term perspective, it is obvious, however, that
throughout the twentieth century and especially during the sexual revolution, many women have been involved in the quest for a more satisfying
lust balance, somewhere in between the extremes of 'love without the ballast
or duty of sex' and 'sex without the ballast of love'. No woman will have
been able completely to withdraw from this development and its inherent
tug-of-war and ambivalence, if only because before the sexual revolution the social code allowed women to express only one side of the lust
balance.

Lust revival

In the latter part of the 1980s, the outlook of leaders in the women's movement was less exclusively outward; that is, less focused on oppression by
men. They developed a more relational view of oppression, a view that
saw oppression as incorporated in the social code as well as within personality structures. Thus the difficulties and pressures connected with the emancipation of women and of emotions came to attract more attention. This
was aptly expressed in the title of the inaugural lecture of a professor of
women's studies: *The Burden of Liberation* (Brinkgreve 1988). Its point of
departure was the insight that 'greater freedom of choice once again
turned out to be a pressure to perform', as the historian Röling summarized
it (1994: 230). Consequently, emancipation (and assertive use of the greater
freedom of choice) was also seen as a learning process in which problems are
expected to occur as a matter of course:

It is the complicated task of a 'controlled letting go', making heavy
demands on affect control, and it is not to be expected that without a
learning process this will proceed spontaneously and 'smoothly'.

(Brinkgreve 1988: 14)

In the latter part of the 1980s, this more reflective outlook coincided with
further emancipation of sexual impulses and emotions. In magazines like
Opzij, more attention was given to themes like 'men as sexual objects',
bought sex for women, women's adultery, SM, positively evaluated passes
and eroticism in the workplace, and also to 'safe sex' (owing to AIDS).
These topics were discussed soberly. When an early attempt at commercia-
lizing this interest was made through the establishment of a Dutch version of
Playgirl, the magazine had the cautious and typical policy of not publishing
'frontal nudes'. It was defended with the argument that:

women have only in the last five years begun to discuss their fantasies.
Male nudity does not eroticize. . . . It is power which makes men eroti-
cally appealing. Hence the popularity of romance novels in which the
male star is a doctor, a successful businessman or an elderly father figure.

(*NRC Handelsblad*, 21 October 1987)

Yet the wave of moral indignation at pornography faded away and in retrospect the anti-pornography movement was characterized as a 'kind of
puritanism' (*Opzij* 9 (1988): 43). From the mid-1980s onwards, a number
of women-made, female-centred pornographic films showing women actively
initiating and enjoying sexual activity appeared on the market (Laan 1994:
163).[7]

In this period, a sexologist relativized the importance of 'intimacy'. She
wrote: 'in many ways, the need for intimacy can be a trap for women',
and after having presented some examples of women who like making
love to strangers, finding sexual pleasure, she concludes:

Indeed, at times there is this double feeling: you *do* want that pleasurable
experience of togetherness, you *do* want to have sex, but you don't bar-
gain for a rather too intimate steady relationship.

(*Opzij* 7–8 (1986): 69)

In 1988, in a special issue of *Opzij* on 'Women and lust', this argument was
supplemented with a strong attack on the traditional lust balance:

Tradition teaches a woman to experience her sexuality as predominantly
relational and intimate. But it is an amputation through traditional
female socialization to represent a sexuality so weakly directed at pleasure and lust.

The article, directed especially at 'career women who live alone', continues first with a plea to have 'sex for the sake of sex, to be erotic and horny but not emotionally committed' and then warns:

> If a woman nevertheless (secretly) needs intimacy in order to enjoy sex, she will be always left with a hangover. After too many hangovers she will stop having this kind of affair. Then, she may help herself, that is, masturbate. That can be gratifying too.
>
> *(Opzij* 1 (1988): 86–7)

In later years, this appreciation for masturbation is supported, although sometimes only half-heartedly because of being merely a copy of what men are used to doing *(Opzij* 2 (1989): 17).

A 'large study of sex and relationships', published in *Opzij* in 1989, comparing female readers of this magazine with a general sample of Dutch women, shows that the emancipation of women and of sexuality run in tandem. It concludes that *Opzij* readers in certain respects had become more like men – a 'masculinization'. They are, for instance, more playfully thinking about keeping up more than one relationship, and they rate having sex (masturbation as well as orgasm) higher on a scale. On the other hand, a 'feminization' is concluded from their pursuit of 'a sex between equals, allowing, even stimulating dedication':

> Traditional 'femininity', including tenderness, foreplay and passion, is not weakened in this process of renewal. On the contrary, men are expected to behave like this too. The renewal can be characterized as eroticizing feminization.
>
> *(Opzij* 1 (1988): 70)

In this period, the Chippendales and similar groups (of male strippers) appeared on the scene, and their success shows that the public titillation of female lust has become a socially accepted fact. However, their coquetry in military uniforms is a continuing variation upon the tradition of the Mills & Boon romance novels in which women need to look up to a man before they are willing to nestle in his arms (cf. van Stolk and Wouters 1987: 136–72). This pleasure in looking up shows how deeply rooted in the personality the longing for (male) protection is, while all the same it is based on the woman's subordination.

Since all the changes described above represent movements in the same direction, it is plausible that from the mid-1980s onward, the difference between men and women regarding their lust balance – ideal and practice – has diminished. There was a certain lust revival, an acceleration in the emancipation of sexuality. The revival was limited, however, as can be demonstrated from the lack of commercial success of magazines aiming at female sexual fantasies, magazines like *Playgirl* and *BEV*: both disappeared after a few issues.

Lust and love revival

In the 1990s, further revival of female lust has been expressed in the success-ful sales figures of mailing businesses and chain stores marketing erotic arti-cles for women, in particular from the sale of vibrators: both in 1993 and 1994 there has been an increase of 25 per cent (*NRC Handelsblad*, 6 April 1995). Owners of videoshops have reported women's growing interest in porno-videos. A 'sexuality weakly directed at pleasure and lust' has become more of a humiliating spectre, while at the same time the sex that prospers in anonymity, sex-for-the-sake-of-sex, evokes far fewer elated reac-tions, and not only in the context of AIDS. A Dutch trend-watcher claims: 'Sex for the sake of sex is out. . . . Sex is once again being perceived as part of a relationship (as it seems to have been before the sexual revolution)' (Kuitenbrouwer 1990: 48–9). And an assertive heading in a book on 'erotic manners' reads: 'Sex for the sake of sex is old-fashioned' (van Eijk 1994). These statements are backed up by research data on young people; they confirm: 'Free sex certainly has not become a new sin, but it is losing popularity.' As an ideal, 'most young people think of love and sexual plea-sure as two sides of the same coin, and this goes for both boys and girls' (van der Vliet 1990: 65). In 1995, 'having strong feelings for each other' sufficed for three-quarters of the Dutch school population (aged 12 years and older) as a precondition to having sex (Brugman *et al.* 1995). This attitude is rein-forced by their parents: 'Many report the presence of a "relationship" to be decisive for their consent to a teenage child wanting to have sex. Some indi-cate that depth and stability of a relationship, more than age or anything else, makes having sex acceptable' (Schalet 1994: 117). Teenagers themselves in no way exclude the possibility of having sex for its own sake, but in the longer run the ideal of lovers being matched to each other, including in bed, seems to have gained strength. This interpretation is supported by an increase in the number of young people between 17 and 24 years old who would consider an act of sexual infidelity to be the end of a relationship; in a 1979 survey, 41 per cent held that opinion and in 1989/1993 this had risen to 63 per cent. This very trend is most spectacular for cohabiting youngsters (by now a 'normal' way of life) from 30 to 65 per cent (Centraal Bureau Van der Statistiek 1994: 15).

In the 1990s, the women's movement joined this trend under the new name of 'power-feminism'. Women's solidarity was no longer axiomatic; women could and did co-operate with men, and this attitude coincided with an increasingly mounted attack on those who still emphasized oppres-sion. This was branded 'victim feminism' and denounced as 'victimism'. The attack was also aimed at romanticizing old harmonious (as well as unequal) relationships and the lust balance of predominantly 'sweet and soft'; by call-ing that 'vanilla sex' a larger variety of tastes is indicated as acceptable.

In the homosexual world as well, pioneers in the cultivation of sex for its own sake have lately expressed an ambivalent if not critical attitude towards this (tilted) lust balance. Opposing the lust profit of 'the streamlined way in which sex was organized, discarded from clumsy introductions and annoying questions', Stephan Sanders (1994: 47, 46, 13, 18) mentions the loss of lust in having sex without passion: 'the continuous coupling . . . of more or less perfunctory fucks – the waiting, the posing desirably, the taking down of the trousers, the panting, the hoisting up of the trousers'. Here 'the suspicion that, despite all his efforts, his grip on his desire had not gained strength, but had rather weakened' is gnawing. This outlook implies the view that in the longer run, the absence of passion or emotional involvement limits the possibility of having a lustful orgasm.

On the whole, the changes of the 1990s can be interpreted as a love or relationship revival. There was an intensified attempt at integrating relational and sexual desires on another level, representing a shift in the ideal lust balance towards 'diminishing contrasts and increasing varieties' (Elias 1994: 460 ff.). This diagnosis is confirmed by other research data showing that 'on the whole, women feel like having sex more often, allow more sexual incentives more easily and have learned to discuss these matters more freely', whereas 'on the whole, men have learned to connect relational satisfaction and sexual gratification' (Straver *et al.* 1994: 154–64).

The emancipation of female sexuality and its counterpart, the bonding of male sexuality, will have certainly been channelled by literature (like feminist publications), by protest activities (like those against sexual violence and harassment) and by changes in the law (like making rape in marriage liable to penalty). But even more significant for explaining this process is the pincer movement that has affected men: they have found themselves between their longing for an enduring intimacy, on the one hand, which became subjected earlier and more strongly to more or less rigorous limitations such as desertion and divorce or the threat of them; and their increasing dependence upon their talent to arouse and stimulate a woman's desires, on the other hand, for satisfying their own sexuality.

REGULARITIES IN PROCESSES OF INTEGRATION AND CIVILIZATION

In this process of integration and civilization of the sexes, and in interconnected changes in the dominant lust balance, a few patterns can be discerned. These are regularities in all integrating and civilizing processes, to be presented in the following sections.

Lust anxiety: social and sexual fear of 'heights' and 'depths'

The first regularity is related to the mechanism of 'identification with the established': identifying with the uneven balance of power between the sexes functions as a psychical impediment in developing a higher-levelled and more integrated lust balance with more sex. It produces a lust anxiety in women: they remain afraid of the 'shame' of becoming more of a sexual subject, of the consequences of repudiating, if only in fantasy, the attitude of subordination. It is a 'fear of freedom'. From the fear of running wild through loosening up, they clam up. Their source of power and identity, the whole of their personality, is still strongly interwoven with the old balance of power between the sexes and also with the old lust balance, the old ratio of relational and sexual desires. In this respect, homosexual women seem more like heterosexual women than homosexual (and heterosexual) men. Many lesbian women report having difficulties in taking sexual initiatives or in seducing their partners:

> In this context, their need to avoid even the slightest ring of dominance, power or male sexual behaviour, and to repudiate any behaviour that could possibly be experienced as an imitation of heterosexuality, is often mentioned as an impediment.
>
> (Schreurs 1993: 333)

From this outlook, the psychical repercussion of the uneven balance of power between the sexes is still a substantial barrier for continued emancipation of sexual impulses and emotions. This barrier might be conceptualized as a fear of social and psychical (including sexual) heights (Wouters 1990: 74–5 and 98). With regard to the men's accommodation process, the counterpart of this barrier might be conceptualized as social and psychical (including sexual) fear of depths, a fear of losing traditional sources of power and identity and of the jealousy and desertion anxieties that are involved, which prevent men from imagining and enjoying the pleasures of a more restrained kind of intercourse with a woman – the more 'civilized' satisfaction which this may bring. An example of someone struggling with this fear of depth comes from an interview with a man who sometimes watches pornographic videos with his wife and who reported being struck by a terrific stab of jealousy when his wife once said: 'It's odd, I'm 31 years old now and yet I only know your dick.' And he continued with an example of what he called the enormous gap between his emotions and his mind:

> For instance, the other day she asked me to lie at her side of the bed, so it would be pleasantly warm by the time she got in. That's what I did, and I don't see any reason why not, but I did feel like an idiot. I thought: 'Luckily my friends can't see me because they would laugh their heads off, Charly impersonating a hot-water bottle.'
>
> (van Stolk and Wouters 1987: 133 and 249)

Lacking data, it must remain an open question how many and to what extent men have suffered from impotence or other forms of loss of lust as an 'accommodation cramp'. However, simply raising this question may suffice to suggest that the distinction between safe sex and emotionally safe sex (Orbach 1994: 165) is significant for both sexes.

Three types: trend-followers, radicals and moderates

Another important regularity follows from the fact that emancipation and accommodation are learning processes in which there are differences in tempo and emphasis, on which basis three different groups can be discerned: there are always trend-followers, radicals and moderates (cf. van Stolk 1991: 59–60). With regard to the lust balance, these three types correspond to the three possibilities or scenarios that are open after the first few preliminary moves on the road of love and sex have been made:

> At that point, the outlines of different possibilities become apparent: one resigns oneself to one's partner's limits and satisfies oneself with what has been accomplished [followers]. The second possibility consists of a continued transgression of boundaries, the path of lust [radicals]. The third solution consists of preserving or reviving sexual tension and challenge in contact with the present partner [moderates].
>
> (Zeegers 1994: 140)

From the sexual revolution onwards, moderates and radicals continued the emancipation of sexuality, whereas trend-followers lagged behind. Confronted with new possibilities, some of these followers actually clammed up. Radicals have continued on the path of lust, whereas moderates have 'learned' to combine their longing for an enduring intimacy with their carnal desires.

One would expect an unequal division of the sexes among the three types, if only because the dangers and anxieties surrounding sex (rape, unwanted pregnancy, etc.) have always been (and are) greater for women than for men. In addition, for many women sex functioned as an important source of power (as a means of temptation, reward and punishment) and identity. On this basis it is to be expected that the fear of giving up that traditional female pattern has been (and is) stronger. However, research into these three types revealed that moderates consist of just as many men as women. Moderates are reported to have developed the kind of sex in which 'lust and proximity are intrinsically connected, and even indulging in lust has the denotation of frankness'. This kind of sex is 'not a personal feature but a characteristic of the interaction with the partner' – that is, of the relationship (Zeegers 1994: 138–40). This means that, as the principle of mutual consent became anchored and expanded both within a relationship and in having sex, the development of such a lust balance of greater uninhibitedness and candour in (sexual) behaviour and feeling has become more strongly a relational process as well as an individual one.

Phases in processes of emancipation, accommodation and integration

Just as the accomplishments of one generation become habitually taken for granted in the next, so the feeling of liberation, inherent in a successful emancipatory struggle, can topple over into its opposite when what was first an achievement becomes a taken-for-granted fact of life: when this happens, a feeling of oppression and of being burdened can become prevalent.

The feeling of liberation prevailed in the 'roaring twenties' and again in the 1960s and 1970s. In those decades, there was a collective emancipation or, to put it differently, the most striking social pressure came from *below*. In such phases of emancipation and resistance, the *gains* in terms of we-and-I feelings are usually emphasized and what prevails is the feeling of liberation from the straitjacket of old authoritarian relationships. In this phase, much of what was once considered to be bad luck is then experienced as injustice.

When collective emancipation chances diminish or even disappear, another phase of accommodation and resignation has begun (for these phases, see Wouters 1986 and 1990). In this phase, the most striking social pressure comes (again) much more unequivocally from *above*. When this occurs, the gains of the emancipation phase have largely come to be taken for granted, and thus the pressures of having to comply with authority relations are emphasized more strongly. The same goes for increased demands such as enlarged knowledge, ability and flexibility in dealing with others and oneself. Complying with these demands had been a precondition for reaping the gains of emancipation, but only when the pressure from above clearly prevails once again do they also come to be experienced as demands. This opens a perspective in which the *loss* of old we feelings and the oppression of we-and-I feelings are emphasized. In this phase, in deliberations as to whether one is confronted with bad luck or injustice and whether it is befitting to react with resignation or resistance, bad luck and resignation will usually get the benefit of the doubt.

In both phases, marriage was one of the institutions involved: while the old Victorian ideal of an elevated spiritual love lost vigour, the demand of always preserving one's marriage lost precedence. Particularly in phases of emancipation, desires and interests of individuals gained importance – a shift in the we–I balance (Elias 1991) in the direction of the I. Moreover, by the 1970s, the social security provided by welfare arrangements had been transformed into an 'equanimity of the welfare state', on the basis of which many women have liberated themselves from the shackles of their marriage (van Stolk and Wouters 1987). In the 1980s and 1990s, as pressures from above gained precedence and collective emancipation chances disappeared, the longing for enduring intimacy has strengthened and intensified – a shift in the we–I balance in the direction of the we. In this most recent phase of accommodation and resignation, this longing will also have gained importance by the trimming down of welfare arrangements, corroding the 'equanimity of the welfare state'.

Seen from a longer-term perspective, these alternating phases appear to change in a particular direction: in a spiral movement, both sides of the we–I balance, liberation as well as the burden of demands, are raised. This is the third pattern or regularity in the connection between changes in prevailing power and dependency relationships and in the dominant lust balance. On the one hand, the spectrum of accepted emotional and behavioural alternatives expanded, but on the other hand, an acceptable and respectable usage of these alternatives implied a continued increase of demands on self-regulation. Although sometimes one side is emphasized and sometimes the other, taken together they are best understood as phases in integration processes of sexes and classes within states (Wouters 1990, 1995a and 1995b).

Intensified tugs-of-war and ambivalence

Coinciding with the spread of less uneven balances of power and of stronger ideals of equality, intimate relationships have become more strongly dependent on the style of emotion management of the partners involved: how to negotiate the terms of the relationship as two captains on the same ship without losing love and respect? At the same time, all kinds of conflict or conflicting needs and interests, formerly a tabooed non-topic, came out into the open and were subject to negotiation. According to traditional ideals, conflicts did not happen – female resignation would prevent them – and if they occurred, then they were seen only as a natural phenomenon, refreshing, like a thunderstorm. Since the 1960s, the art of 'conflict management' has developed, and marriage or living intimately together has become a conflict-prone balancing act (Mahlmann 1991: 327).

As more egalitarian rules take time to 'sink in', both men and women have increasingly become subjected to a tug-of-war between old and new ideals (and power resources) and to related feelings of ambivalence. Most men and women seem to be egalitarian 'on the surface' and traditional 'underneath'. Most men react in accordance with the dynamics of established–outsider relationships: they do not want to accommodate and do not easily perceive the 'civilized' pleasures of a more egalitarian relationship. Therefore, they will use the 'gender strategy' of appealing to a woman's *old* identity underneath, trying to restore it, whereas most women will appeal to a man's *new* identity, trying to reinforce it and make it sink in. To put it differently: 'Sex and love are no longer given facts but talents to be exploited' (Schnabel 1990: 16). Therefore, the art of obliging and being obliged as well as the art of escaping or sublimating these pressures have developed to increasingly higher degrees. Recent discussions of issues like sexual harassment, pornography, rape in marriage and date-rape, can be understood as a common search for ways of becoming intimate and of keeping at a distance that are acceptable to both women and men. Precisely because of the sensitivity and caution needed to proceed in such a way, erotic and sexual consciousness and tensions have expanded and intensified, stimulating a further sexualization of love and an erotization of sex. This quest for an exciting and satisfying lust balance, avoiding the extremes of emotional wildness and emotional numbness, has also stimulated the emotional tug-of-war and ambivalence to a higher tension-level. That is so, if only because the increased demands on emotion management will have intensified both the fantasies and the longing for (romantic) relationships characterized by greater intimacy, as well as the longing for easier (sexual) relationships in which the pressure of these demands is absent or negligible, as in one-night stands. This ambivalence, together with an increasingly more conscious and calculating[8] emotion management as a source of power, respect and self-respect, is characteristic of processes of the decreasing segregation and increasing integration of classes and of sexes. This forms another, fourth pattern or regularity in the connection between changes in figurations and in lust balances: as long as those integration processes continue, these ambivalent emotions may be expected to accumulate and intensify, including both longings that make up the lust balance.[9] This is why the body, nudity and sex are becoming increasingly prominent in the media (for Germany, see König 1990), and why this trend is likely to persist; they contain the promise of natural physicality and of a harmoniously combined attention for both person and body in intimate activity. It may be expected that as the integration of the sexes continues to proceed, heightened sensitivity to this promise will accumulate as well, together with erotic consciousness and erotic tensions. However, because in the same process the ideal and longing to be known and loved body and soul, will mount as well, both longings will remain connected to each other in heightened ambivalence. Overall, this boils down to intensified longings, more contradictory desires, and thus, on the whole, less satisfaction or gratification . . . unless people (once again) manage to deal with these contradictions in playful ways.

ACKNOWLEDGEMENTS

I would like to thank Jon Fletcher and Stephen Mennell for improving my English and for their stimulating suggestions. Thanks also to Tom Inglis, Richard Kilminster, Peter Stearns and Bram van Stolk, whose creative remarks helped me to improve the text.

NOTES

1 This development seems to reverse Victorianism: 'Victorians sought to control the place of sex in marriage . . . by urging the desexualization of love and the desensualization of sex' (Seidman 1991: 7).
2 Cf. Blom (1993); Hatfield and Rapson (1994); Komter (1985); Kooy (1968, 1983); Zessen and Sandfort (1991); and Zwaan (1993). Besides the problem of distinguishing between changes in the lust balance as a dominant ideal and as a practice, there is an additional complication: studies of sexuality usually do not pay much attention, if any, to the kind of relationship in which it occurs; and vice versa, studies of loving relationships usually do not take a systematic interest in sex.

Both kinds of research are even reported as attracting different kinds of respondents (Schreurs 1993: 332).

3 My thanks to Bram van Stolk who initiated this study and presented me with his notes and photocopies. I would also like to thank Jon Fletcher; without his stimulating advice, this article would have remained behind the one-way mirror surrounding Dutch society.

4 In 1973, Erica Jong had her large audience dream about the 'zipless fuck': 'the incident has all the swift compression of a dream and is seemingly free of all remorse and guilt; because there is no talk of her late husband or of his fiancée; because there is no rationalizing; because there is no talk at *all*. The zipless fuck is absolutely pure. It is free of ulterior motives. There is no power game. . . . No one is trying to prove anything or get anything out of anyone. The zipless fuck is the purest thing there is. And it is rarer than the unicorn. And I have never had one' (Jong 1973: 14).

5 In 1974 Anja Meulenbelt, probably the foremost Dutch feminist, also contributed to this development by announcing her love affair with a woman under the title 'Homosex en feminisme' in *Opzij* 3: 7–9.

6 In 1976, one of two lesbian women was reported to have said: 'We are interviewed because of being lesbians, because we make love to women . . . whereas this is the perfectly normal result of seeing yourself as important and of refusing to live in oppressive conditions any longer' (*Opzij* 10: 4–6). In 1980, in a report entitled *Women and Sexuality: Ten Years after the Sexual Revolution*, the author (Gerda de Bruijn) excuses herself for being 'obliged' to discuss male sexuality: 'Because most women still [*sic!*] prefer to make love with men, we cannot talk about "her" sexual gratification without referring to "his" modelling of sexuality.'

7 In her study, Ellen Laan compared women's responses to the 'regular' man-made film and the 'woman-made film': 'Contrary to expectation, genital arousal did not differ between films, although genital response to both films was substantial. Subjective experience of sexual arousal was significantly higher during the woman-made film. The man-made film evoked more feelings of shame, guilt, and aversion' (Laan 1994: 49).

8 Arlie Hochschild (1994: 3–13) has observed the rise of a calculating attitude in American advice literature for women, in books with titles such as *Having It All*, *The Cinderella Complex* and *The Total Woman*. She evaluates this attitude negatively and typifies it as 'the commercial spirit of intimate life': 'modern advice books reaffirm one ideal (equality) but undermine another (the development of emotionally rich social bonds)'. On these grounds she refers to Max Weber: 'The ascetic self-discipline which the early capitalist applied to his bank account, the late twentieth-century woman applies to her appetite, her body, her love. The devotion to a "calling" which the early capitalist applied to earning money, the latter-day woman applies to "having it all".'

9 The increasing tension between these longings is likely to be heightened by a relentless and less religiously inspired curiosity for what was placed behind social and psychical scenes in former centuries, for both sex and death: the denial of endurance in relationships.

BIBLIOGRAPHY

Ang, Ien (1983) 'Mannen op zicht', *Tijdschrift voor Vrouwenstudies* 15, 4(3): 418–34.
Bailey, Beth (1994) 'Sexual revolution(s)', in David Farber (ed.) *The Sixties: From Memory to History*. Chapel Hill, NC, and London: University of North Carolina Press, pp. 235–62.

Blom, J. C. H. (1993) 'Een harmonieus gezin en individuele ontplooiing', *BMGN* [Berichten en Mededelingen betreffende de Geschiedenis der Nederlanden] 108(1): 28–50.

Brinkgreve, Christien (1988) *De belasting van de bevrijding*. Nijmegen: Socialistische Uitgeverij Nijmegen.

Brugman, Emily, Goedhart, Hans, Vogels, Ton and van Zessen, Gertjan (1995) *Jeugd en seks 95. Resultaten van het nationale scholierenonderzoek.* Utrecht: SWP.

Bruijn, Gerda de (1980) *Vrouw en seksualiteit. Tien jaar na een seksuele revolutie.* Literatuurrapport 13. Zeist: Nisso.

Calcar, E. van (1886) *Gelukkig – ofschoon getrouwd. Een boek voor gehuwden en onge- huwden*, trans. from the English. Haarlem: Bohn.

Centraal Bureau van der Statistiek (1994) *Sociaal-culturele berichten 1994–1995. Trends in de leefsituatie van Nederlandse jongeren 1979–1989/1993.* Voorburg/ Heerlen: CBS.

Daalen, Rineke van and Stolk, Bram van (1991) 'Over revolutie en onwetendheid. Seksuele ervaringen en klachten van jongeren', in Peter van Lieshout and Denise de Ridder (eds) *Symptomen van de tijd. De dossiers van het Amsterdamse Instituut voor Medische Psychotherapie (IMP), 1968–1977.* Nijmegen: Socialis- tische Uitgeverij Nijmegen, pp. 34–54.

Dekker, Joost (1987) 'Voluntary control of sexual arousal: experimental studies on sexual imagery and sexual history as determinants of the sexual response', PhD dissertation, University of Utrecht.

Dowling, Colette (1981) *The Cinderella Complex: Women's Hidden Fear of Independ- ence.* New York: Pocket Books.

Eijk, Inez van (1994) *Bij jou of bij mij? Erotische etiquette.* Amsterdam: Contact.

Elias, Norbert (1991) *The Society of Individuals*, ed. Michael Schröter. Oxford: Blackwell.

Elias, Norbert (1994) *The Civilizing Process*, trans. Edmund Jephcott. Oxford: Blackwell.

Fisher, W. A. and Byrne, D. (1978) 'Sex differences in response to erotica: love versus lust', *Journal of Personality and Social Psychology* 36: 117–25.

Frenken, Jos (1976) *Afkeer van seksualiteit.* Deventer: Van Loghum Slaterus.

Fromm, Erich (1942) *The Fear of Freedom.* London: Routledge & Kegan Paul.

Garcia, L. T., Brennan, K., DeCarlo, M., McGlennon, R. and Tait, S. (1984) 'Sex differences in sexual arousal to different erotic stories', *Journal of Sex Research* 20: 391–402.

Groenendijk, H. (1983) 'Vrouwelijke seksualiteit uit het kader van pornografie', *Tijdschrift voor Vrouwenstudies* 15, 4(3): 352–71.

Hatfield, Elaine and Rapson, Richard L. (1994) 'Historical and cross-cultural per- spectives on passionate love and sexual desire', *Annual Review of Sex Research* 4: 67–97.

Heiman, J. R. (1977) 'A psychophysiological exploration of sexual arousal patterns in females and males', *Psychophysiology* 14: 266–74.

Hochschild, Arlie Russell (1994) 'The commercial spirit of intimate life and the abduction of feminism', *Theory, Culture and Society* 11(2): 1–24.

Jong, Erica (1973) *Fear of Flying.* New York: Signet Books.

Komter, Aafke (1985) *De macht van de vanzelfsprekendheid.* The Hague: VUGA.

König, Oliver (1990) *Nacktheit: Soziale Normierung und Moral.* Opladen: West- deutsche Verlag.

Kooy, G. A. (ed.) (1968) *Sex in Nederland.* Utrecht: Het Spectrum.

Kooy, G. A. (ed.) (1983) *Sex in Nederland.* Utrecht: Het Spectrum.

Kuitenbrouwer, Jan (1990) *Lijfstijl. De manieren van nu.* Amsterdam: Prometheus.

Laan, Ellen (1994) *Determinants of Sexual Arousal in Women: Genital and Subjective Components of Sexual Response*. Amsterdam: University of Amsterdam, Faculty of Psychology.

Mahlmann, Regina (1991) *Psychologisierung des Alltagbewußtseins. Die Verwissenschaftlichung des Diskurses über Ehe*. Opladen: Westdeutsche Verlag.

Ministerie van Sociale Zaken en Werkgelegenheid (1984) *Nota met betrekking tot het beleid ter bestrijding van sexueel geweld tegen vrouwen en meisjes*. The Hague: Ministerie van Sociale Zaken en Werkgelegenheid.

Mosher, D. L. and White, B. B. (1980) 'Effects of committed or casual erotic imagery on females' subjective sexual arousal and emotional response', *Journal of Sex Research* 16: 273–99.

Orbach, Susie (1994) *What's Really Going On Here?* London: Virago Press.

Röling, H. Q. (1990) 'Samen of alleen: initiatief en overgave in "Wij willen weten" (1938–1985)', *Amsterdams Sociologisch Tijdschrift* 17(2): 85–102.

Röling, H. Q. (1994) *Gevreesde vragen. Geschiedenis van de seksuele opvoeding in Nederland*. Amsterdam: Amsterdam University Press.

Sanders, Stephan (1994) *De grote woede van M*. Amsterdam: Bezige Bij.

Schalet, A. Townsend (1994) 'Dramatiseren of normaliseren? De culturele constructie van tienerseksualiteit in de Verenigde Staten en Nederland', *Amsterdams Sociologisch Tijdschrift* 21(2) (October): 113–47.

Schnabel, Paul (1990) 'Het verlies van de seksuele onschuld', *Amsterdams Sociologisch Tijdschrift* 17(2): 11–50.

Schreurs, Karlein (1993) 'Sexualität und Bedeutung der Geschlechtszugehörigkeit bei lesbischen und heterosexuellen Paaren. Ergebnisse einer empirischen Studie in den Niederlanden', *Zeitschrift für Sexualforschung* 6(4): 321–34.

Seidman, Stephen (1991) *Romantic Longings: Love in America, 1830–1980*. New York and London: Routledge.

Sigusch, V. and Schmidt, G. (1970) 'Psychosexuelle Stimulation durch Bilder und Filme: geschlechtsspezifische Unterschiede', in G. Schmidt, V. Sigusch and E. Schorsch (eds) *Tendenzen der Sexualforschung*. Stuttgart: Enke, pp. 39–53.

Stearns, Peter N. (1994) *American Cool*. New York: New York University Press.

Stolk, Bram van (1991) *Eigenwaarde als groepsbelang. Sociologische studies naar de dynamiek van zelfwaardering*. Houten: Bohn Stafleu Van Loghum.

Stolk, Bram van and Wouters, Cas (1987) *Frauen im Zwiespalt. Beziehungsprobleme im Wohlfahrtsstaat. Eine Modellstudie. Mit einem Vorwort von Norbert Elias*. Frankfurt am Main: Suhrkamp.

Straver, Cees (1980) *Kijken naar seks*. Deventer: Van Loghum Slaterus.

Straver, Cees, Heiden, Ab van der and Vliet, Ron van der (1994) *De huwelijkse logica. Huwelijksmodel en inrichting van het samenleven bij arbeiders en anderen*. Leiden: NISSO/DSWO Press.

Swidler, Ann (1980) 'Love and adulthood in American culture', in Neil J. Smelser and Eric H. Erikson (eds) *Themes of Work and Love in Adulthood*. London: Grant McIntyre, pp. 120–47.

Vennix, Paul and Bullinga, Marcel (1991) *Sekserollen en emancipatie*. Houten/ Antwerpen: Bohn, Stafleu & Van Loghum.

Vliet, Ron van der (1990) 'De opkomst van het seksuele moratorium', *Amsterdams Sociologisch Tijdschrift* 17(2): 51–68.

Wolfe, Tom (1976) *Move Gloves & Madmen, Clutter & Vine*, New York: Farrar, Straus & Giroux.

Wouters, Cas (1984) 'Vrouwen, porno en seksualiteit', *Tijdschrift voor Vrouwenstudies* 5(2): 246–50.

Wouters, Cas (1986) 'Formalization and informalization: changing tension balances in civilizing processes', *Theory, Culture and Society* 3(2): 1–18.

Wouters, Cas (1990) *Van minnen en sterven. Informalisering van de omgangsvormen rond seks en dood.* Amsterdam: Bert Bakker.

Wouters, Cas (1992) 'On status competition and emotion management: the study of emotions as a new field', *Theory, Culture and Society* 9: 229–52.

Wouters, Cas (1995a) 'Etiquette books and emotion management in the 20th century: Part One – The integration of social classes', *Journal of Social History* 29(1): 107–24.

Wouters, Cas (1995b) 'Etiquette books and emotion management in the 20th century: Part Two – The integration of the sexes', *Journal of Social History* 29(2): 325–40.

Zeegers, Wil (1994) *De zonnige zijde van seks. De nawerking van positief beleefde seksualiteit.* FSW, Rijksuniversiteit Leiden: DSWO Press.

Zessen, Gertjan van and Sandfort, Theo (eds) (1991) *Seksualiteit in Nederland: seksueel gedrag, risico en preventie van aids.* Amsterdam: Swets & Zeitlinger.

Zwaan, Ton (ed.) (1993) *Familie, huwelijk en gezin in West-Europa.* Amsterdam/Heerlen: Boom/Open Universiteit.

Part V
Emotions and health

14 Emotions, pain and gender

Gillian Bendelow and Simon J. Williams

INTRODUCTION

Like emotions, pain lies at the intersection of mind and body, biology and culture. Medical theories of pain, however, have traditionally been dominated by its physiological aspects. This is clearly demonstrated by *specificity theory,* the basis of which was classically described in 1664 by Descartes, who proposed that a specific pain system carries messages from pain receptors in the skin to a pain centre in the brain. The location of the centre is thought to be contained in the thalamus and the cortex is assumed to exert an inhibitory control over it. Although there have been modifications and refinements with the emergence of physiology as an experimental science in the nineteenth century, the proposition none the less remains basically unchanged.

Medicine has produced a taxonomy of pain syndromes, with over 250 classifications, which can roughly be divided into four main categories, namely deep tissue damage (e.g. arthritis), peripheral nerve damage (e.g. amputation), root damage (e.g. arachnoiditis) and, finally, idiopathic pains, such as the majority of low back pain cases and migraines, in which there is no sign of tissue damage and no agreed cause (Melzack and Wall 1984).

Specificity theory cannot adequately explain this latter category. Although *physiological* specialization can be identified through particular neurones in the nervous system which conduct patterns of nerve impulses that can be recorded and displayed, *psychological* specificity cannot be demonstrated in the same way as no neurones in the somatic projection system are indisputably linked to a single, specific psychological experience. Melzack and Wall (1965, 1984) have challenged the assumptions of specificity theory, emphasizing affective and evaluative dimensions as well as sensory ones. Since 1962, they have developed and refined the *Gate-Control theory*, which suggests that psychological and cognitive variables (heavily influenced by sociocultural learning and experiences) have an impact on the physiological processes involved in human pain perception and response. The widespread acceptance of Melzack and Wall's Gate-Control theory, along with other influences such as the hospice movement, has shifted the pain paradigm and increased the emphasis on cultural and psychological components and the need for a multidisciplinary approach.

Emotions have rarely been taken seriously within the psychological rubric of pain perception and most research in this field uses experimental methods involving the infliction of a noxious stimulus to demonstrate psychophysical laws and to establish thresholds of pain (see Hardy *et al.* 1954; Otto and Dougher 1985; Feine *et al.* 1991). There is little reference to the need to broaden out the definition of pain from the Cartesian proposition, which inevitably acts to divorce mental from physical states and tends to attribute single symptoms to single causes. These methods have been criticized for isolating subjects from the contexts in which they live (Bates 1987: 49). In contrast, as Turner (1989) argues, the diversity and flexibility of both theoretical and methodological approaches within the sociology of health and illness are highly appropriate to the analysis of pain as an ongoing structure of lived experience:

> a focus on the sociology of the body inside medical sociology would suggest new, or at least innovative, areas of enquiry, for example, into the complex inter-dependencies between self-image, personal identity, social interaction and body-image; it would also suggest alternatives to behavioural or informational models of pain.
>
> (1989: 5)

As we have argued elsewhere (Bendelow 1993a; Bendelow and Williams 1995), the notion of pain having a substantial emotional component, literally the obverse of pleasure, is in fact a much older conceptualization than that of pain being a physiological sensation. Indeed it can be traced back to Plato's (429–347 BC) deliberations of extremes and opposites in *The World of Forms* in which he declares pleasure and pain to be the twin passions of the soul, the results of the interactions between earth, air, fire and water. Subsequently, Aristotle (384–322 BC) developed the pain/pleasure dichotomy, describing them as basic moral drives guiding human action, and held that the pain experience was negative passion, which had to be conquered by reason. He believed that pain was conveyed by blood to the heart, but excluded it from his classification of the five senses, describing it as a *quale*[1] of the soul: a state of feeling and the epitome of unpleasantness. Literature, theology and philosophy abound with considerations of the nature and purpose of pain, as in Tillich's *Systematic Theology*, Vols 1–3 (1950–63); or Kierkegaard's *Works of Love* (1962 [1847]). The pleasure/pain dichotomy is constantly evoked and reinforced, as epitomized by de Montaigne:

> Our well-being is only freedom from pain. That is why the philosophical school which has given the greatest importance to pleasure has also

reduced it to mere absence of pain. Not to suffer is the greatest good man can hope for.

(de Montaigne 1959 [1592]: 44)

At the turn of the century, in frank condemnation of the dominance of the school of thought which regarded pain as mere sensation, the philosopher Marshall (1895) laid much emphasis on the strong negative affective quality which motivates some kind of activity to alleviate pain. In other words, we are compelled to do something about it and to act effectively in order to relieve it, beyond a simple reflex action; as Proust says, 'pain we *obey*'. Thus, the affective processes become parallel with sensory processes, yet it remains the case that emotional aspects of pain are rarely acknowledged or studied.

However, within the newly emerging arena of the sociology of pain, new approaches to the field have been developed which can conceptually encompass the complexities of emotion. For example, Foucauldian analyses of pain-relief in childbirth and in dentistry have drawn attention to the shift from the anatomical to the psycho-social space since the mid-twentieth century (Arney and Neill 1982; Nettleton 1989), and other sociological and anthropological work has analysed theodicies and narratives of pain, which legitimate human suffering and endow it with biographical meaning (Herzlich and Pierret 1987; Kleinman 1988; Williams 1990).

Freund (1990) has emphasized the relevance of the sociology of emotions to the study of health and illness, arguing that the Durkheimian legacy of the non-reducibility of 'social facts' to biological 'facts' has resulted in a lack of acknowledgement of the body within sociology, but that this imbalance can be redressed by the development of

> an existential-phenomenological perspective which emphasizes subjectivity and the active expressive body [and which can be] used to bridge the mind–body–society splits that characterise both fields . . . a focus on the emotionally expressive, embodied subject, who is active in the context of power and social control, can provide a useful approach for studying distressful feelings, society and health.
>
> (Freund 1990: 452)

The development of the sociology of emotions, which is centrally concerned with the *social* contexts in which emotions take place and are managed, raises fundamental issues for the mind–body relationship. According to Hochschild (1983), it is common practice amongst social scientists either to ignore emotions completely or to subsume them under other categories. As she states:

> social psychologists believe the exquisite care they take to 'avoid' discussing feeling, in order to focus ever more intently and narrowly on cognition, increases the scientific character of the work.
>
> (Hochschild 1983: 201)

Hochschild's central concept of emotional management directly challenges mind/body and emotional/physical divides, and, in turn, other dichotomies such as individual/societal, instrumental/expressive and masculine/feminine. The research described in this chapter explores the relationship between emotions and pain with a particular focus on gender and the lived body.[2]

Essentialist differences in emotional development have been theorized by feminist psychologists (Chodorow 1974; Gilligan 1982), and feminist philosophers have stressed the linkages in the dominant rationalist ideologies in western thought between the 'lower' status of emotions and nature with bodily functioning, and women's bodies in particular (Martin 1987; Bordo and Jagger 1989; also see Seidler in this volume). Gender is also, of course, crucial to theories of emotional labour and the division of emotion work; something which many chapters in this volume address (Hochschild 1983, 1992; Jackson 1993; Duncombe and Marsden 1993 and this volume). The role of gender is also of prime importance in terms of the links with the theoretical and methodological contributions to the sociology of health and illness that have been made by feminist scholars over the last fifteen years. Much of this work is grounded in ethnographic and humanistic traditions, the essential feature being to emphasize the subjective (Oakley 1989; Smith 1988; Harding 1991), and an explicit agenda involved in employing a phenomenological methodology is that it aims to reveal the 'lay' voice rather than that of the 'expert' or professional. By this means, it is hypothesized that the discussion of feelings and emotions is more likely to take place.

RESEARCHING PAIN AND GENDER

The fieldwork took place through access to a health centre in an inner-city area of North London which has a very mixed social profile. The sample conveys a reflection of experiences of people in an inner-city area that has a mixture of both deprivation and gentrification, in housing and other services, and a varied ethnic mix.[3] Permission for access to the surgery having been given, two stages of fieldwork were carried out over a period of nine months from 1989 to 1990.

First, a questionnaire was designed to attempt to examine the beliefs about health, illness and pain of a wider population, and to engender themes which would be examined in more depth by a sub-sample. Key questions addressed general health beliefs, experiences of illness and pain, the role of emotions in pain perception, the perceived ability of men and women to cope with pain, and the importance (or not) of other variables such as race and class in shaping pain experiences. The research questions were not confined to chronic pain, encompassing any experience the subjects themselves defined as pain, either in the past or in the present. In all, 107 men and women agreed to fill in a self-completing questionnaire which included detailed information about ethnic background, occupation, household status and tenure. From this survey data, two major themes emerged in terms of statistically significant gender differences in pain perception: namely the role of emotions in the process and the social expectations of the ability of women and men to cope with pain. Using these themes the second stage of the fieldwork was developed and eleven men and women from the larger sample volunteered to participate in an informal, semi-structured, in-depth interview to probe the complexities of attitudes and beliefs about the nature of pain.

The interviews began by going back to the questionnaire and asking for more detail about the most painful experience the interviewee could remember, and this gave rise to a 'pain narrative' in which the theme of physical/emotional pain and the separation or interlinking of those two were explored, often without any prompting.

In order further to elicit beliefs about the conceptualization of pain, visual images of people in pain were used at this point, with the specific purpose of evoking emotional responses and reactions. The sequence of six pairs of images consisted of a selection of paintings and photographs collected from various art and photographic galleries, which portrayed men and women (and in one case, children) in a wide range of social circumstances. Although some of the images conveyed physical pain, many of them were deliberately ambiguous, depicting scenes infused with emotional suffering and open to broad interpretation. The inclusion of visual imagery in the research design resists the tradition of the social sciences, generally, and medical sociology in particular, to embed themselves in scientific models. Aside from Goffman's exceptional *Gender Advertisements* (1976), there is a notorious reluctance to acknowledge the ways in which the social order is represented and endorsed by art in the tradition of Berger's *Ways of Seeing* (1964). In contrast, art history has used theories from social science, particularly Marxist and feminist critiques (see Fischer 1964; Nochlin 1971; Pollock 1982). The exploratory use of images to replace vignettes in this fashion elicited rich and evocative data on pain beliefs (for a fuller discussion of this methodology, see Bendelow 1993b).

Having described how the research was designed to incorporate subjective assessments of pain, we turn now to an analysis of the data and the two main themes which emerged, namely, the role of emotions in definitions and conceptualizations of pain, and, secondly, the gendering of pain beliefs.

THE CONCEPTUALIZATION OF PAIN

A central aim of the study was to examine the role of emotions and feelings in pain perception and to explore how mind/body dualisms impinge on conceptualizations of pain. One of the questions in the survey asked respondents to describe the most painful experience they could remember and to rate it on a scale between one (mild) and six (severe). Predictably, nearly all of the responses were rated between four and six, but although

258   *Gillian Bendelow and Simon J. Williams*

the types of pain described were extremely diverse, they concentrated almost exclusively on physical trauma, encompassing accidents, injuries, illnesses, back pain, childbirth and migraine. There were no significant gender differences here, although men were more inclined to be represented in the accidents and injury category than women. Only three women and one man described pain of an emotional or psychological nature, these being the death of a mother, marital and partnership break-ups, and being thrown out of the parental home.

Asking about feelings and emotions in a questionnaire is beset with difficulties. Somewhat crudely, respondents were asked whether they thought that anxiety, depression and fear had an effect upon pain perception, and significant gender differences were found. A considerable number of the respondents did not fill in any of the three sections of this question, despite completing the rest of the questionnaire. The fact that the missing cases comprised twice as many men as women reinforced the differing gendered emphasis, suggesting that the men in the sample were more likely to resist including emotional components in conceptualizations of pain. This became a major theme to be explored in the interview and, in stark contrast, all the interviewees acknowledged or made reference to the existence of 'emotional pain' as a concept. The terms mental, emotional and psychological were used repeatedly and interchangeably as the following examples show:

> Pain itself – it's quite hard to remember *physical* pain – I think probably *mental* pain is the worst – it's hard to say and I can't remember what I put down but I think *mental* pain is worse than *physical* – the *physical* is hard to remember, it goes, but the *mental* stays there.
>
> (Male, salesman, aged 26, white Irish)

> I don't know, in some ways it might be easier to be in *physical* pain than *mental* pain, especially like with people with schizophrenia, they're often described as being in *mental* pain, aren't they, but usually it's a *physical* thing, there's more chance that the doctor or someone can cure [it].
>
> (Male, housing clerk, aged 50, white British)

> It's very *psychological* pain – if you don't think about it and take your mind off it, it will go away or it's not as bad, I don't think about it. *Emotional* pain is something that I've felt quite a lot – in a way I think it's worse than *physical* pain – that's tangible and you know what's causing it and you can put your finger on it – well it hurts there, that's the reason, but *emotional* pain – I mean I don't think anyone can explain why human beings have emotions. But because people are capable of loving a great deal, hating a great deal – if someone you love does something nasty out of spite, well that can be worse than any *physical* pain.
>
> (Female, student, aged 18, mixed race)

I think you can see *physical* pain as a result of *emotional* trauma . . . like you asked how you see things in your life affecting your health and one thing I put was things going well within the primary relationship and – I've recently split up from my partner in the last few weeks and I know that some of the *emotional* pain I've had from that has been experienced *physically* in terms of um – really aching inside all around the stomach and – I'm sure that's an *emotional* thing but I can feel it *physically* . . . I think that – it may be different for different people but I know that *emotional* pain and stress manifest themselves in *physical* ways in me and I can recognize my stress responses and I do get sort of aching inside and I come out in cold sores. On one occasion I came out in an incredible itchy rash and as soon as you start dealing with the stress that's provoking that, then it stops. There's probably something in between that, it's a two-step thing . . . but the *emotional* pain goes on longer – I think it's somehow worse than a *physical* pain because that is usually comprehensible, logical and there's a certain amount of control – you can get your head round it. I'd rather go through all the horror of smashing up my leg and all the being in hospital than two months of what I've just been through.

(Female, health adviser, aged 34, white British)

Of course there is *mental* pain as well but only in its *true* sense pain is *physical* – I mean they're not the same thing – I mean there's *mental* pain and there's *physical* pain but they're not the same thing – I mean the pain that I've known has been purely *physical* sort of things. I mean the other sort of pain comes through problems but it's not related to the *physical* part. I suppose the few times I've been in jail I would say it's painful but not *physically* so.

(Male, registered heroin addict and unable to work, aged 40, white British)

As these quotes suggest, there appeared to be a stigma attached to emotional or psychological pain and, for the men more than the women, pain with a pathological physical cause seemed more respectable and authentic. Women were more likely to have a holistic approach and acknowledge emotional vulnerability. The relative informality and increased personal contact of the interview gave rise to a broadening and expansion of the definition of pain and the experiences included. As well as emphasizing emotional and psychological components, spiritual and existential aspects were also encompassed, as the following quote illustrates. The male interviewee, a black British musician, aged 36, is responding to one of the pain images:

It's pain, but I have a sort of dual approach to this – since we've begun I've held this and I know you want me to answer around the definition that you're not defining, around my own definition . . . my problem is to do with things like physical, which is like you cut yourself, like my hand – or the emotional or possibly the spiritual which is the three – it's in that area that I'm having problems so if you can look at pain on those three levels, then yes. But we can't establish between us while we're talking about what we're trying to define together. We can't even take a piece of paper and try to map out, at least for me, what this area is, it's a difficult thing to do. But I think you can experience pain, therefore, on a spiritual level, a mental spiritual level – anguish on a mental level, on a physical level and an emotional level. And although they are holistically one, I would separate them. So if I was a doctor and somebody was suffering from mental pain which was then coming out of the body through things like arthritis or who knows – then that would need a course of treatment and I would say 'Oh you're in pain, take this tablet', but if it's spiritual anguish it would need another treatment, emotional the same thing – you'd need love. We all need love, we all need care, we all need everything.

In the transition from questionnaire to interview, four men and four women changed their classification of the most painful experience from something physical to much more of an emotional component. For example, the following interviewee, an unemployed white actor, aged 24, had previously described an episode of prolonged toothache as his worst experience of pain in the questionnaire. In the interview, however, he claimed that he had felt unable to mention an ongoing condition he had been experiencing over the last few months, which caused him much more pain and anguish. He revealed that he had been experiencing 'panic attacks', which he described as a feeling of 'depersonalization':

I felt totally separate from whatever was going on – it's like an inner terror, it is like a physical pain at times, it's like a vice on my temples and an incredible pressure on my head that it does produce a headache but essentially it's just a brooding feeling within the skull.

He had sought treatment through his doctor, and had been referred to a psychologist but was very reluctant to accept that there might not be a physical cause. Although he was using tranquillizers for symptomatic relief, and pursuing alternative treatments such as acupuncture and homeopathy, he felt that he should have been sent for a brain scan, and hoped that a chemical imbalance might explain the torment he was experiencing.

The ambiguity and 'broadening out' of definitions of pain was illustrated by the way in which pain was not necessarily always seen as negative. It could, for example, be seen as a sign of health, a 'signal function', providing a system of warning the body, or even as being productive, as in successful childbirth. Positive qualities of pain perception were associated with acute, short-lived, invariably physical aspects, although the notion that character and personality could be 'strengthened' by having to cope with emotional hurts emerged recurrently.

A central issue here was that of control, linked to having knowledge and information, and the associated sense of powerlessness in its absence. The more chronic and terminal pain was, the more negatively it was perceived as it was linked with depression, poor self-esteem and mental illness. Explanations were often sought, involving self-blame, as in the case of a female, white British, retired nurse, aged 69, who was in continual pain from a fractured skull, following a hit-and-run accident:

> Before my accident I was a carefree, very 'with it', I could always sort of think what the day was and what I was going to do this time next week, on Tuesday I must get my order ready for my groceries and what-not. Now, I don't know from one day to the other what the day is and what I've got to do – I look think oh it's two o'clock and I've made no lunch and things like that – I've lost all my preciseness – it's all gone by the board, I'm just an old, an old has-been now I feel.

In the following example, a white South African male ex-journalist, aged 55, who had received various forms of treatment for cancer over the last five years, including the amputation of an arm and a leg, described how the attitudes of even the most well-meaning of medics could be undermining:

> One thing that worried me about the Bristol approach was that deliberately or accidentally it seemed to encourage the attitude that patients were in some way responsible for their illness, that they had brought it upon themselves. I've been thinking about that a lot and I do acknowledge that in the past I have neglected my own health and been casual about it but to say that I had wanted in some strange way to be ill seems iffy. I think there are many factors involved. There is the economic factor – I've been unemployed on and off for a long time. There's the question of ignorance – having come from a privileged background where I never had to cook I'm bad at cooking for myself . . . there are enough problems in coping with the pain without worrying about the stigma.

Beliefs about pain as a form of punishment may develop, as in the case of a 56-year-old Irish woman, who was struggling to keep her cleaning job as well as providing full-time care of her husband, who was afflicted with Alzheimer's syndrome, and needed constant supervision in their cramped fifth-floor flat. She considered herself to be in continual pain, physical, emotional and especially spiritual, from the burden of coping in nightmare conditions. However, she rationalized this pain as a punishment ordained by God, and used her Catholic faith both to explain and sustain her predicament. Another male respondent, aged 26, had developed a complex belief system around religion and race and felt tormented and persecuted thus:

> I feel that all the pain I've suffered comes back to the fact that basically I'm a cross-breed, I don't mean in terms of colour but I'm meant to be

Irish but I'm not really, not pure . . . I suppose I'm the only one in the family that feels that – I've said it to them, I've even said to my mum – she didn't like it but she's had a lot of problems and I said to her one day that it's all to do with the Jews. My mum's real mother died when my mum was only 17, she was Jewish – the grandad's been married twice since, he's still alive and in good health but she died of cancer and I said to my mum one day, the reason you're having problems with your legs and your knees now is because of the Jews, because of the curse upon them – because going back to religion again, because they crucified Christ. But if I said that to a Jewish person they'd take offence and I don't mean to offend them, I'm not anti-Jewish but I think a Jew should be a Jew and a Catholic – well that's just religion . . . but people should be what they are, there's no sense of identity any more, like patriotism is a dirty word. I think people should be given back a sense of identity as something to even fight for if it came to it. When I say to people, I blame the Jews, I don't mean to er . . . I think it's a curse that follows people around and now I think it's following me and I blame a lot of the problems that I have – but you've got to be careful what you say to people and sometimes you bottle things up rather than say it.

The informal and supportive nature of the interview appears to have elicited these intensely personal accounts and extended the biomedical definitions of pain which would never have been accessed by the questionnaire format.

PAIN AND GENDER

The questionnaire in this study asked whether there were any differences in men's and women's ability to 'cope' with pain. Over half the sample (two-thirds of the women and a third of the men) indicated that they believed women to be 'superior' to men in this respect. Other studies have shown an even higher bias towards women's perceived endurance; for instance, a national study by Nurofen (1989) of 265 married or heterosexual cohabiting couples across Britain revealed that 86 per cent of women and 64 per cent of men in the sample believed that women are better able to tolerate pain than men.

In the interview sub-sample, only one man thought there were no differences in the pain-coping capacities of men and women, and the rest of the sample opted in favour of women (although two of the women and five men had originally indicated in the questionnaire that they thought there were no differences). Again, these issues could be explored more fully in the interviews. Although the responses could be described as 'essentialist', they were sophisticated, combining both biological and sociocultural explanations. For instance:

Women are made to suffer pain because we have periods and childbirth. Whatever the social climate, women end up child-rearing therefore they don't have the 'privilege' of giving in to pain and sickness.

> (Female, full-time childcare, aged 36, white British)

Nature has built women that way to cope with everyday pressures – raising a family, running a home and so on.

> (Female, full-time childcare, aged 33, black British)

Repeatedly, the view was expressed by both women and men alike that the combination of female biology and the reproductive role served to 'equip' girls and women with a 'natural' capacity to endure pain, both physically and emotionally. Many of the men expressed a sense of awe, at times almost of reverence, at the idea of childbirth, seeing it as the 'ultimate' in pain experience.

Alternatively, it was felt that childhood socialization actively discouraged emotional expression in boys, and adult males felt an obligation to display stoicism. Several male respondents felt that expressing pain would brand them as 'sissy' or effeminate, and would imply that they were homosexual (there was a tacit assumption that gay men are able to express their feelings and that it is socially acceptable for them to do so). Both men and women put forward the view that for men pain of any sort is 'abnormal', being outside of their expectations, and subsequently they are less able to deal with it:

Men are not allowed socially to express pain as much, they're supposed to be stronger. We're allowed to cry and they're not . . . although women have more breakdowns than men, men don't allow it to come out, they hide it until it's unbearable whereas a woman will usually say 'I can't cope' long before.

> (Female, student, aged 18, mixed race)

The average man always thinks he's tougher than he is but is not so good when it comes to coping with pain when it happens.

> (Male, interior designer, aged 38, white British)

Men will sort of try and battle it out, whereas women will give in and take a pain-killer. As a boy I was always told that the good Indian suffers in quiet but in fact the feeling is that women actually cope better, have a bigger threshold.

> (Male, freelance copywriter, aged 24, white British)

Whilst no claims to generalizability are being made here, data of this nature support the arguments identified earlier about the gendering of emotional development across the nature/culture, reason/emotion divide. It is to issues such as these that we now turn in the discussion.

DISCUSSION

As we have argued throughout this chapter, an *embodied* approach to pain as an ongoing structure of lived experience is, we suggest, able to transcend many former dichotomous modes of western thought, thereby reconciling mind with body, biology with culture, reason with emotion, and championing the (biographical) voice of the 'lifeworld' over the dominant (dispassionate) voice of medicine.

People in pain need to find *meaning* for their symptoms, however inappropriate or anti-therapeutic this may seem from an orthodox biomedical viewpoint (Priel *et al.* 1991). Without such meaning, feelings of isolation and despair may develop. This biographical search for meaning, in turn, calls for the development of ever more sensitive qualitative methodologies which, in contrast to so-called 'objective measures', capture the emotional and cultural significance of pain in complex, subtle and sophisticated ways through a commitment to lived experience and the 'mindful body'.

As the findings of our study suggest, issues of gender mesh closely with these arguments. Whilst all the interviewees acknowledged the existence in some form or other of 'emotional' pain, physical pain, in the form of acute, readily observable symptoms, elicited more legitimacy, sympathy and respect. Men, however, were more likely to separate out these definitions, to ascribe a 'hierarchy of respectability' to different types of pain, and were more reluctant to consider emotional pain as 'real' pain. Women, in contrast, although making similar distinctions, tended to operate with more holistic, integrated notions of pain; meanings which, again, were difficult to access using anything other than qualitative methods.

Another particularly striking feature of our study was the strongly gendered notion of men's and women's ability to 'cope' with pain. Whilst findings from experimental research suggest that women have lower pain thresholds, our study suggests a very different picture; one in which, irrespective of gender, women, rather than men, are seen to have a superior endurance. As we have seen, these views seemed to be underpinned by biological principles, yet still embraced sociocultural issues such as gendered roles and differential patterns of childhood socialization. The salient point here seems to be that female hormonal and reproductive functioning, together with the role of motherhood, were strongly linked to the capacity for emotion management, thus equipping girls and women with a 'natural' capacity to endure pain which was lacking in boys and men.

Again, the links between female bodies and emotions become apparent here as male socialization is seen actively to discourage men from being allowed to express pain, whether physical or emotional. For males, pain is much more obviously a state of 'abnormality', making their bodies *dys*-appear, in contrast to the 'natural' expectation of females. Coping capacities, for women, are seen to encompass affective as well as sensory components, through more integrated notions of the 'mindful' body. These assumptions about female coping are, in turn, linked to wider structural divisions, particularly the public and the private domains, in which women, historically, have been tied to the domestic sphere and more readily associated with the 'natural' world of 'lower' bodily functions such as child-birth and menstruation. By comparison, men are more involved in the public world of culture and 'higher' mental process. As Martin (1987: 17) comments, 'it is no accident that so-called "natural" facts about women, in the form of claims about biology, are often used to justify social strati-fication based on gender'.

Thus, emotion work is equated with women's work, including their per-ceived capacity to 'cope' with pain, and their greater readiness to talk about feelings generally. Feminist psychologists have also emphasized that female childhood socialization encourages caring for others and the devel-opment of imagination and empathy for human pain, suffering and distress (Gilligan 1982; Ruddick 1990). In addition, women's ontological security and sense of identity may be less threatened by the admission of being in pain than is the case for men, for whom the psychological structure of masculinity is predisposed to inhibit the admission of vulnerability.

To conclude, we would suggest that, despite the so-called 'natural' assumptions made about female biology, the attribution to men and women of differential capacities for experiencing, expressing, understanding and responding to pain is primarily linked to gender-differentiated processes of socialization and emotion management. This, in turn, draws attention to the various ways in which the experience of embodiment may be different for boys and girls (Chodorow 1974; Martin 1987). Physical experience of the body, in other words, is modified by the social categories through which it is known. All theories about its care, its lifespan, its abilities, its functions, its ability to withstand pain, emanate therefore from a culturally processed and located idea of the (gendered) body. Pain, as we have argued, lies at the heart of these matters. In the immortal words of one of our (male) respondents:

> Women have more *awareness* – a more intimate and responsible instinct to their biology – all we do is shave!

NOTES

1 Old word meaning emotional quality.
2 In stressing the issues of gender, we recognize that gender does not, of course, operate in isolation and is cross-cut by other social structural characteristics such as social class and 'race', resulting in other forms of discrimination, some of which are touched upon in the study; see G. Bendelow, *Pain and Gender: A Sociocultural Study* (Harlow, Essex: Addison Wesley Longman, forthcoming).
3 In this particular area of north-west London, there is a large Irish population, many of whom are third-generation and have British nationality, but prefer to describe themselves as Irish. Similarly, there are many members of the community

who are second- or third-generation, with parents or grandparents who originally emigrated from the Caribbean. Many of the study respondents who described themselves as 'mixed race' emerge from intermarriages between these two cultures.

BIBLIOGRAPHY

Arney, W. and Neill, J. (1982) 'The location of pain in natural childbirth: natural childbirth and the transformation of obstetrics', *Sociology of Health and Illness* 7: 375–400.

Bates, M. (1987) 'Ethnicity and pain: a bio-cultural model', *Social Science and Medicine* 24(1): 47–50.

Bendelow, G. (1993a) 'Pain perceptions, emotion and gender', *Sociology of Health and Illness* 15(3): 273–94.

Bendelow, G. (1993b) 'Exploring gender and pain through visual imagery', in C. Renzetti and R. Lee (eds) *Researching Sensitive Topics*. London and Thousand Oaks, CA: Sage, pp. 273–94.

Bendelow, G. and Williams, S. J. (1995) 'Transcending the dualisms: towards a sociology of pain', *Sociology of Health and Illness* 17(2): 139–65.

Berger, J. (1964) *Ways of Seeing*. Harmondsworth, Mx: Penguin.

Bordo, S. and Jagger, A. (eds) (1989) *Gender/Body/Knowledge: Feminist Reconstructions of Being and Knowing*. New Brunswick, NJ, and London: Rutgers University Press.

Chodorow, N. (1974) *The Reproduction of Mothering*. Berkeley, CA: University of California Press.

Duncombe, J. and Marsden, D. (1993) 'Love and intimacy: the gender division of emotion work', *Sociology* 27: 221–41.

Duncombe, J. and Marsden, D. (1998) '"Stepford wives" and "hollow men"? Doing emotion work, doing gender and "authenticity" in intimate heterosexual relationships', in G. Bendelow and S. J. Williams (eds) *Emotions in Social Life: Sociological Themes and Contemporary Issues*. London: Routledge.

Feine, J., Bushnell, M., Miron, D. and Duncan, G. (1991) 'Sex differences in the perception of noxious heat stimuli', *Pain* 44: 255–63.

Fischer, E. (1964) *The Necessity of Art*. Harmondsworth, Mx: Penguin.

Freund, P. (1990) 'The expressive body: a common ground for the sociology of emotions and health and illness', *Sociology of Health and Illness* 12(4): 452–77.

Gilligan, C. (1982) *In Another Voice: Psychological Theory and Women's Development*. Cambridge, MA: Harvard University Press.

Goffman, E. (1976) *Gender Advertisements*. Hong Kong: Macmillan Press.

Harding, S. (1991) *Whose Science? Whose Knowledge? Thinking from Women's Lives*. Ithaca, NY: Cornell University Press.

Hardy, J., Woolf, M. and Goddell, H. (1954) *Pain Sensations and Reactions*. New York: Williams & Williams.

Herzlich, C. (1973) *Health and Illness: A Social Psychological Analysis*. London and New York: Academic Press.

Herzlich, C. and Pierret, J. (1987) *Illness and Self in Society*. Baltimore, MD, and London: Johns Hopkins University Press.

Hochschild, A. (1983) *The Managed Heart: The Commercialization of Human Feeling*. Berkeley, CA: University of California Press.

Hochschild, A. (1992) *The Second Shift: Working Parents and the Revolution at Home*. London: Piatkus.

Jackson, S. (1993) 'Even sociologists fall in love: an exploration of the sociology of emotions', *Sociology* 27(2): 201–20.

Kierkegaard, S. (1962 [1847]) *Works of Love: Some Christian Reflections in the Form of Discourses*. London: Collins.

Kleinman, A. (1988) *The Illness Narratives: Suffering, Healing and the Human Condition*. New York: Basic Books.

Marshall, R. (1895) *Pain, Pleasure and Aesthetics*. London: Macmillan.

Martin, E. (1987) *The Woman in the Body*. Milton Keynes, Bucks: Open University Press.

Melzack, R. and Wall, P. (1965) 'Pain mechanisms: a new theory', *Science* 150: 971–9.

Melzack, R. and Wall, P. (1984) *A Textbook of Pain*. London: Churchill Livingstone.

Montaigne, Michel Eyquem de (1959 [1592]) *In Defense of Raymond Sebend*, trans. Arthur Beattie. New York: Frederic Ungar Publishing.

Nettleton, S. (1989) 'Power and pain: the location of fear in dentistry and the creation of a dental subject', *Social Science and Medicine* 29(10): 1183–90.

Nochlin, L. (1971) *Realism*. Harmondsworth, Mx: Penguin.

Nurofen (1989) *Pain Relief Study*. London: King's Fund.

Oakley, A. (1989) 'Interviewing women: a contradiction in terms', in H. Roberts (ed.) *Doing Feminist Research*. London: Routledge & Kegan Paul.

Otto, M. and Dougher, M. (1985) 'Sex differences and personality factors in responsivity to pain', *Perceptual and Motor Skills* 61: 383–90.

Pollock, G. (1982) 'Vision, voice and power: feminist art history and Marxism, *Block* 6: 6–9.

Priel, B., Rabinowitz, B. and Pels, R. (1991) 'A semiotic perspective on chronic pain: implications for the interaction between patient and physician', *British Journal of Medical Psychology* 64: 65–71.

Ruddick, S. (1990) *Maternal Thinking*. London: Women's Press.

Smith, D. (1988) *The Everyday World as Problematic: A Feminist Sociology*. Milton Keynes, Bucks: Open University Press.

Tillich, P. (1968) *Systematic Theology*. Welwyn, Herts: Nisbet.

Turner, B. (1989) 'The body in sociology', *Medical Sociology News* 151: 9–15.

Williams, R. (1990) *A Protestant Legacy: Attitudes to Death and Illness among Older Aberdonians*. Oxford: Clarendon Press.

Williams, S. J. and Bendelow, G. (1996) 'The "emotional" body', *Body and Society* 2(3): 125–39.

15 Social performances and their discontents
The biopsychosocial aspects of dramaturgical stress

Peter E. S. Freund

INTRODUCTION

'Stage fright' is a potential occupational hazard for an actor in the theatre or for a social actor arriving for a job interview. Performing and monitoring one's own performances and those of others thus can be stressful whether on stage or in the theatre of life. This chapter develops and refines earlier observations on what I have called dramaturgical stress (Freund 1982, 1990; Freund and McGuire 1995). I shall develop these observations through the use of spatial metaphors, viewing dramaturgical activities in the context of psychosomatic space and social-physical spaces. Spatial metaphors can help to incorporate into theorizing such diverse elements as movement, activities of extension–withdrawal, boundaries and informational flow. They also provide a way of linking mind, body and society, enabling us to analyse embodied actors, their activities and the relational contexts in which they occur.

I begin by examining the use of spatial metaphors in some of Erving Goffman's work and conceptualize the maintenance of individual and/or group identity and informational preserves as involving the building and maintenance of boundaries and the regulation of informational flow across such boundaries – in a sense, a geography of emotions and emotional relationships. Dramaturgical stress emanates from threats to self–other or group boundaries, or to the security of informational preserves – threats, in short, to ontological security (Laing 1965; Giddens 1984). I then turn to the embodied aspect of emotions and social relationships. This is followed by a discussion of emotional communication, psychosomatic space as well as dramaturgical stress in intra-psychosomatic space. Finally, I examine dramaturgically stressful encounters in social-physical space and their relationships to an actor's social space and the forms of social control imposed on him or her. The chapter concludes by addressing issues involved in linking dramaturgical stress to health.

THE GEOGRAPHY OF EMOTIONS AND EMOTIONAL RELATIONSHIPS

Goffman's *Presentation of Self in Everyday Life* (1959) is his earliest and most comprehensive attempt to develop a metatheory and theory of social life using dramaturgical metaphors. This work views dramaturgical strategies as means of information control through which individual actors, small groups, institutions and even societies manage the style in which information is presented and expressed, and the flow of information across the boundaries of their informational preserves. Actors, for instance, seek to delve into the secrets of individuals, groups or institutions while at the same time protecting personal and team secrets.

Spatial metaphors in Goffman's work describe ways in which space is used to sustain performances, maintain appearances and in general manage the flow of information about individual actors, groups or institutions. Front stage and back stage, for instance, demarcate territories – and informational preserves. In works such as *Frame Analysis* (1974), the 'frame' is the spatial metaphor through which we locate and interpret activities by 'framing' them, placing 'brackets' around them, and so on.

There is a geography of self–other (and even boundaries within the territory of the self – internal 'splits') and of intra- and inter-group relationships that threads its way through *The Presentation of Self* and can be found in other works (even in *Asylums* (1961)). In *Relations in Public* (1971), for example, Goffman looks at actors as 'vehicular units' manoeuvring social-physical spaces, discusses the 'insanity of place' and utilizes Jakob von Uexkull's concept of subjectively experienced space (*'Umwelt'*). Goffman's geography includes physical barriers that control the flow of information. Thus an increasingly wide range of activities is carried out behind the scenes of everyday life (for example, the expression of intense, inappropriate and socially disruptive emotion (Newton 1995)).

Goffman introduced a sensitivity to space into sociological analysis by looking at the dramaturgical uses of space but did not make space a 'master' metaphor, because, in fact, it was the metaphor of the theatre that prevailed in his early work (Silber 1995: 332). None the less, for our purposes, we shall use space as 'master' metaphor in order to look at mind, body and society relationships and at the use of space for organizing information about self and others. The organization of biopsychosocial and physical space is utilized by individuals as a way of sustaining a performance, or, in other ways, to establish boundaries and to regulate the flow of information.

Dramaturgical work thus involves creating and maintaining boundaries between informational preserves, regulating the 'flow' of information across boundaries, reading other actors' expressions, and sometimes attempting to 'penetrate' their informational preserves.

Boundaries that act as barriers to perceptions may be established not only in physical and social space but through the expressive activities of the body. Both establishing boundaries and levels of permeability – i.e. degrees of openness to the world – and responding to anxieties concerning boundaries which, for instance, delineate territories of the self, may be expressed somatically. Thus, while establishing a boundary to protect one 'psychologically' from the threat of 'ontological insecurity', gestural-postural and internal neuro-hormonal activities represent ways in which the fear of threats or the methods of coping with potential threats are embodied.

Expressive activities (facial expressions, postures and gestures) help to demarcate and clarify the relationship of body to environment and environment to body (Lyon 1994). As Wentworth and Yardley (1994: 28) observe:

> Human biology and subsequent life experiences leave individuality suspended on a continuum between differentiation and engulfment by the social complex between stark, alienated individuality and absorption of self into others' experience.

Dramaturgical activities such as emotion work regulate the psychosocial and experienced bodily boundaries between self and others. They regulate, among other things, the permeability of these boundaries and what information passes through them.

The simultaneously symbolic *and* somatic management of self–other boundaries has been overlooked in the sociology of emotions (especially in encounters where actors are co-present). Clark (1990), for example, in her excellent essay on the micropolitics of social place looks at emotional strategies for negotiating one's place. Yet to be 'put in one's place', for instance, by being humiliated, involves more than just a symbolic exchange and may be accomplished by literally restricting persons to a certain physical location or by the postures, gestures and facial expressions that will be assumed by actors in relationship to each other in social space. While place does not equal physical location and certainly one's social place is not synonymous with a physical place or position, actors in encounters move through and use socially produced space in particular ways, assume postures and gestures *vis-à-vis* each other that are in keeping with their respective places, or use their bodies to show resistance to how they are placed. Thus, for instance, being 'put down' may be experienced and/or resisted not only psychologically (as in 'psychological' notions of alienation which 'measure' alienation in purely cognitive terms) but somatically-spatially as well.

Information about groups, institutions, oneself and others is managed dramaturgically through the establishment and regulation of boundaries in psychobiological, social and physical space, by, for instance, segregating them in space. Of course, information about self, others, groups, etc., is also regulated by scheduling performances and by collectively and intrapsychically 'rewriting' history so that it is congruent with current definitions of an individual's or group's self-definition (Berger and Luckmann 1967).[1]

In a sense, many dramaturgical-emotional relationships can be represented topographically – as a 'map' of relationships within the embodied self and between the embodied self and others. Located in a sociophysical place, the feelings that underlie emotions are experienced positionally – that is, in terms of merging and establishing boundaries in one's relationship with others. The structures of feelings are shaped by activities occurring within the context of socially organized emotional 'spaces'. Goffman's use of spatial metaphors to describe this space and of the politics of social communication are illustrative of one way to conceive of the 'topography' of 'external' and 'subjective' social-emotional, psychological, physical and biological space. Dramaturgical strategies of impression management, the reading of what others either intentionally or 'unconsciously' make visible to us, are part of this 'topography' that affects our conscious and unconscious subjective relationship to self and others. The display and concealment from others (and from oneself) of emotions and the use of dramaturgical space interact with emotional modes of being and psychosomatic space.

MIND–BODY AND PERFORMANCES

Some emotions are visibly linked to physiological activity – as in the case of 'coarse' emotions (Scheff 1985). Furthermore, the physiological 'responses' can be read. In the case of anger, for instance, it can involve forms of 'bodily mobilization' to cope with a threat or an emergency (Lazarus 1991). In other emotions (e.g. sadness), the physiological aspect may not be visible and easily identified. In the case of such emotions (e.g. pride), Franks (1987) argues that it would be difficult to locate any internal sensations. While this may be true, since emotions have an 'outside, relational thrust', they may also be accompanied by motoric expressions – in the form of facial expression, posture, or gestures. Thus, Plessner's observation that 'Joy without expansive and extending feelings in the chest region is not joy' (Plessner as cited in Buytendijk 1974: 179) may have some basis.

It is possible that potential somatic aspects accompanying feelings of, for instance, pride have not been systematically studied. The 'sinking feeling' that accompanies feelings of disappointment might have a physical aspect if we looked for it, assuming, of course, that we looked in the right places (Lazarus 1991: 58). Clinical studies such as Gottschalk *et al.* (1993) and George *et al.* (1995) using modern imaging techniques have examined the links between cerebral activity and such feelings as hopelessness, hope, sadness and happiness. Despite the use of sophisticated technologies, these studies are crude and above all done on inactive, decontextualized mind-bodies. Yet Franks (1987: 227) admits 'there is a bodily aspect of emotion that is not to be reduced to sensation' – one that needs to be more clearly identified.

Thus emotions are not just cognitions nor are they clearly locatable in any specific sensation or biochemical change. Lazarus (1991: 59) argues:

> We need the idea of *embodiment*, which expresses that our entire being, including glands, muscles, visceral organs and brain are actively engaged in an emotion, and if we dispense with it, a crucial distinction is lost, even if that distinction ultimately comes down to a continuum from little to much, a just-noticeable difference that is almost arbitrary when it is small but important when it is large.

Emotions are a 'fusion' of mutually modulating cognitive-physiological and behavioural aspects (most 'visible' in so-called coarse emotions). Thus, for instance, respiratory patterns are influenced by neurochemical (e.g. neuro-muscular) changes induced through movement and expressive activities. Activities such as speaking, for instance, require the modulation of respiration and in turn speaking may influence physiological functions such as blood pressure, for instance (Lyon 1994).[2] Respiration figures prominently in metaphors describing emotional relationships ('Don't hold your breath', 'You leave me breathless', 'Stop breathing down my neck').

It is not merely appraisal (an 'internal' activity) that is involved; bodily activities such as movement can help make body metaphors, for instance, an emotional-physical reality (McGuire 1996). Barbalet (1994) argues it is possible that in addition to appraisal, bodily actions and relationships are in themselves sources of emotion. Thus, 'in spatially moving her body, an actor may achieve a modification or change in emotional experience' (Barbalet 1994: 120). Situations which involve co-presence occur in a 'field of bodily activities' in which bodily activities may be 'geared into' or 'detached from' others. Discomfort or distress may thus be generated not only by the appraisal of self and others but by the psychosomatic postures (or modes of being; Freund 1990) one is maintaining and from the con-textualized embodied experience of other actors' psychosomatic expressive activities. Emotions are thus embodied not merely in one's subjectivity or in an internal biochemical milieu but also in motoric activities, such as pos-ture, gesture, etc., and are embedded in the field – the social-psycho-biological-physical spaces – of social relations. Franks (1987) is thus correct in emphasizing bodily gestures, not just the 'internal' biochemical milieu.

Ways of attending to our bodies and others' embodied presence thus involve not simply cognitive coding–decoding of information but engaging the other person (Csordas 1993) – a relation of moving bodies in space (as in a situation between two people dancing). The bodiliness of anger is not just found in inner states (e.g. biochemical), but is an aspect of how we act towards that with whom and/or which we are angry (Crossley 1995: 143). Anger is communicated through and by the body and our daily encounters involve 'carnal interchanges' (Crossley 1995: 145) through which we relate to each other biopsychosociologically, through mutually attuned or antagonistic gestures and postures expressive of involvement or detachment. These may be, I believe, fruitfully conceptualized in spatial metaphors.

Radley (1984) argues that the 'psychosocial' characteristics of coronary-prone behaviour are embodied and embedded in a social context. Thus, such behaviour may be indicated in facial, postural and movement styles – through uses of the body. Body techniques (which are a part of one's repertoire of dramaturgical strategies) such as raising one's arms outward in prayer, may encourage a more open breathing pattern with accompanying subjectively experienced changes. Children reach outward to be embraced or to embrace, and such postures have 'affective correlates' (Lyon 1994: 105, note 28). Getting and feeling close – as opposed to keeping one's distance – are accomplished through bodily activity and linked to one's subjective experience of self and others.

Such styles are modes of engaging others (or keeping one's distance) – that is, emotional modes of being (Freund 1990). One's neuromuscular activity, such as a particular distribution of muscular tonicity, is an inseparable part of these modes, which, among other things, prepare a person for anticipated activity (Radley 1984: 1229). Such modes of being intensify, dampen, ebb and flow, in fields of action – social contexts which include, of course, others and their psychosomatic presentations. Feelings (e.g. fatigue) that may be expressed in such activity thus must be understood as emerging in the 'fields of action' or social contexts in which persons act (Radley 1984).

EMOTIONAL INFORMATION AND PSYCHOSOMATIC SPACE

It is recognized among cognitive psychologists that appraisals – interpretive activities – may be characterized by an 'automaticity'. Some interpretive activities are carried out 'automatically', rapidly 'below the threshold of wide-awake awareness' (Schneider 1995).[3] Giddens (1984) suggests levels of consciousness that range from discursive consciousness where motives, etc., can be put into words, through practical consciousness (somewhat akin to Freud's pre-conscious), to finally unconscious process. Giddens is rightly uncomfortable with Freud's metaphors which reify parts of the psyche – making them into little homunculi. He (as I do) prefers the more 'process'-oriented phenomenological and ethnomethodological approaches. Levels of consciousness in these perspectives are modes of attending to, turning towards, or moving away from the world, and interpreting it. I would argue that the 'speed' at which one grasps, perceives and interprets activity is an important dimension for differentiating levels and 'types' of consciousness. Furthermore, the agency that is apprehending the world is not a disembodied mind but an embodied actor.

Emotions, at least in primates, function as 'rapid' and efficient modes of information-'processing' (Wentworth and Yardley 1994). They rapidly focus on and co-ordinate information perceived on a number of 'simultaneous' levels. Our emotions are ways of perceiving wholes, or *Gestalten*, of expressed verbal–non-verbal information. Hence their information appears as intuited because they derive from a number of levels and are 'processed' rapidly. Since some emotional communications and responses occur more 'automatically' than others, some expressions are easier 'consciously' to modify than others (Bull 1995). Thus the 'startle reflex' is very hard to feign and to 'inhibit'.

There is the possibility that some emotional communication may not involve cognition – at least not in the usual sense of the term. Thus it is possible to be afraid without understanding why (Krohne 1990). This is not just a feature of practical consciousness. One researcher provides an example:

> Think of stepping off a curb and jumping back when you suddenly hear the blast of an onrushing car's horn. You jump before you have time to figure out why. We think that is because the amygdala senses the horn before the cortex can explain it.
>
> (As cited in Waldholz 1993: AI)

Here there is a kind of 'body consciousness' that does not involve 'higher' cortical functions (the cortex, especially the frontal cortex, is seen by some as the cerebral seat of consciousness).

It is worth noting in this context that people – or more precisely their bodies – may respond to stressors even when they are not consciously aware of them (Krohne 1990). Thus a behaviourally comatose patient 'responds' to the presence of a visitor or nurse by increases in blood pressure (Lynch 1979). In a sense, our bodies can respond to situations in ways that our conscious minds do not. For instance, as Shilling (1993: 126, note 3) points out:

> Bodies are not just affected by various forms of work, though, but can act as a corporeal conscience which has the potential to affect people's willingness to engage in certain tasks. This is illustrated by Gusterson's analysis of nuclear physicists. As a physicist who refused to work on nuclear weapons explained: 'There's this thing in my stomach. My head understands the reasons to work on the weapons, for deterrence and so on, but when I think about doing this work, I feel this thing in my stomach.' Physicists who continued to work on nuclear weapons programmes did not necessarily avoid this 'rebellion of the body', but had learned to treat their bodies as machines 'prone to malfunction'.

It may be that a 'pre-linguistic knowledge' of feelings (Newton 1995: 122) may take the form of somatic responses. Leder (1984) suggests that our bodies express and respond to the existential situations in which they are embedded. Such a language of the body does not, for instance, express a feeling of being overwhelmed by the world in one fixed way of 'speaking', but as with generative grammar, which makes written and spoken language possible, we are able to produce an indeterminate number of ways of saying things. Cultural and social conditions will, of course, influence how our body speaks. In the case of 'coarse emotions' (like fear, anger, etc.), ways of communicating or responding to feelings may be more fixed and embedded in specific organismic response (it would appear that neither a general nor a specificity theory of the physiological expression of emotion is adequate but both have elements of truth to them).[4]

Emotion work as a dramaturgical strategy may, of course, involve consciously managing emotional expression or reshaping one's feelings (Hochschild 1979). Yet as Wentworth and Ryan (1990) argue, much emotion work on bodily expression can occur in the space of a short temporal lag (one or two seconds) between emotion as a cognitive-brain event to its expression in aspects of bodily behaviour.

The 'appraisal' activities of mind–body can occur on a number of different levels of consciousness and include our experience of others' psychosomatic expression – such as the position of their body in space. Emotional communication can be seen as a reciprocal signalling in which co-present actors 'co-ordinate' subjective states (for example, moods) and accompanying expressive activities.

Feelings and emotions among other things 'motivate', or, more accurately, move, us. Mind–body may open to others or may close boundaries, readying to fight or resist. Feelings of alarm, for instance, may involve responses and expressions in the form of shallow breathing, rigid body postures and expression (tight lips, tightness of voice, tentative contact, averted gaze, etc.) (Griffith and Griffith 1994). Involved in these somatic expressions (which may 'feed back' to influence mood and feeling; Lyon 1994: 95) are whole complexes and configurations of hormonal, neurological and muscular activity (Griffith and Griffith 1994).

In her analysis of somaticized symptoms such as 'nerves', Duffie (1996) argues that such psychosomatic expressions are the result of an impaired existential balance that 'intersects' on levels of psyche, physiology and culture. Drawing on existential phenomenological sources, she argues that space is the site of conscious embodied experience. Moods affect the character of this space and relatively open or closed modes of psychosomatic being correspond to either positive or negative emotional styles. Open 'apertures of being' characterize being ecstatic, in love, joyful, etc. Constricted modes of being accompany fear or anxiety.

Griffith and Griffith (1994: 66) argue there are two basic emotional postures – those of mobilization and those of tranquillity. While this classification oversimplifies, it is possible to speak of emotional modes of being (Freund 1990) that involve heightened arousal and bodily 'closure' or 'openness' in relationship to the world. Postures of mobilization include activities such as hiding, guarding, 'walling off', ignoring, etc. (Griffith and Griffith 1994: 68). Postures of embracing and 'walling off', for example, may, furthermore, coexist at any given time in oscillation (e.g. ambivalence), moving towards and away from the world. Under certain conditions, 'opposing' postures may be 'evoked' simultaneously. Such situations, according to Griffith and Griffith, may include 'double bind' social situations in which response to such dilemmas involves stressful efforts to silence psychosomatic expressions of distress. They observe:

> Detailed interviews of patients suffering from somatoform symptoms have shown that the bodily experience of such a dilemma is that of mobilizing the body for action (e.g., an aggressive emotional posture), while expressing a contradictory emotional posture (e.g., a warm welcoming with smiles and attentive listening, belying privately held seething). In essence, the body receives two conflicting directions for organizing its physiological readiness to act.
>
> (Griffith and Griffith 1994: 61)

Such states of 'push me–pull you' psychosomatic posturing are responses to contradictory dramaturgical demands and represent an acute form of dramaturgical stress. Such stress is the result of one way of responding to social situations in which there is a profound disjuncture between the ways in which one desires to present oneself and the social context which demands an 'opposite' style of self-presentation and does not allow the actor to leave the field. Under such conditions the body, Griffith and Griffith argue, may cope with such a 'push me–pull you' situation through 'spontaneous' expressions of so-called somatoform or psychosomatic symptoms.

Individuals develop 'coping' strategies in distressful situations – particularly in those situations of heightened dramaturgical stress in which a 'sincere' or authentic performance that belies distress is demanded. This coping is accomplished by compartmentalizing psychosomatic space, by dissociating feelings (e.g. gut feelings) from 'conscious' feelings, thus convincing oneself that 'all's well'. Such a splitting may involve a dissociation between bodily activities of expression and 'internal' function such as blood pressure – akin to what has been called 'schizokinesis' (Lynch 1985). I have used the term 'emotional false consciousness' to describe the social consequences of such a 'splitting' (Freund 1990). Emotional false consciousness occurs when emotion work disrupts the body's equilibrium and our ability to interpret embodied feelings. Such false consciousness involves a split between bodily expressions and an awareness of internal psychosomatic sensations, on the one hand, and continued heightened physiological reactivity to distressful situations, on the other (Freund 1990). It is as if the levels of consciousness come to be more or less permanently split between bodily appraisals and cognitive appraisals of situations.

An effective social performance (one that, for instance, appears sincere) may be accomplished through subjectively redefining relationships ('It is not his fault, he had a hard day at work', 'If I tried harder, he might not be so angry'). Such strategies may work for the short term but, on another 'level' of psychosomatic space, continue to produce feelings of ontological insecurity. These feelings are apprehended as 'free-floating' since one has 'written' or redefined the source of the threat out of one's wide-awake consciousness.

Newton (1995) argues that people collusively and collectively reproduce oppressive and distressing structures. This notion is not part of discourses on stress (Newton 1995). Indeed situations produce individuals who collude as their own agents of social control to reproduce distressing arrangements. Following this argument, one might say that to some degree social differentiation may be accompanied by subtle physiological differences. Certainly this has been shown in primates (Weiner 1992; Sapolsky 1989, 1990). It is possible that under certain conditions such responses may become fixed and in turn affect the production of feelings (e.g. depression). (Under what conditions such responses might come to be sedimented as part of a creature's psychosomatic activity is another issue.) Actors who experience depression are less likely to offer resistance (though, of course, might not be able to function at all eventually), thus facilitating the social reproduction of oppressive social relationships. As Shilling (1993) observes in his review of my analysis of the 'emotional body':

> Freund's analysis not only examines some of the mechanisms by which society shapes our experiences of health and illness, but also has implications for how these experiences 'react back' upon social classifications and social relations. As Freund argues, the appearances and experiences of bodies 'act as concrete manifestations and prototypes of "ideas" about socially appropriate bodies' which can help sustain social divisions and inequalities.

> (Shilling 1993: 117)

The splitting of consciousness in psychobiological space, for instance, facilitates the smooth functioning of hierarchical relationships, even while they produce distress. Furthermore, such splitting, or chronically 'disavowing' one's 'heart', may also serve to blur the boundaries between self and other and affect one's ability to clearly 'experience' social situations, hence contributing to making the blaming of the victim process more viable. There is a breakdown in one's ability to experience situations accurately as oppressive. Karasek and Theorell (1990: 114) point out that there is some evidence linking the 'denial' of feelings to coronary heart disease. Such splitting may produce costs that the actor meets in the form of psychosomatic symptoms of illness, symptoms that 'leak' out to communicate the fact that distress none the less continues to be experienced by the embodied actor – though not 'consciously'.

Hochschild (1979, 1983) has shown how one may learn to respond to situations by redefining one's feelings about them. Here, given the different levels of consciousness on which we operate, there is the possibility that feelings may be reworked only on one level of consciousness and not perhaps on the level of 'somatic' or body 'consciousness', thus 'short-circuiting' the signal function of emotion (Hochschild 1983). As Bendelow and Williams (1995: 151) observe, emotions 'lie at the juncture between mind, body, culture and biology and are often considered crucial to our survival by their signal function in relation to danger'.

THE THEATRE OF INNER PSYCHOSOMATIC SPACE

The psychosomatic aspect of dramaturgical stress is not confined to encounters of co-presence in which it is evoked. It can be 'carried' out of the social space in which encounters occur, into an actor's inner psycho-somatic space. Here previous and anticipated stressful encounters may sink below or rise to the surface in the stream of our consciousness.[5]

Distressful, humiliating events are reviewed, evoked, recalled, replayed and rewritten. (For a discussion of rewriting history – in the form of biography, autobiography or 'collective' history – see Berger and Luckmann 1967.) Future scenarios are anticipated and encounters rehearsed in the theatre of our embodied mind. Accompanying somatic aspects (such as forms of 'arousal') are amplified or dampened or 'split' in the course of the narratives that unfold 'in' our heads. In these internal conversations (which may be also accompanied not only by neurohormonal arousal but by motoric and other activity) we amplify, subdue, refine or 'recast' arousal states. We thus 'past-urize' and 'futurize' the dramatic activities and encounters of everyday life in the space of our imagination. The somatic aspect of such activity can be demonstrated by our capacity to place ourselves into subjective states that will influence our internal biochemical milieu and our 'outward' expression. This capacity is highly developed in humans. The yogic manipulation of *prana* (breathing) exemplifies this human capacity to regulate blood pressure, for instance, to some degree (Wentworth and Ryan 1994).

Emotions as modes of preparation for action regulate attention and motivation as well as being a medium for social communication (Wentworth and Ryan 1994). They help us 'process' sensory information quickly and thus are very important 'tools' in helping us engage with or detach ourselves from social and physical environments. The strength or permeability of self–other or self–environmental boundaries is a function of our feelings. Emotions are also biochemical ways in which our bodies 'talk' to *themselves* and in humans communicate information to self and others. In the mind's eye emotional encounters are reviewed, anticipated, and so on, in tandem with ebbs and flows in the internal biochemical milieu and in the expressive activities of the body.

A 'universal' experience that accompanies embodiment is a sense of containment.[6] This experience that our bodies are 'three-dimensional' containers emerges in our encounters with the external world of objects and persons who resist us, give way, or whatever.

From the beginning, we experience constant physical containment in our surroundings (those things that envelop us). We move in and out of rooms, clothes, vehicles and numerous kinds of bounded spaces. We manipulate objects, placing them in containers. In each of these cases there are repeatable spatial-temporal organizations. In other words, these are typical schemata for physical containment.

(Johnson 1987: 21)

Thus, many of our cognitive schemata emerge out of bodily activities as we engage the environment. Similarly, our ways of apprehending feelings, the basis of emotion, emerge in encounters with others. One might argue that there are *structural* isomorphisms on the level of meaning in our experience of the world of physical *and* of social 'objects' (McCarthy 1984). Of course, how 'contained' we feel depends on sociocultural factors such as forms of social control and the status relationships in which we find ourselves.

Initially our encounters with others consist of non-verbal gestures, touching and mirroring the other's expression (such as engaging in activities in which we align our rhythms with the bodily expressiveness of others) (Johnson 1987). Our experience of physical containment leads us to develop an 'inside–outside' orientation (the degree and quality of this experience will vary socioculturally). Gradually, our interaction with others also leads us to develop a sense of self and of emotional boundaries that emerge out of others' responsiveness or non-responsiveness. Such experiences form the ground of our sense of ontological security or insecurity (Laing 1965). Various feelings of bodily emotional and spatial boundedness are the basis of such metaphors as 'I feel vulnerable', 'I feel surrounded by friends', 'I'm touched by your expression of concern', or 'I feel smothered by your love'. A sense of boundedness may also include a sense of being trapped 'inside' oneself, unable to express feelings. In contrast, the opening of boundaries experienced as a result of feelings, such as 'I'm overflowing with joy', is often expressed in a bodily idiom.

The 'civilizing process' (Elias 1978, 1982a, 1982b) involves the increasingly complex emotional work and labour demanded for 'functioning' in various social situations. Emotional skills of display, the management of our subjective states, and the 'reading' of others' expressions come to be more pervasively used, refined and developed. The continued development and use of these 'skills' result in a heightened reflexivity, a sharper self-consciousness and a growing inner space of imagination, and hence more room in 'postmodern' societies for brooding, reflecting, etc. The enlargement of internal psychological space – the theatre of our mind – is accompanied by an increased sense of self–other boundaries.

The firmer, more comprehensive and uniform restraint of the affects characteristic of this civilizational shift, together with the increased internal compulsions that, more implacably than before, prevent all spontaneous impulses from manifesting themselves directly and motorically in action, without the intervention of control mechanisms – these are what is experienced as the capsule, the invisible wall dividing the 'inner world' of the individual from the 'external world' or, in different versions, the subject of cognition from its object, the 'ego' from the 'other', the 'individual' from 'society'. What is encapsulated are the restrained instinctual and affective impulses denied direct access to the motor apparatus. They appear in self-perception as what is hidden from all others, and often as the true self, the core of individuality.

(Elias 1978: 258)

Elias (1978: 258–9) argued that while the brain is located within the physical confines of the skull, distinctions between 'inner' and 'outer' – that is, spatial metaphors – when applied to personality, are problematic. Thus, however real the experience of boundedness may seem to the person, there is no real 'wall'. In other words, physical space is not the same as psychological space in which boundaries are 'in the mind' ('intuited', to use Elias's phrase). It is important to recognize these limits to the use of spatial metaphors, given the well-developed ability among humans to express psychological states physically (Freund 1988, 1990). Emotion work and a sense of being contained in a vessel can be embodied, for instance, in particular distributions on the 'surface' of the body of muscular tonicity and in neurohormonal changes in the internal milieu. Increased autogenic capacity to influence the workings of the body may thus accompany the increased sense of boundedness and reflexivity that is generated by the 'civilizing process'.

With the civilizing process and the forms it takes under particular social and economic systems (capitalism, patriarchal arrangements and so on), dramaturgical skills such as emotion work become more pervasive, refined and developed. The civilizing process thus creates a greater inner 'space' of imagination: more 'room' to brood, regret, anticipate – that is, to 'futurize' and 'past-urize'. The enlarged stage of the mind is paralleled by an increased sense of self–other boundaries. However, such increased ability to manage feelings and motoric expressions such as facial expressions may also blur boundaries between one's own feelings and those demanded by a situation. The increased reflexivity allegedly characteristic of 'postmodern' actors may have somatic aspects (including consequences for our health).

DRAMATURGICAL STRESS IN SOCIOPHYSICAL SPACE

Since performing is a part of social life in all societies, some dramaturgical stress is present everywhere.[7] Yet in a 'dramaturgical' society, one in which the manipulation of appearances is an important skill and a highly complex and self-conscious act, not only are emotions and bodily expressions very much controlled, but the very activity of manipulating appearances is, in itself, more stressful. It takes energy to contain feelings and actions (Jourard

1964) and to manage emotional communication, while monitoring that of others. Under what social conditions does such stress become particularly intense and chronic?

It has been suggested that dramaturgical stress is heightened 'when an individual perceives his chosen face or performance in a given situation to be inconsistent with the concept of self he tries to maintain for himself and others in that situation' (Cockerham 1978: 49). Stress may be generated by 'the task of managing an estrangement between self and feeling and between self and display' (Hochschild 1983: 13). In short, under those conditions, in which one's ontological security is threatened, the response to a breach of boundaries, the stress of keeping informational spheres apart and performances credible, and of managing and maintaining the flow of information in psychological, social-physical space, becomes highly stressful.

Some actors are in social places that make them particularly vulnerable to such stress. These include those who occupy subordinate places in various institutional contexts and those whose strongly held self-definitions are potentially stigmatizable.

Persons in subordinate positions may lack 'status shields' (Hochschild 1983) to protect their psychobiological and social space (Freund 1990). As Franks concluded:

> Borrowing from Mead's theory of the perception of objects, I noted the central role resistance plays in constructing an ontology in the person. It was then suggested that persons were granted the capacity to resist violation through social rank and status shields making them less vulnerable to depression and anxiety.
>
> (1989: 169)

An inability to protect the boundaries of self and to counter the resistance or intrusion of others thus leads to depression and anxiety. A person's social position will determine the resources he or she has to protect the boundaries of the self and how that person will come to define himself or herself.

Subordinate status combined with the forms of social control that prevail in a situation (such as the imposed and stressful emotion work demanded of them) requires that intense feelings be suppressed, denied, relegated to another sphere and in other ways managed. This makes such actors vulnerable to dramaturgical stress and renders stress more 'intense'. Responses to such intense stress may be somaticized (Kleinman 1988).

Feeling off-balance and other expressions of psychosomatic stress can be linked to one's sense of ontological security about one's social place. Asymmetric relationships such as those between rich and poor or male and female may produce anxiety about place and hence about the maintenance of boundaries (Duffie 1996).

Over thirty years ago, Franz Fanon, the Algerian psychiatrist, wrote about the connections between racial and colonial domination and psychological and physical well-being. In the following passage, he linked muscular tension and illness in Algerians to their powerlessness in the face of French colonial authority:

> This particular form of pathology (generalized muscular contraction) had already called forth attention before the revolution began. But the doctors described it by portraying it as a congenital stigma of the native, an 'original' part of his nervous system where, it was stated, it was possible to find the proof of a predominance of the extra-pyramidal system in the native. The contracture is in fact simply the postural accompaniment to the native's reticence and the expression in muscular form of his rigidity and his refusal with regard to colonial authority.
>
> (Fanon 1963: 293)

Since it was not possible for the colonized Algerians to express anger openly towards colonial authority, their anger was held in, but manifested itself in the form of muscular tension. Note also that the effects of a social problem (colonial rule) were viewed by the colonial doctors as an inherited, individual problem. The individual could not leave the social space of a racist encounter and thus somatically expressed a resistance that could not be shown. The particular form and distribution of muscular tonicity represented a way in which the body was used to create an 'impermeable' boundary between self and other. This muscular 'armouring'[8] keeps others and their claims on one out of one's psychological space.

Sociological minorities may often experience dramaturgically stressful encounters. Those who must cope with a social stigma by concealing their identity under a cloak of 'normal' appearances face special stresses. For example, in our society the widespread fear of homosexuality (homophobia) pressures homosexuals to hide their true selves in order to survive psychological and social expectations, yet trying to 'pass' as heterosexuals may place them under considerable dramaturgical stress. In addition to the self-hatred that comes from internalizing anti-gay values and the repressed anger that results from discrimination, they may suffer from the constant fear of disclosure. 'Closets' are the refuge of the powerless, but the use of this refuge has its price. 'Closets are a health hazard' was a slogan first used by the physicians marching in the 1981 'Gay Freedom Day Parade' in San Francisco.

There are many other situations in which people are pressured into various closets. For instance, there are many social pressures for 'appropriate' appearances that demand that one inhibit one's self-presentation: women are forced to hide their competence under the veil of appropriate feminine roles; salespeople must project an ever-smiling façade.

Not all closets are equally stressful, nor are all situations that demand a 'split' between self-presentation and feelings. Thus, one may more easily distance oneself from work situations than from those that involve intimate, 'primary' group relationships – such as family or sexual-romantic situations.

This can be illustrated by some 'ideal-typical' situations in family space. This, of course, is not to say that both work and familial encounters do not possess similar structural features that make them both in differing degrees stressful.

In the dramaturgical work required to hide or redefine distressing feelings, new tensions are created which must also be hidden from the audience (Newton 1975: 128). Threats to ontological security occur when masks 'crack', or threaten to do so, or when masks and feelings fuse, which then leads to a 'short-circuiting' of one's feeling and the development of a 'false' self (Newton 1995; Laing 1965). The ontologically insecure person sees his/her 'inner' self as always potentially visible to others and hence feels vulnerable (Laing 1965: 108).

Stress-related emotions such as anxiety, dread, anger and fear, according to Kemper (1990), arise from the anticipation that a more powerful person will invade or encroach upon a person's self or space. If the person sees him/herself as responsible for the distress-producing situation, the anxiety is turned inward, producing feelings of dread.

In their discussion of 'somatic symptoms' noted in people who live in 'totalitarian' societies, Griffith and Griffith (1994: 55) observe:

> In nontotalitarian, Western societies, we find remarkably similar examples of somatic symptoms that have been fostered within micropolitical systems of abusive families, where a child sexually abused at home hides the abuse at school and church, even defending her father as if he were a wonderful parent; or where a wife is physically beaten at home by her husband but hides the abuse even from friends or coworkers, believing that she cannot or should not escape and will only suffer more if she were to disclose.

Thus micropolitical circumstances as well as those that occur in oppressive macropolitical contexts may require a distressful 'containment' of feeling that can be expressed only somatically. Work, family and other settings are some of the social spaces in which such encounters occur.

One example of 'micropolitical' directives that 'bind the body' can be found in situations in which sexual abuse or gendered violence occurs. Griffith and Griffith (1994: 55–6) present a case of a woman who was sexually abused but had to contain her distress while routinely encountering her abuser in the micropolitical context of familial space.

> In meeting with Jana alone, however, the story widened. With specific questioning about possible abuse, she told how during the summer, while out of school, she stayed at home with her stepfather on days that her mother worked. When they were alone, the stepfather had sexually fondled her and warned her not to tell anyone. She had not spoken out of fear that she would not be believed, that she would be punished by him, or that the revelation would threaten her mother's new marriage.

She was terrified that he would touch her again but spoke to no one.
Instead her body began jerking violently out of control.

Such a situation is a prototypical one for women who must live with their
abuser and dramaturgically conceal their distress. Such situations created
what Griffith and Griffith describe as 'unspeakable dilemmas'. They observe
that children who are victims of sexual abuse when seen in emergency rooms
often 'present' symptoms of seizures that are non-epileptic in origin (Griffith
and Griffith 1994: 55). Gendered violence of different sorts, from sexual
abuse and rape to domestic violence or the threat of such abuse, threatens
the person's psychophysical boundaries, social status and hence ontological
security. The feelings that accompany such a threat or the source of such
threats cannot be acknowledged; that is to say, they must be dramaturgically contained through the organization of psychobiological and social-
physical space.

The double-bind communication found in many families in which contradictory demands are imposed with no possibility (or perceived possibility) of
leaving the social space in which they are made, is characteristic of dramaturgically stressful situations. Double-bind communication, as Laing[9]
argued in his analysis of family communications, can function as a means
of social control and most adversely affect those in vulnerable positions.
Their sense of reality, feelings and sense of self are 'sacrificed' for purposes
of maintaining certain family appearances.

Such a micropolitical situation (though one that is not as emotionally
intense) may, to different degrees, characterize other social situations such
as those found in workplaces. As more and more people work in corporate
and bureaucratic settings, a great deal of control over the presentation of
self becomes an important part of their work skills. To get along, manners
and politeness become tools for the efficient and effective accomplishment of
work. The emotion work involves both repressing 'undesirable' emotions,
such as displays of anger, and forcing oneself to appear happy and enthusi-
astic, even when one does not feel that way.

The proportion of jobs providing services has increased in our economy.
Those that involve some form of selling (e.g. sales clerk or stockbroker) or
provide emotional services such as friendliness or reassurance (e.g. social
worker or flight attendant) have especially increased (Hochschild 1983).
These service jobs demand elaborate skills in self-presentation and in managing one's emotions (both of which entail emotion work).

In his description of the white-collar stratum that has replaced the more
entrepreneurially oriented middle class, Mills (1956: xvii) noted that the
management of one's personality has increasingly become an essential
work skill 'of commercial relevance and required for the more efficient
and profitable distribution of goods and services'. This demand for 'pleasing
personalities', particularly in the face of job conditions that are anything
but pleasing, can be highly stressful and often requires workers to deny

their emotional responses to those stressors.[10] The following provides an example:

> Researchers placed blood pressure and pulse monitors on participants in one study and correlated the changes in these stress indicators with activities and social pressures throughout the day. The case of one hospital aide exemplifies workplace stress.
>
> Her peak reading at the office – a diastolic pressure of 77 – came in the morning when she was mediating a dispute between two secretaries. . . . She hit this level again just before lunch when she was in that perennial secretarial bind: politely taking orders from someone who annoys you.
>
> In this case, it was a patient, a tense, well-dressed suburban matron convinced that something was wrong with her despite repeated tests showing she was healthy. . . . At that moment, there were two real emergencies going on – doctors were rushing in and out of the office to consult about a woman near death on an operating table, and a cardiac patient from another hospital needed to be transferred by helicopter to the medical centre. In the midst of all this, Collins spent 15 minutes negotiating appointments for the matron; her voice remaining pleasant, but her diastolic pressure peaking and her pulse hitting 90.
>
> (Tierney 1988: 81)

A study of bank employees found that when the emotional and physical appearances demanded of workers conflicted with their own sense of self, they began to experience self-artificiality. Bureaucratized structures, particularly those with commercial goals, are most likely to produce this tension between the public face and private self (Karasek and Theorell 1990: 33; Jackall 1977). The rude customer who 'is always right', the demand for geniality in the face of social isolation within the office, the interpersonal competitiveness and the hierarchical pressures, all produce dramaturgical stress in the workplace (Freund 1982).

Workplace relationships – like those in the 'private' sphere – are intertwined with gendered, racial and ethnic micropolitical inequality. Heightened dramaturgical stress occurs when the situation of one's social status and the demands for emotional-social control create threats to one's ontological security. These threats emanate from one's positional vulnerability (e.g. a lack of status shields) and from the attendant difficulty in maintaining one's self-definition and self–other boundaries, while being 'open' to the world at the same time. Such insecurity or the means of coping with it may come to be embodied, though not necessarily on the level of 'wide-awake' consciousness.

The expression of 'disruptive' feelings and emotions in the workplace and other 'public' settings in contemporary society is increasingly relegated to the private sphere (or to the enclaves of a therapist's office). There is a tendency in modern society to 'privatize' impulses and feelings – particularly sexual ones (Elias 1978). One might say that intense displays of anger, fear, anxiety and other kinds of distress are pushed 'behind the scenes' of everyday life (allowed under controlled 'out of context' circumstances only in the commoditized or bureaucratic setting of a professional's office). They are dramaturgically 'closed' and the spaces available for 'back stages' shrink.

Physical containment may support emotional containment (Newton 1995: 84, note 16).[11] Since we cannot escape the co-presence of colleagues in work-places, or family members in homes, we are cautious in expressing 'disrup-tive' emotions. Thus our performance takes place at our location not only in social space but also in social-physical space. These influence our dramatur-gical competence, the availability of 'back stages' and our levels of security about our psychological space and hence levels of dramaturgical stress.

The social organization of physical space is related to dramaturgical com-petence. The social status of actors influences their degree of control over this organization. Spatial arrangements provide access to back stages, and means of segregating audiences, which in turn influence the quality of dramaturgical stress. This makes it easier, for instance, to sustain a consis-tent presentation of self and effective performance. The organization of space also influences the degree of surveillance to which an actor's perfor-mance is subject and hence 'levels' of stress. Again, actors in subordinate places are relatively more likely to find themselves in places where they are subject to maximum surveillance. This is certainly often the case in work spaces but is also characteristic of family space. Parents have more privacy than children. On another level, access to bodily space is also related to one's social status. Non-reciprocal touch, such as the right to be searched, provides an example of ways in which body 'privacy' and control over bodily boundaries may be violated.

Newton (1995: 42) has argued that work-related stress might reflect a 'containment of emotion' (resulting from the 'binding' practices that Griffith and Griffith (1994) discuss) that 'arises between employer and employee, superior and subordinate or men and women'. These conditions create par-ticularly high levels of dramaturgical stress for those occupying subordinate or vulnerable positions in social space. Newton (1995) argues that much of the stress discourse is silent about the relationship between stress and social stratification.

The inability of a 'subordinate' individual to cope emotionally is seen as a personal failure, not as a systemic one. Stress research seldom challenges the emotion and feeling rules demanded by institutional arrangements (Newton 1995). 'Ventilation' of distressful feelings must not occur in the encounters that evoke them but at best in therapeutic spaces (Newton 1995), most often in the context of commoditized and bureaucratized relationships. As indicated earlier, when individuals cope 'successfully' with dramaturgical stress, this coping may produce other 'costs' for them.

While 'coping' as individuals, they are at the same time less likely to alter stress-producing situations. Thus, as I argued, 'effective' emotional coping –

through, for instance, splitting – 'disconnects' a person from the signal function of his or her emotions. This disconnection allows the person to be conscious of the stress, while on the other hand the body continues to manifest stress responses. At the same time, such coping functions as a means of social control.

There is evidence that physiological changes – some of which may contribute to ill health or disease – are linked to social status:

> a wide-ranging pattern of physiological changes is associated with subordinate rank. This characteristic pattern is conserved on the whole in different vertebrate species. It entails the adrenal-cortical and gonadal steroids, levels of adrenal catecholamine-synthesizing enzymes, indoleamines, raised LDL [low-density lipoprotein] to HDL [high-density lipoprotein] ratios, the progression of atherosclerosis and some measures of immune function. These physiological patterns change as the social status of the animal is altered. They are a 'function of rank'.
>
> (Weiner 1992: 176)

The activities involved in establishing and maintaining hierarchies – such as activities of social control – have physical consequences (Weiner 1992: 195). The organismic consequences of these activities may, in turn, in themselves, serve to function as means of social control.

Sociocultural situations in which such dramaturgical work is done influence the intensity, quality and 'quantity' of emotional demands as well as how actors will respond to them. Two features of these situations – the form of social control that prevails and the relative social positions of the actors performing with each other – are particularly relevant.

Those likely to be in subordinate or 'stigmatized' social positions (such as women, members of sociological minority groups, workers in lower-class service occupations) are particularly vulnerable to dramaturgical stress. This is not only because they may face heightened and often conflicting emotional demands but also because, as with other demands that are made on individuals with relatively less social power, they lack resources and options for coping or resisting them.

DRAMATURGICAL STRESS AND HEALTH

To what extent do the somatic aspects of stressful experience influence health? Weiner (1992: 150) concludes:

> The tentative conclusion is that ill health results from a change in the normal rhythms of a subsystem incited by stressful experience. Disease, by contrast, occurs when stressful experience interacts with a preexisting regulatory disturbance or with structural change.

Ill health (illness) may have no visible organic causes but takes somatic forms such as insomnia, hyperventilation, or irritable bowel syndrome.

Disease (such as coronary heart disease), on the other hand, has a 'clear' biological basis. The disruptions or 'perturbations' of a bodily function may act to 'directly' produce ill health. Distress such as anxiety (due to threats to one's psychological, social and physical space which engender insecurity) may be accompanied by somatic experiences (fatigue, body-aches, trembling, restlessness, and so on). 'Folk' diseases such as *nervios* are somatized expressions of distress (Duffie 1996). It is also possible that a structural change in the body such as that created by coronary heart disease may interact with stress to produce rhythmic disturbances in the functioning of the heart. (This is not to say that on some level structural changes, such as arteries constricted by plaque, may not be related to sociocultural factors such as diet.) The point is, however, that stressful experiences do not linearly produce disease in most cases but act as a co-factor in persons predisposed to a disease (Weiner 1992). It is very important to note that the distinctions between ill health and disease in this context do *not* suggest that some physical problems are 'psychological' and others physical. On the contrary, as Weiner argues, reconceptualizations in the field challenge such distinctions and the sharp division between ill health and 'somaticized' expressions and organic disorders. It is simply that in disease a more complex 'web of causation' prevails, with stress acting in conjunction with a number of other co-factors (including possible genetic vulnerabilities of other origin).

Therefore, the relationships between ill health, disease and stress (including dramaturgical stress) are neither linear nor uni-causal. Most analyses (including Weiner's) focus on the internal milieu and on single neuro-hormonal rhythms. I have suggested here and elsewhere (Freund 1988, 1990) that a conception of the body actively engaged with its internal and external environment is needed. This conception includes, among others, neuro-hormonal *and* neuromuscular activity. Weiner (1992: 283) himself concludes:

> Integrative concepts have been needed in the field of stress research and theory in order to describe and capture the nature of functioning organisms in their daily, ever changing mutual interactions with other organisms in the physical world.

Such a conception may help us to understand how, given their unique predispositions and history of experiences, 'organisms' may either respond to stress in ways that allow them to remain 'healthy', or be transformed from a state of health to a state of illness and/or disease (Weiner 1992: 284).

One factor that significantly mediates the impact of stress on the body is the degree of somatic vulnerability, or, to use Buytendijk's metaphor, the degree to which the body is 'open to the world'. Infants who are biologically maturing in social wombs are more plastic and hence their psyche-soma is more open to the world (Weiner 1992: 50). In the case of bereavement, for instance, children and elderly persons are somatically more sensitive to such experiences because the state of their endocrine and immune system varies with their age (Weiner 1992).

According to Weiner (1992), 'perturbations of the organism' are partly a function of 'disordered' communication exchange. Such exchange occurs 'within and between cells and organs, between them and the brain, and between the brain and the environment' (Weiner 1992: 284). In this communication exchange what is missing in the nexus between brain and environment is the active body, which communicates mood, intentions, etc., and which attends to the environment (what Csordas (1993) calls 'somatic modes of attention'). Such 'exchanges' occur when we draw closer to, engage with, move away from, attend to, brace ourselves against, others in a social field of their active bodies.

Wentworth and Yardley (1994: 28) propose that

> Human biology and subsequent life-experience leave individuals suspended on a continuum between differentiation and engulfment by the social complex: between stark, alienated individuality and absorption of self into others' existence. This ontological, dialectical suspension between poles has been represented as the 'conflict' between the individual and society that we have all felt by degree. Hobbesian, Marxian, and Freudian portrayals of the human condition found this 'conflict' essential to their theoretic. And so too here. The experience of this dialectic between engulfment and individuation keeps an individual's psychology emerging, by sustaining our proper sensitivity to the world of others.

Dramaturgical strategies regulate the psychosocial-biological and physical boundaries, their relative permeability or impermeability, and in general the flow of information across them. The ability to manage these boundaries is essential to our ontological security. (Ontological security and health may be intimately connected; Antonovsky 1987.)

Weiner (1992) suggests that the principles underlying information exchange at various levels are homologous. While open to dispute, this direction seems worth pursuing. Indeed I have argued that, like responses to information, its regulation – 'information exchange' – can be understood using integrative concepts in the form of spatial metaphors. Such concepts help us to link various 'levels' of information exchange in biopsychological, social and physical space and to understand the changing interaction of embodied actions.

Foss and Rothenberg (1987) develop an info-medical (as opposed to bio-medical) model which attempts to bridge mind, body, society separations by viewing them as different levels of communicative activity. Weiner's perspective seems similar. Several decades ago Moss (1973) suggested that disordered communication, produced by what he called informational incongruity (such as between an actor's expectation and reality), would affect the body by 'tuning' the nervous system to respond in such a way as to influence immunity and hence vulnerability to disease. The problem with these approaches (and I suspect mine) is how symbolic and biological messages are linked. By treating both biological messages (e.g. neuro-hormonal activity) and symbolic messages as 'information', it is easy to gloss over basic qualitative differences between these different types of information and the ways in which one kind of information is transformed into another. The same issue would apply in trying to determine the degree of homology between biopsychological and social-physical space. While the degree of homology between psychosomatic, social and physical spaces is problematic, the spatial metaphors in this chapter may help unite individual performances in the form of emotional conduct, embodiment and social-cultural context. How helpful these metaphors are is a matter of theoretical debate and empirical study.

ACKNOWLEDGEMENTS

My thanks to Miriam Fisher for her usual patient editorial help and to Sue Goscinski for her excellent typing.

NOTES

1 It is, of course, clear that time and its social organization can help to establish boundaries between various self-definitions and keep performances from being discredited. Scheduling activities so that different audiences are segregated and social worlds do not collide is an example (Goffman 1959). The rewriting of one's biography over time is another. Time, like space, may be used by actors as a dramaturgical resource.

2 Repetitive motor activity increases serotonin production. Hence compulsive handwashing or jogging can be seen as bodily practices that help to reduce anxiety and increase feelings of security (Jacobs 1994). Of course, it might be argued that it is in their symbolic aspect that such practices enhance a sense of ontological security by symbolically constructing and affirming order. None the less, while this is certainly one aspect of such repetitive activities, it does not preclude their also influencing the internal psychobiological milieu.

3 For instance, if an anomalous playing card (e.g. a four of spades that is red) is briefly shown (on a tachistoscope), either it may be read as a four of hearts (thus the interpreter without being 'aware' of it changes the *Gestalt* on the card to fit his/her presuppositions) or the anomaly is not noticed (Bruner and Postman 1949).

4 The idea of a 'pre-linguistic' knowing body, embedded in and engaging the world, can be found in Merleau-Ponty's work (e.g. Merleau-Ponty 1962).

5 In healing, McGuire (1996: 16) points out, the body is melded with processes such as imagination, memory, language and symbolization.

6 I am aware that the universality of the experience of containment might be questioned. Indeed, the degree and quality of containment experienced by an actor may be influenced by, for instance, gender (e.g. Chodorow 1978). Yet given the resistance offered by the social-material world, and the capacity to take the role of the other and hence to undergo self-reflexivity, the possibility of experiencing oneself as bounded in space is universal.

7 Simply conversing with another person raises blood pressure; conversing with a person of a higher status raises it even more (Lynch 1979).

8 The notion of muscular armour (which is 'character' armour embodied) was first developed by Wilhelm Reich (e.g. Reich 1976).

9 The notion of double-bind communication finds its roots in the works of Gregory Bateson and has been applied to the study of 'pathogenic' communication in families (e.g. Laing and Esterson 1965). Double-bind communication sends opposing emotional messages. Thus, for instance, verbal claims ('I love you') may be contradicted by a body-language that says the opposite. Double binds may also be communicated by moving towards someone to embrace them and, while embracing them, pulling away. Actors may not always be able to articulate what is inauthentic about a performance or in the case of a double bind may be prohibited from noticing anything wrong. The inhibition imposed on challenging or even appearing to 'notice' such splits allows such communication to serve as a means of social control. However, this is at the expense of the ontological security of those 'against' whom such communication is directed.

10 Karasek and Theorell (1990) define high-strain work situations as those that combine high levels of demand (stressors) with low decision latitude. These adverse psychosocial conditions are more characteristic of lower-status jobs than of executive or professional positions. It can be argued that from a dramaturgical vantage point, many lower-status jobs may combine high levels of *emotional* demands with low levels of control over one's presentation of self.

11 In their discussion of psychosocial job demands, Karasek and Theorell (1990: 63) observe: 'Of course, we are explicitly trying to differentiate physical and psychological stressors, but there are problems in doing even this. For example, "static physical loading" – holding the body's mass in an uncomfortable position, such as when painting a ceiling – is associated with many of the same psychophysiological responses as purely psychological demands.' Thus one may argue that the stress of a psychosomatic posture that one must hold in a situation may be similar in its impact on the body to a bodily posture that must be sustained under certain circumstances in physical space.

BIBLIOGRAPHY

Antonovsky, A. (1987) *Unravelling the Mystery of Health: How People Manage Stress and Stay Well.* San Francisco, CA: Jossey-Bass.

Barbalet, J. M. (1994) 'Ritual emotion and body work: a note on the uses of Durkheim', in D. D. Franks (ed.) *Social Perspectives on Emotions*, Vol. 2. Greenwich, CT: JAI Press, pp. 111–23.

Bendelow, G. and Williams, S. (1995) 'Transcending the dualisms: towards a sociology of pain', *Sociology of Health and Illness* 17(2): 139–65.

Berger, P. and Luckmann, T. (1967) *The Social Construction of Reality.* Garden City, NY: Doubleday.

Bruner, J. S. and Postman, L. (1949) 'On the perception of incongruity: a paradigm', *Journal of Personality* XVIII: 206–25.

Bull, Peter (1995) 'Non verbal communications', in M. Argyle and A. M. Colman (eds) *Social Psychology.* London: Longman, pp. 354–73.

Buytendijk, F. J. (1974) *Prolegomena to an Anthropological Physiology.* Pittsburgh, PA: Duquesne University Press.

Chodorow, N. (1978) *The Reproduction of Mothering.* Berkeley, CA: University of California Press.

Clark, C. (1990) 'Emotions and micropolitics in everyday life: some patterns and paradoxes of place', in T. Kemper (ed.) *Research Agendas in the Sociology of Emotions*. Albany, NY: State University of New York Press, pp. 305–33.

Cockerham, W. (1978) *Medical Sociology*. Englewood Cliffs, NJ: Prentice-Hall.

Crossley, N. (1995) 'Body techniques, agency and intercorporeality: on Goffman's *Relations in Public*', *Sociology* 29(1) (February): 133–49.

Csordas, T. (1993) 'Somatic modes of attention', *Cultural Anthropology* 8(2): 135–56.

Duffie, M. K. (1996) 'Intrapsychic autonomy and the emotional construction of bio-cultural illness: a question of balance', in J. Subedi and E. B. Gallagher (eds) *Society, Health and Disease*. Upper Saddle River, NJ: Prentice-Hall, pp. 47–71.

Elias, N. (1978) *The Civilizing Process*, Vol. 1, *The History of Manners*. New York: Urizen Books.

Elias, N. (1982a) *The Civilizing Process*, Vol. 2, *State Formation and Civilisation*. New York: Pantheon Books.

Elias, N. (1982b) *Power and Civility*. New York: Pantheon Books.

Fanon, F. (1963) *The Wretched of the Earth*. New York: Grove Press.

Foss, L. and Rothenberg, K. (1987) *The Second Medical Revolution: From Biomedicine to Infomedicine*. Boston, MA: New Science Library.

Franks, D. D. (1987) 'Notes on the bodily aspect of emotion: a controversial issue in symbolic interaction', in *Studies in Symbolic Interaction: Research Annual*, Vol. 1 (of 8 vols), ed. N. K. Denzin. Greenwich, CT: JAI Press, pp. 219–33.

Franks, D. D. (1989) 'Power and role taking: a social behavioralist's synthesis of Kemper's power and status model', in *The Sociology of Emotions: Original Essays and Research Papers*, ed. D. Franks and E. D. McCarthy. Greenwich, CT: JAI Press, pp. 153–77.

Freund, P. E. S. (1982) *The Civilized Body: Social Domination, Control and Health*. Philadelphia, PA: Temple University Press.

Freund, P. E. S. (1988) 'Bringing society into the body: understanding socialized human nature', *Theory and Society* 17: 839–64.

Freund, P. E. S. (1990) 'The expressive body: a common ground for the sociology of emotions and health and illness', *Sociology of Health and Illness* 12(4): 452–77.

Freund, P. E. S. and McGuire, M. (1995) *Health, Illness and the Social Body*, 2nd edn. Englewood Cliffs, NJ: Prentice-Hall.

George, M. S., Ketter, T. A., Paravh, P. I., Horwitz, B., Herscovitch, J. and Post, R. M. (1995) 'Brain activity during transient sadness and happiness in healthy women', *American Journal of Psychiatry* 152(3) (March): 341–51.

Giddens, A. (1984) *The Constitution of Society*. Cambridge: Polity Press.

Goffman, E. (1959) *The Presentation of Self in Everyday Life*. Garden City, NY: Doubleday Anchor.

Goffman, E. (1961) *Asylums*. Garden City, NY: Doubleday Anchor.

Goffman, E. (1971) *Relations in Public*. New York: Harper & Row.

Goffman, E. (1974) *Frame Analysis*. New York: Harper & Row.

Gottschalk, L. A., Fronczek, B. and Montes Buchsbaum, E. (1993) 'The cerebral neurobiology of hope and hopelessness', *Psychiatry* 56 (August): 270–81.

Griffith, J. L. and Griffith, N. E. (1994) *The Body Speaks*. New York: Basic Books.

Hochschild, A. (1979) 'Emotion work, feeling rules and social structure', *American Journal of Sociology* 85: 551–75.

Hochschild, A. (1983) *The Managed Heart: The Commercialization of Human Feeling*. Berkeley, CA: University of California Press.

Jackall, R. (1977) 'The control of public faces in a commercial work situation', *Urban Life* 6(3): 277–302.

Jacobs, B. L. (1994) 'Serotonin, motor activity and depression-related disorders', *American Scientist* 82(5): 456–63.

Johnson, M. (1987) *The Body in the Mind*. Chicago: University of Chicago Press.

Jourard, S. N. (1964) *The Transparent Self*. New York: Van Nostrand.

Karasek, R. and Theorell, T. (1990) *Healthy Work: Stress, Productivity and the Reconstruction of Working Life*. New York: Basic Books.

Kemper, T. D. (1990) *Social Structure and Testosterone*. New Brunswick, NJ: Rutgers University Press.

Kleinman, A. (1988) *The Illness Narratives: Suffering, Healing and the Human Condition*. New York: Basic Books.

Krohne, H. W. (1990) 'Personality as a mediator between objective events and their subjective representation', *Psychological Inquiry* 1(1): 26–9.

Laing, R. D. (1965) *The Divided Self*. Baltimore, MD: Penguin Books.

Laing, R. D. and Esterson, A. (1965) *Sanity, Madness and the Family*. New York: Basic Books.

Lazarus, R. S. (1991) *Emotions and Adaptations*. New York: Oxford University Press.

Leder, D. (1984) 'Medicine and paradigms of embodiment', *Journal of Medicine and Philosophy* 9: 29–43.

Lynch, J. (1979) *The Broken Heart*. New York: Basic Books.

Lynch, J. (1985) *The Language of the Heart*. New York: Basic Books.

Lyon, M. L. (1994) 'Emotion as mediator of somatic and social processes: the example of respiration', in *Social Perspectives on Emotions*, Vol. 2, ed. D. D. Franks. Greenwich, CT: JAI Press, pp. 83–108.

McCarthy, E. (1984) 'Towards a sociology of the physical world: George Herbert Mead on physical objects', in *Studies in Symbolic Interaction*, ed. N. K. Denzin. Greenwich, CT: JAI Press: pp. 105–21.

McGuire, M. (1996) 'Religion and healing the mind/body self', forthcoming in *Social Compass*.

Merleau-Ponty, M. (1962) *Phenomenology of Perception*. New York: Humanities Press.

Mills, C. W. (1956) *White Collar*. New York: Oxford University Press.

Moss, G. E. (1973) *Illness, Immunity and Social Interaction*. New York: Wiley.

Newton, T. (1995) *Managing Stress: Emotion and Power at Work*. London: Sage.

Radley, A. R. (1984) 'The embodiment of social relations in coronary heart disease', *Social Science and Medicine* 19(11): 1227–34.

Reich, W. (1976) *Character Analysis*. New York: Pocket Books.

Sapolsky, R. M. (1989) 'Hypercortisolism among socially subordinate wild baboons originates at the CNS level', *Archives of General Psychiatry* 46: 1047–51.

Sapolsky, R. M. (1990) 'Stress in the wild', *Scientific American* 252: 116–23.

Scheff, T. (1985) 'Universal expressive needs: a critique and a theory', *Symbolic Interaction* 8: 241–62.

Schneider, D. (1995) 'Attribution and social cognition', in M. Argyle and A. M. Colman (eds) *Social Psychology*. London: Longman, pp. 281–306.

Schutz, A. (1962) *Collected Papers*, Vol. I. The Hague: Martinus Nijhoff.

Shilling, C. (1993) *The Body and Social Theory*. London: Sage.

Silber, I. F. (1995) 'Space, fields, boundaries: the rise of spatial metaphors in contemporary sociological theory', *Social Research* 62(2) (Summer): 322–55.

Tierney, J. (1988) 'Wired for stress', *The New York Times Magazine* (15 May).

Waldholz, M. (1993) 'Study of fear shows emotions can alter "wiring" of the brain', *Wall Street Journal* (29 September): AI.

Weiner, H. (1992) *Perturbing the Organism: The Biology of Stressful Experience*. Chicago: University of Chicago Press.

Wentworth, W. M. and Ryan, J. (1990) 'Balancing body, mind and culture: the place of emotion in social life', in *Social Perspectives on Emotions*, ed. D. D. Franks. Greenwich, CT: JAI Press, pp. 25–46.

Wentworth, W. M. and Ryan, J. (1994) Introduction, in *Social Perspectives on Emotions*, Vol. 2, ed. D. D. Franks. Greenwich, CT: JAI Press, pp. 1–17.

Wentworth, W. M. and Yardley, D. (1994) 'Deep sociality: a bioevolutionary perspective on the sociology of human emotions', in *Social Perspectives on Emotions*, Vol. 2, ed. D. D. Franks. Greenwich, CT: JAI Press, pp. 21–55.

16 'Getting the job done'

Emotion management and cardiopulmonary resuscitation in nursing

Liz Meerabeau and Susie Page

INTRODUCTION

It has become almost a truism in sociology that the body has been neglected and recently 'rediscovered'; for example, through the work of Turner (1984). Frank (1991) attributes the growth of interest in the body to the influence of feminist theories, Foucault, and debates on modernity/postmodernity. As Scott and Morgan (1993: 19) state:

> The body and its close companion, the emotions, are after all the very matter of everyday experience. In dealing with the body and the emotions we are dealing with that which is closest to us, as researchers or as readers, with our very sense of being in the world.

We may want to draw here a distinction between the (reasonably healthy) body which is a 'matter of everyday experience' and the sick body. Since one of the reasons that sociologists of health and illness have often produced a rather disembodied sociology has been a reluctance (whether from squeamishness or ethical qualms) to observe the messier aspects of medical care (Frank 1990), perhaps nurses such as ourselves are in a good position to remedy this.

In this chapter, we will use an analysis of nurses' accounts of cardiopulmonary resuscitation (CPR) to reflect upon the increasing literature on emotions and embodiment in nursing, and the emotions which CPR aroused in retrospect, of which laughter was the most notable. The chapter draws on our clinical experience, plus a series of five taped debriefing sessions held with nursing personnel on a cardiology ward, within twenty-four hours of their participating in an arrest (Page 1992). Seven staff nurses, seven students and one ward sister were involved.

Cardiopulmonary resuscitation

A cardiac arrest is best described as a sudden cessation of cardiac activity. Unless prompt and effective measures are taken by nursing and medical personnel, that is to say, cardiopulmonary resuscitation (CPR), death is inevitable. The original intention of this procedure was as a curative measure for relatively healthy individuals following (witnessed) catastrophes such as drowning and electrocution. Yet since its inception the use of this therapy has been expanded to most situations in which there is cessation of heartbeat or respiration and it is true to say that resuscitation is now routine therapy (Omery and Caswell 1989). It is also a first aid measure, in which a trained lay person may be expected to perform as well as (or better than) a doctor or nurse.

Significantly, however, a CPR event has been described by a professor of cardiology (Vincent 1991) as dramatic, undignified, often inappropriate, poorly understood and of uncertain long-term outcome. The procedure is not without risks, and potentially exposes victims to serious injury and questionable outcomes, including chest abrasions, defibrillator burns and broken ribs (Sawyer Sommers 1991). Not surprisingly perhaps, preparation of nursing and medical personnel for such an event is fraught with difficulties, not least because the reality of the event frequently bears little resemblance to how it is presented in a training situation. It is widely acknowledged to be a highly stressful and 'most-dreaded' event for the majority of those who may be involved (Manderino *et al.* 1986; O'Donnell 1990; Smith 1992) and generates considerable anxiety. Such anxiety may be manifest in several ways at just the moment when a calm and controlled approach to the rapid employment of a complex array of physical and cognitive skills is required. A cardiac arrest is a dramatic event, but the technology used is not particularly advanced, nor long-lasting (most adult CPRs last five to ten minutes). It is also notable for taking place 'on stage' (Goffman 1971), and if it occurs on the ward other patients are likely to be auditory if not visual witnesses.

Nurses are required to start resuscitation procedures on all patients unless specifically told otherwise by medical colleagues. Whilst the subject is clearly open for negotiation between patient, family and the different health care personnel involved, nurses nevertheless sometimes find themselves undertaking resuscitation procedures they feel are highly inappropriate (Rundell and Rundell 1992). Sanctity of life versus quality of life issues underpin the do-not-resuscitate/resuscitate debates; the emotions engendered by such circumstances have to be suspended whilst the body work of a resuscitation is under way. This management and commodification of feelings to suit the public (paid) arena represent an aspect of what Hochschild (1983) terms emotional labour.

EMOTIONAL LABOUR AND CARING

Fineman (1993: 1) considers that emotions have generally been 'written out' by students of organizations, whereas he argues that their management and mobilization are pivotal to organizational life. There is a growing literature in nursing on the linked concepts of emotional labour and caring, both of which are briefly considered here. Nurses generally are heavily involved in emotional labour (Smith 1992; James 1984, 1992; Hochschild 1983) because, in addition to the physical care they are required to deliver, there is an expectation that emotions will be controlled. As Lawler (1991: 126) states: 'Such emotional control is part of the nurse's "professional" approach, that is learning how to do body care and perform other nursing functions in a manner typical of the occupation.' This emotional control/labour may also be seen in the commitment which nurses are exhorted to demonstrate towards their patients whilst at the same time avoiding 'over-involvement'. Dunlop (1986) likens this to a tightrope walk between closeness and distance with the inherent risk of tipping either way, although there are signs that in the 'new nursing', a philosophy involving partnership with patients and greater informality, nurses may feel able to loosen this control (e.g. Savage 1995).

The concept of emotional labour is closely linked in nursing to that of care. Several nursing writers have explored how caring is enacted in a technological environment, the intensive care unit in which nursing practice is inextricably interwoven with technology (Ray 1987; Cooper 1993; Walters 1995). Less experienced nurses are distracted by the equipment (in Walters's term, borrowed from Heidegger (1962), it is present to hand, not ready to hand). Ray argues for the equal importance of nursing competence and humanistic caring; Cooper considers that the greatest challenge is to confront the dehumanizing impact of the technologized environment on both doctor and nurse, to 'temper the insults of technology with care' (1993: 30).

Apart from the nursing literature on caring as an embodied action, there is also a more abstract literature about caring (Leininger 1988; Watson 1988), which Barker *et al.* (1995) critique as 'new age nursing'. Several authors, such as Dunlop (1986), have argued that this nursing theory has, like sociology, become disembodied; it 'etherealizes the body' and removes the 'mess and dirt of bodily life' (Dunlop 1986: 664).

Doing dirty work: pollution and body work in nursing

The 'mess and dirt of bodily life' are well represented in the anthropological literature on nursing. This literature may be seen as a way for nursing to reclaim a previously stigmatized subject (women's knowledge and work). For example, James (1992) compares domestic carework with that in hospices, and Murcott's work (1993) on how women manage their infants' excretion has parallels with Lawler's (1991) interest in how nurses manage body products, a topic which she claims is 'on the fringe of respectability' (1991: v). The absence of discussion of these issues within preparation for nursing practice echoes their absence in social discussion since the 'civilizing' of the body began in the sixteenth century (Elias 1978). Since this work is not openly discussed it is not publicly displayed and as such becomes invisible, which poses problems for articulating the breadth of the nurse's role and its knowledge base (Reed and Procter 1993).

Much of the anthropologically informed nursing literature (Wolf 1988, 1989; Lawler 1991; Littlewood 1991; Savage 1995) uses Douglas's work on pollution and marginality (Douglas 1966, 1975). Perhaps the most fully developed position has been that of Lawler (1991) who draws on anthropology and phenomenology to develop what she terms somology, an account of how nurses help to reconcile the person and the lived, often damaged body. The nurse is viewed as a mediator of pollution; to share or care for the pollution of another to whom one is not intimately bound is a restatement of humility or love (Dunlop 1986). As Littlewood (1991: 185) states:

> Caring is manifest in the act of protecting the body marginals, helping to define 'self' and 'not self'; it is the mediation between meaning of illness and meaning of disease.

Pollution is matter out of place, but people, such as the sick and dying, can also be out of place, or marginals who transgress codes. The issue of marginality and ambiguity is an important one in the context of cardiopulmonary resuscitation, as will now be discussed.

Death and dying

There is a considerable literature on death and dying, much of which examines the process over time; for example, Glaser and Strauss (1965), Sudnow (1967), James (1984). There is, however, little literature on how sudden death is managed, or the anomaly of the newly dead body. Strauss *et al.* (1982: 254) describe 'sentimental work' as 'any kind of work where the object being worked on is alive, sentient, reacting' and claim that it is important not to violate the rather basic rules of human interaction, which can lead to feelings of biological and psychological invasion. They argue that work is less complex when the object is inanimate; however, the newly dead body, although literally an inanimate object, has a marginal, ambiguous status. Wolf (1988) and Lawler (1991) give examples of nurses who continue to see the newly dead not as a body, but as the person they looked after. Lawler (1991: 189) quotes one nurse as saying 'He's still sort of there, it's still him', although nurses viewed bodies that were dead on arrival differently. Our understanding of the body is interwoven with personhood, although the latter concept is difficult to translate into action, particularly at the margins of life.

James (1984) gives an example of the gentle humour used by nurses as they lay out the corpse. Lawler (1991: 191) states that nurses are aware of the expectation that the dead body should be handled with respect, but that often their composure deserts them and they recount untoward incidents as 'dead body stories'; for example, if the body groans as it is turned. Such happenings frequently give rise to uncontrollable laughter, which is not the everyday type, but nervous and often due to uncertainty and even fear. As will be explored later, laughter may reflect several different or even mixed emotions; Lawler (1991: 191) quotes one interviewee who says: 'If you were serious and didn't laugh, didn't joke, then you would spend a lot of your time crying.'

Wolf (1991), in her study of nurses' experiences of giving post-mortem care to patients who have donated organs, also highlights issues of duality in relation to caring for the newly dead. The emotional workload in caregiving whilst procuring organs from transplant donors is taxing in the extreme; indeed, the very possibility of organ transplantation eliminates the chance of a 'peaceful' death for some patients and thus presents a conflict for some nurses. The situation is particularly complex as donors move from machine-supported life (although technically brain dead) to being 'dead dead' following organ procurement. Thus nurses care for legally dead patients who are not clinically dead until their organs are removed. The incongruity of this situation is recognized by those involved as they care for the living/dead: life and death coexisting in one patient. In CPR, the status of the body is perhaps even more ambiguous than in the newly dead, since the person may or may not be regarded as dead, as doctors and nurses continue to work on them and hope for resuscitation.

Sanitized theory and the messiness of practice

The recalcitrance of the body is not of course confined to CPR, but is a recognized if little discussed aspect of nursing; for example, the high incidence of back injuries in nurses indicates that handling the physical body is not something which can be made easy simply by using techniques for safe lifting. Similarly, CPR appears simple in theory, but can be difficult to put into practice. As one student commented after attending an arrest:

> I don't think that the experience that we get practising on the dummies in the School of Nursing . . . I didn't find any good at all. I don't think it was at all like [the real thing].

When asked about the relationship between taught theory and practice two staff nurses commented:

> I remember going to a lecture where we were given criteria of things to look out for [then lists these] but the chances are they might only have one of those things . . . and it's never as it is in textbooks.

> [Y]ou can write it down in a textbook and say this is what happens, this is what you need to do but as [the other respondent] said, you don't get it in textbooks, things happen in different orders . . . people do things differently.

It appears that the theory does little to prepare nurses for the sheer physicality and intimate proximity of the body work that may be involved in

CPR. Chest compressions in order to maintain some cardiac output and mouth-to-mouth ventilation in order to put oxygen into the lungs are acknowledged essentials although administering these to a plastic (training) doll is radically different from doing them to a clammy, choking individual. (In fact, in the ward where the study was undertaken, no attempts were made to use mouth-to-mouth resuscitation, perhaps owing to a distaste for intimate and possibly unpleasant contact.) Furthermore, what is often not mentioned is the possibility of encountering alarming colour changes in the patient, hearing odd noises and dealing with vomit, urine and sometimes blood during the process. For example, Kiger (1994) quotes a student who was shocked by the 'blue bits and pale bits' and the 'gargly' noise which a patient made. This constitutes some of the 'dirty' work of nursing the body referred to by Lawler (1991) as pollution management. The following extract, given after a particularly stressful resuscitation, captures some of this 'dirty' work and was accompanied by laughter.

> We had been told he was fine and then he comes up blue and gasping on no oxygen.

> I've never seen someone with so much ascites and fluid. I mean he was really enormous. . . . He was obviously really gasping for it. He was hardly on the bed when he started to vomit and his eyes started to go slightly . . . so of course he went sideways . . . I couldn't get his legs up.

> We had an airway there but we wouldn't have been able to use it actually. He was vomiting.

> A Hoover would have been better at the time, you just couldn't do anything.

EMOTION WORK

One of the hardest tasks in debriefing was the identification of positive feelings. Ellis (1991: 35) suggests that this may be a general finding; talking about negative emotions may be interesting or easier, whereas positive emotions other than perhaps ecstasy are less acute and more diffuse. First, as the following extract suggests, the participants seemed unaware of or loath to admit the value of their actions, even after a successful resuscitation.

> Susie: So what did you think was the most effective thing that was done nursing-wise?

> Silence.

> Susie: Why do you think she survived? Was it attributable to your actions?

Jane: Luck. I don't know. Going back . . . do we know why the curtains were drawn?

Second, the conversation tended to focus on the worst aspect of the event rather than the best and the tangible feelings of anger and tension in some of the accounts made it difficult to progress; staff appeared at times stuck with their feelings, especially after an unsuccessful resuscitation. Feelings of failure may be exacerbated since staff tend to overestimate the chance of success in CPR (Wagg *et al.* 1995).

Susie: What do you make of that?

Clare: It was a shambles from start to finish. [*General agreement.*] It was the worst arrest I have ever seen . . . the worst arrest I have ever had the misfortune to be at.

Susie: How did you feel after the event?

Clare: Just unbelievable, really bad.

Elaine: It was a long night.

Susie: Can you explain why you felt so bad?

Clare: Just everything we tried to do we couldn't. It just went wrong from start to finish from the minute . . . I mean, what a way to go, it's not very nice at all and he was conscious throughout most of it . . . and then the fact that we couldn't contact his wife.

Elaine: I think I felt really inadequate afterwards.

Frequently the extreme agitation felt during a resuscitation event handicapped nurses and resulted in 'de-skilling' or inefficient practice. As one staff nurse put it: 'In the stressful situation your brain just goes completely y'know.' The following excerpt provides an apt illustration of the point – this time it appears to have affected one of the medical staff. (Ambubagging is a procedure undertaken via a mask and oxygen flow for assisting maintenance of respiratory function.)

Anita: Just went out to see what was happening really . . . just loads of people round the bed. . . . [I] connected the oxygen [*giggles*] . . . 'cos the oxygen wasn't connected . . . 'cos he [the doctor] was Ambubagging . . . I just looked [*giggles*] and thought he's Ambubagging and it's not connected to the oxygen.

Mary: I remember on my first arrest up here I was running around trying to find an oxygen cylinder yet we've got piped oxygen and I just didn't think [*laughter*]. . . . I was running up and down the ward with a cylinder!

Anita: You just die afterwards don't you?

Mary (*laughing*):   Yeah.

The emotional control required in the actual emergency situation contrasted with the outpouring of emotion that occurred for some within the debriefing sessions. Repetition may have helped to make sense of the experience and/or disperse individual and shared feelings of guilt or failure if 'poor practice' was being recounted. It made the chronological description of events difficult to orchestrate. Conversely, a few participants went to great lengths *not* to convey any emotions they may have felt in relation to the event. They chose instead to focus on non-personal issues such as equipment problems or the performance of others (usually doctors). In that particular context, expression of feeling appeared to be eschewed by some in order to maintain an image of professional competence, a point of considerable importance within the (still) hierarchical structure of nursing, and a coping mechanism in itself. It is possible that trained staff may find it more difficult to discuss a perceived lack of competence in front of students.

Several staff said that talking about a previous arrest had helped:

Mary: I felt a lot calmer with this one because we had all talked about it and we knew a bit more whereas usually your hands start shaking and the adrenaline's pumping and you think 'Oh my God' at first but then you think . . . I started laughing, I kept thinking here we go again . . . [*laughter*] 'cos like even my nerves were different because you pick up on so much. Because I felt as though I'd learnt a lot from last time we all talked about it . . . and that it's not only me that sometimes feels a prat afterwards [*laughter*] 'cos you always think back and dread everything that has gone on [*agreement*] . . . and you know for a fact that it's not only you!

Susie: And what about talking about it like this?

Fiona: It's good. . . . It helps you . . . just talking about it gets rid of any . . . I don't know . . . if you're feeling . . . pent-up emotions . . . if you're feeling, gosh, shocked by it all, sometimes it's calming just to talk through it and analyse what you have been doing and . . . emm . . . you don't dread the next one . . . perhaps as much. I used to get terribly upset about arrests and I don't get as upset as I used to. I feel I'm emotionally coping a lot better.

Anger

Although anger was expressed in most of the accounts, it was particularly marked after one failed resuscitation attempt. The emotion of anger has seldom been explored in the theoretical or empirical literature in nursing

(Thomas 1990). Where it is addressed it is usually seen as something nurses may encounter in others, as a manifestation of the grieving process, or in clients suffering from mental ill health, and something which requires 'managing'. Indeed, like laughter, anger has an historical legacy associating it with madness, making it something to be contained (Thomas 1990). The general absence of anger from the nursing literature may be related to its deemed inappropriateness to nursing practice, or to sanctions within a predominantly female profession on who may express it. For anger, certainly within the psychology literature, is seen as gendered (Sharkin 1993; Stearns 1992).

The sociocultural literature addresses the interpersonal nature of anger, and associates it with a variety of other emotions such as shame and guilt; it may also be linked with laughter. Davies (1984) and Pache (1992) highlight the use of laughter, which was apparent in all debriefings, as a strategy for hiding or suppressing anger. Sullivan (1953, cited in Thomas 1990) links the emotions of anger and anxiety; when an individual's expectations of others are not met, anxiety is produced, and anger may ward off this anxiety. Certainly in the debriefing session which was so overshadowed by anger, the nurses concerned had important expectations of themselves as well as others, such as medical staff at the scene and nursing staff on other shifts, who should have checked the resuscitation equipment. Moreover, the marked differences in power and status between medical and nursing staff were felt acutely during that arrest; Kemper (1978) suggests that such felt deficits of power and status may give rise to several distressing emotions, including anger.

Laughter

Despite the expression of negative feelings such as anger, laughter occurred frequently throughout the accounts, particularly when harrowing aspects of a CPR event were being recalled or when 'less than perfect' practice was conveyed (or confessed). Perhaps this should not surprise us; Ellis (1991: 37) considers that emotions are often intertwined, ambivalent or contradictory, and different emotions may be felt simultaneously. The following quotes are taken from a debriefing session in which such an admission was being made. (The established procedure recommends that the person who finds an arrested patient *shouts* for help but *stays* with the patient whilst *one* other person telephones for the emergency team.) This departure from taught theory may, once again, be related to the anxiety engendered by the situation but it is recounted here to illustrate the use of laughter in the 'telling'.

Susie: So what happened?

Clare: This time I found the patient. She was my patient. Her eyes were starting to roll back . . . I went in and thought, ohhh . . . she

> can't be . . . do you think she is? She is, she is, she must be. . . . And then I thought somebody has probably not phoned the twos [emergency telephone number], I'll go and phone the twos and as *I'd* gone, *she'd* gone to phone the twos [*laughter*].

Elaine: I said to you 'I'll phone the twos' and you thought I said 'you phone the twos'.

Clare: I thought you said 'you phone the twos' [*laughter*]. So I went off and we were both phoning the twos!

Elaine: And it was engaged when you phoned! [*laughter*]

The sociological literature on humour gives us some help in understanding this laughter, although Fox (1990) considers that humour is a generally neglected area, and much of the literature (e.g. Fox 1990; Zijderveld 1983; Mulkay 1988) tends to concentrate on jokes and what may be a rather masculine approach to humour. The humour expressed in this study is what Mulkay (1988) termed applied humour; it is fairly unstructured, arises out of the situation, and would not transplant easily. Zijderveld (1983) suggests laughter is a way of dissolving the dissonance between the reality of everyday practice and ideal practice; it helps people to cope with situations over which they may have no control, and is thus a triumph *vis-à-vis* reality (ibid.: 40). In particular, Zijderveld argues that 'black' humour erases the boundary between the couth and the uncouth, the proper and improper, and is therefore particularly prevalent in ambiguous situations (such as the newly dead) or where pollution occurs both figuratively, owing to the transgression of boundaries, and literally. Other examples are given by Koenig (1988), who in a study of plasma exchange technology describes nurses dissolving in uncontrollable laughter when the machine spurted blood everywhere, and Lella and Pawluch (1988), who refer to medical students' accounts of others' (never their own) jokes about the bodies they were dissecting.

Zijderveld is particularly fruitful in helping us to understand this area. At first, he states, our feelings are hurt, and then laughter covers up our embarrassment. However, he is less convincing when he draws on linguistic theory to argue that black humour is a rather abstract play with words and that 'the blood in anecdotes is never bloody' (1983: 23); in the incident described by Koenig above, the blood is very bloody, and the pollution is literal. Zijderveld draws on Plessner (1961) to argue that the tragic and comic are often hard to distinguish; both laughing and crying are on the borderline, where 'the body-one-has is taken over by the body-one-is' (1983: 28), and the 'crying or laughing body has taken control of the mind', particularly in situations when we do not know how to react meaningfully and adequately (ibid.: 29). As is often said, we don't know whether to laugh or cry, and as Lawler's interviewee, cited earlier, said, if you didn't joke you would spend a lot of your time crying.

Strong (1979: 187), drawing on Goffman (1971), argues that humour is to be expected in back-stage areas such as these group discussions. From a purely professional perspective such laughter may appear highly inappropriate, although it is recognized as a useful method in the emotional processing required to learn from experience (Boud *et al.* 1985). This laughter may be construed not as humour, but rather as being due to embarrassment (Babcock 1988; Edelmann 1985). Kuzmics's (1991) discussion of embarrassment draws heavily on Elias (1982, 1983) and Goffman (1972), the latter of whom sketches a somewhat ahistorical programme for the study of embarrassment, and suggests that it derives primarily from the unrealized expectations placed on someone else, or the self. However, Goffman is surely incorrect in claiming that embarrassment results in a state of 'affectual inhibition' since that would leave no room for the laughter expressed here. A gender/power element is also missing; it may be that laughter about failures in practice is a feature of less powerful groups, and an alternative to expressing anger. Edelmann (1985) identifies 'jokework' as one of the tactics for handling embarrassment; Fox (1990: 443) and Coser (1962) consider that humour defuses incongruities, but then leaves situations unchanged.

The embarrassment may be all the greater the more solemn or more serious the nature of the activity; it may be that the collapse of composure is not the result but the cause of the embarrassment. Many of us may have experienced the urge to giggle at a funeral; one of us (Liz Meerabeau) has found herself having to avoid the gaze of her sister (another giggler) when, in the process of arranging a funeral, the unctuous performance of a young undertaker was undercut by the off-stage sound of a hammer on a pinewood box. Lawler (1991) states that an exploration of embarrassment is fundamental to a sociological understanding of the body, although in her work much of the discussion is about the management of embarrassment in body care, and many of the situations were embarrassing at the time rather than in retrospect, as here.

Laughter, which was evident to a greater or lesser degree in every account, may have served additional functions, such as catharsis and relief, a contribution to group/team cohesion (Dwyer 1991), a barrier to more questioning, the maintenance of stress within manageable bounds and a distancing from the threat of death. Whatever its purpose, and Zijderveld (1983) claims that it may sometimes have no purpose at all, laughter and the use of humour are certainly a standard way of coping amongst nurses, doctors and patients as they deal with their emotions and responses amidst uncertainty, anxiety and death experiences (Coser 1960, 1962; Lawler 1991; Savage 1995; Koenig 1988; Mallett 1993; Astedt-Kurki and Liukkonen 1994; Harries 1995). Nurses' anxiety in the face of death has been interpreted as strongly related to the 'unknownness' of death and the implications for their own mortality (Kiger 1994; Austin Hurtig and Stewin 1990). Moreover a sudden death and the chaos of a cardiac arrest represent for many 'the bad' in nursing as opposed to the rewarding aspects or 'the good' in facilitating a peaceful end (Kiger 1994), although ironically sudden death from cardiac arrest may be how many of us think we would like to go.

DEATH, DRAMA AND INDIGNITY

To warrant a full-blown cardiac arrest procedure, many patients have effectively already 'died', for a CPR event is a moment where self-sustainable life has been lost and valiant attempts are being made in order to try to regain it. The aim is to restore an efficient cardiac output within two to four minutes, or brain damage (resulting from an inadequate oxygen supply) will be irreversible.

Attitudes towards death, whether personal or acquired from nursing/ medical education, have to be 'managed' in the face of required action; the ability to do this is variable. Within a CPR event health care professionals are not only attempting to prevent death, but actually converting death to life and thus challenging death's irreversibility and life's boundaries. Omery and Caswell (1989) claim that the (zealous) use of resuscitation has not only changed the meaning associated with death, it has also changed the meaning associated with life. As such it can bring on emotional responses for which probably no other treatment can claim such responsibility.

The pursuit of life in the face of death has led the outcomes from a cardiopulmonary resuscitation to be seen in nursing/medical terms as *success or failure*,[1] success being a restoration of cardiac function and failure being death. This reflects societal attitudes and those of mainstream medicine which see death as a defeat, the 'point zero' at which individuals lose control over themselves and their bodies (Giddens 1991). The game appears to be to gain victory and control over death, which adds an exquisite tension to the actions and emotions required of the health care staff since performance may be directly related to outcome. The pressure to perform well is considerable despite the potential for dissonance between preferred professional outcomes and those of the patient.

Susie: What's your lasting impression you will take away from this one?

Elaine: When I went home I thought God y'know, we saved him, he lived. But afterwards, immediately afterwards, when he was quite stable we were asking him if he was OK, could he remember anything and he said, 'Oh, it would have been a nice way to go', because he's had a very sad history, he's been on his own for quite a long while. I thought that bit was really sad.

The apparent professional predilection for life at all costs may be derived from twentieth-century fears of death. Death, through its medicalization, is no longer seen as a natural phenomenon but as a threat to life. In some

health care contexts it is a 'business lost', a shameful thing, an embarrassment, even dirty and indecent and as such it is disarticulated from human
dignity (Madan 1992). Walter (1991) argues that death may be more of a
taboo for doctors (though not, perhaps, nurses) than for the general population. A 'negative outcome' from a CPR event is, on the whole, to be
avoided and elaborate procedures are in place to assist this. Death is
made difficult to achieve through the advent of technology, aptly demonstrated by the equipment required at a resuscitation event and the sometimes
lengthy and energetic activities of the health care staff. Muller and Koenig
(1988) state that while staff exercise their power to keep someone alive,
they suspend the definition of dying. Any dignity associated with death
(or indeed life) is removed as the body is subjected to pummelling, pushing
and shoving, electric shocks and a variety of invasive procedures. Certainly
the drama and indignities of a resuscitation event diminish the spectre of
death and may be themselves another coping mechanism in the face of
'failure'.

Yet nurses see a lot of death. They are probably the only occupational
group who deal with the body before and after death and often have an
established relationship with the person who has died (Lawler 1991).
Nurses have a unique role in assisting the individual, sick or well, in the performance of those activities contributing to health or its recovery, or to a
peaceful death (Henderson 1969). They therefore have an implied responsibility for the quality of the patient's experience of dying and, unlike doctors,
they do not generally undertake dissection in their training, and therefore do
not experience the same distancing from and objectification of the body
(Lella and Pawluch 1988; Frankenberg 1994). The circumstances of death
around a CPR event may be seen as 'counter-cultural' and therefore stressful to many. This is particularly so as the construct of dignity, although
generally poorly clarified, assumes great importance in the delivery of
nursing care, especially when people are helpless or unconscious (Mairis
1994). (The concept is referred to in the statutory/professional guidelines
for nurses; for example, United Kingdom Central Council 1994a, 1994b;
and even the *Patient's Charter,* Department of Health 1990).

Dignity regained

Death carries many rituals in all societies. A hospital is no exception, with
nurses having to perform the last offices: wash and lay out the body, deal
with relatives, complete the appropriate documentation, and accompany
the body to the morgue (Wolf 1991). Walsh and Ford (1989: 105–6)
deride the rituals of washing and applying clean linen, and the concealment
of the body during removal, together with the drawing of the other patients'
curtains. The felt need to show respect means that the situation and the
body are handled with dignity and seriousness. Thus although dignity may

have been lost in the process of dying it may be retrieved in death via appropriate actions and the assumption of 'suitable' emotions.

Whilst this time may offer a valued opportunity for 'closure' of the nurse–patient relationship (Smith 1992), it is yet another arena for emotional management. Those involved in a resuscitation attempt have to move abruptly from 'assaulting' the body in an action-packed scenario to treating it with care and deference within a matter of minutes: at best an emotional pendulum if not a minefield. The common thread throughout is the hands-on, dirty, mess-clearing body work necessary alongside the emotional labour. Not surprisingly the onset of laughter at this time is not uncommon and although considered inappropriate may obscure other potentially disabling emotions in respect of getting done what needs to be done (Lawler 1991).

Understandably perhaps, 'death experiences' for many nurses are problematic, occurring as they do in a wider societal framework, which may be changing (McNamara *et al*. 1995) but which is still marked by apprehension, avoidance, embarrassment and secrecy towards death. This is perpetuated by the bureaucracy of making hospitals primarily responsible for death management (McNamara *et al*. 1995; Bauman 1992). Interestingly death within the hospice movement, although underpinned by a different philosophy and far removed from CPR activities, reverses the definition of death as 'bad'. The terminology of winning and losing is equally reversed. A 'good death' (or one that has been won) in a hospice is one that incorporates the dying person's physical, psychological, social and spiritual needs and where there is an awareness of, an acceptance of and a preparation for death (McNamara *et al*. 1995), what Seale (1995: 612) terms the 'heroic script of aware dying'; a situation which bears little resemblance to a cardiac arrest situation.

CONCLUSION

The process of cardiopulmonary resuscitation and nurses' accounts of their experiences of participating in such events have been used as a vehicle to explore the existence of some fundamental dualisms. The seemingly tenuous relationship between taught CPR theory and the reality of practice has been highlighted. It is a situation in which the skills, knowledge and experience of the nurse are rigorously and publicly tested since a positive performance and outcome are highly prized. The responsibilities of the nurse are significant and the assumption of appropriate emotions is all-important. The difficulties in achieving these may be compounded by bigger questions regarding the appropriateness of the procedure itself.

Not surprisingly the role of anxiety in inhibiting performance is considerable and the reactions afterwards vary from sadness to laughter, from emotional outpourings to tight-lipped professional control. The difficulties, dangers and draining nature of this emotional work are submerged beneath the business of body work and practicalities of 'getting the job done'. The unpredictability of the event and the proximity of death result in unique tensions classified in terms of good or bad, success or failure, desirable versus undesirable.

The medicalization of death and its amenability to human manipulation (Madan 1992) are evident in the moves from life to death and death to life during a resuscitation. Each stage requires feelings and actions that befit the moment, the see-saw between indignity in CPR and dignity with last offices providing a key example. Issues of power and control over the body in both its living and dead states weave their way throughout as resuscitation spans the field of ethical, moral, spiritual, physiological, professional and economic debate. Nurses surely deal with both the sacred and the profane.

ACKNOWLEDGEMENT

We would like to thank Barbara Harrison for her helpful comments on this chapter.

NOTE

1 In reality the notion of success requires qualification because more than 50 per cent of resuscitated patients go on to die as a result of neurological sequelae and more than 20 per cent of survivors sustain severe brain damage (Liss 1986). Only about 10–20 per cent of those undergoing CPR in acute general hospitals live to be discharged (Wagg *et al.* 1995), with few returning to previous lifestyles (Omery and Caswell 1989).

BIBLIOGRAPHY

Astedt-Kurki, P. and Liukkonen, A. (1994) 'Humour in nursing care', *Journal of Advanced Nursing* 20: 183–8.
Austin Hurtig, W. and Stewin, L. (1990) 'The effect of death education and experience on nursing students' attitude towards death', *Journal of Advanced Nursing* 15: 29–34.
Babcock, M. (1988) 'Embarrassment: a window on the self', *Journal for the Theory of Social Behaviour* 18(4): 459–83.
Barker, P., Reynolds, W. and Ward, T. (1995) 'The proper focus of nursing: a critique of the "caring" ideology', *International Journal of Nursing Studies* 32(4): 386–97.
Bauman, Z. (1992) *Mortality, Immortality and Other Life Strategies.* Cambridge: Polity Press.
Boud, D., Keogh, R. and Walker, D. (1985) *Reflection: Turning Experience into Learning.* London: Kogan Page.
Cooper, M. C. (1993) 'The intersection of technology and care in the ICU', *Advances in Nursing Science* 15(3): 23–32.
Coser, R. (1960) 'Laughter among colleagues: a study of the functions of humour among the staff of a mental hospital', *Psychiatry* 23: 81–95.
Coser, R. (1962) 'Laughter in the ward', in *Life in the Ward.* East Lansing, MI: Michigan State University Press, pp. 84–9.

Davies, C. (1984) 'Commentary on Anton C. Zijderveld's trend report on "The sociology of humor and laughter"', *Current Sociology* 32(1), 142–57.

Department of Health (1990) *The Patient's Charter*. London: HMSO.

Douglas, M. (1966) *Purity and Danger*. Harmondsworth, Mx: Penguin.

Douglas, M. (1975) *Implicit Meanings*. London: Routledge & Kegan Paul.

Dunlop, M. J. (1986) 'Is a science of caring possible?' *Journal of Advanced Nursing* 11: 661–70.

Dwyer, T. (1991) 'Humour, power and change in organizations', *Human Relations* 44(1): 1–19.

Edelmann, R. (1985) 'Social embarrassment: an analysis of the process', *Journal of Social and Personal Relationships* 2: 195–213.

Elias, N. (1978) *The Civilizing Process*, Vol. 1, *The History of Manners*. Oxford: Blackwell.

Elias, N. (1982) *The Civilizing Process*, Vol. 2, *State Formation and Civilization*. Oxford: Blackwell.

Elias, N. (1983) *The Court Society*. Oxford: Blackwell.

Ellis, C. (1991) 'Sociological introspection and emotional experience', *Symbolic Interaction* 14(1): 23–50.

Fineman, S. (1993) *Emotions in Organizations*. London: Sage.

Fox, S. (1990) 'The ethnography of humour and the problem of social reality', *Sociology* 24(3): 431–46.

Frank, A. (1990) 'Bringing bodies back in: a decade review', *Theory, Culture and Society* 7(1): 131–62.

Frank, A. (1991) 'For a sociology of the body: an analytic review', in M. Featherstone, M. Hepworth and B. S. Turner (eds) *The Body: Social Process and Cultural Theory*. London: Sage.

Frankenberg, R. (1994) 'What is power? How is decision? The heart has its reasons', in I. Robinson (ed.) *Life and Death under High Technology Medicine*. Manchester: Manchester University Press, pp. 188–208.

Giddens, A. (1991) *Modernity and Self-Identity*. Cambridge: Polity Press.

Glaser, B. and Strauss, A. (1965) *Awareness of Dying*. Chicago: Aldine.

Goffman, E. (1971) *The Presentation of Self in Everyday Life*. Harmondsworth, Mx: Penguin.

Goffman, E. (1972) *Interaction Rituals*. Harmondsworth, Mx: Penguin.

Harries, G. (1995) 'Use of humour in patient care', *British Journal of Nursing* 4(17): 984–6.

Heidegger, M. (1962) *Being and Time*. New York: Harper & Row.

Henderson, V. (1969) *The Nature of Nursing*. London: Collier Macmillan.

Hochschild, A. R. (1983) *The Managed Heart: The Commercialization of Human Feeling*. Berkeley, CA: University of California Press.

James, N. (1984) 'Postscript to nursing', in C. Bell and H. Roberts (eds) *Social Researching: Politics, Problems and Practice*. London: Routledge & Kegan Paul.

James, N. (1992) 'Care = organisation + physical labour + emotional labour', *Sociology of Health and Illness* 14(4): 488–509.

Kemper, T. (1978) 'Toward a sociology of emotions: some problems and some solutions', *American Sociologist* 13(1): 30–41.

Kiger, A. M. (1994) 'Student nurses' involvement with death: the image and the experience', *Journal of Advanced Nursing* 20: 679–86.

Koenig, B. (1988) 'The technological imperative in medical practice: the social creation of a "routine" treatment', in M. Lock and M. Gordon (eds) *Biomedicine Examined*. Dordrecht: Kluwer, pp. 465–96.

Kuzmics, H. (1991) 'Embarrassment and civilization', *Theory, Culture and Society* 8(2): 1–30.

Lawler, J. (1991) *Behind the Screens: Nursing, Somology and the Problem of the Body*. Melbourne, Australia: Churchill Livingstone.

Leininger, M. (1988) 'Leininger's theory of nursing: cultural care, diversity and universality', *Nursing Science Quarterly* 1: 152–60.

Lella, J. and Pawluch, D. (1988) 'Medical students and the cadaver in social and cultural context', in M. Lock and M. Gordon (eds) *Biomedicine Examined*. Dordrecht: Kluwer, pp. 125–53.

Liss, H. P. (1986) 'A history of resuscitation', *Annals of Emergency Medicine* (15 January): 65–72.

Littlewood, J. (1991) 'Care and ambiguity: towards a concept of nursing', in P. Holden and J. Littlewood (eds) *Anthropology and Nursing*. London: Routledge.

McNamara, B., Waddell, C. and Colvin, M. (1995) 'Threats to the good death: the cultural context of stress and coping among hospice nurses', *Sociology of Health and Illness* 17(2): 222–44.

Madan, T. N. (1992) 'Dying with dignity', *Social Science and Medicine* 35(4): 425–32.

Mairis, E. D. (1994) 'Concept clarification in professional practice – dignity', *Journal of Advanced Nursing* 19: 947–53.

Mallett, J. (1993) 'Use of humour and laughter in patient care', *British Journal of Nursing* 2(3): 172–5.

Manderino, M. A., Yonkman, C. A., Gangong, L. H. and Royal, A. (1986) 'Evaluation of a cardiac arrest simulation', *Journal of Nursing Education* 25(3) (March): 107–11.

Mulkay, M. (1988) *On Humour: Its Nature and Its Place in Modern Society*. Cambridge: Polity Press.

Muller, J. and Koenig, B. (1988) 'On the boundary of life and death: the definition of dying by medical residents', in M. Lock and M. Gordon (eds) *Biomedicine Examined*. Dordrecht: Kluwer, pp. 351–74.

Murcott, A. (1993) 'Purity and pollution: body management and the social place of infancy', in S. Scott and D. Morgan (eds) *Body Matters: Essays on the Sociology of the Body*. London: Falmer, pp. 122–34.

O'Donnell, C. (1990) 'A survey of opinion amongst trained nurses and junior medical staff on current practices in resuscitation', *Journal of Advanced Nursing* 15: 1175–80.

Omery, A. and Caswell, D. (1989) 'Ethical perspectives. (Brain resuscitation)', *Critical Care Nursing Clinics of North America* 1(1) (March): 165–73.

Pache, I. (1992) 'Maybe there is some anger behind that laughter: humor and laughter in a multicultural women's group', *Working Papers on Language, Gender and Sexism* 2(1): 87–97.

Page, S. (1992) 'Debriefing following cardiopulmonary resuscitation: towards a strategy for reflective practice?', unpublished BEd (Hons) thesis, South Bank University, London.

Plessner, H. (1961) *Lachen und Weinen*. Berne: Francke Verlag.

Ray, M. A. (1987) 'Technological caring: a new model in critical care', *Dimensions of Critical Care Nursing* 6(3): 166–73.

Reed, J. and Procter, S. (1993) *Nurse Education: A Reflective Approach*. London: Edward Arnold.

Rundell, S. and Rundell, L. (1992) 'The nursing contribution to the resuscitation debate', *Journal of Clinical Nursing* 1: 195–8.

Savage, J. (1995) *Nursing and Intimacy*. London: Scutari.

Sawyer Sommers, M. (1991) 'Potential for injury: trauma after cardiopulmonary resuscitation', *Heart and Lung* 20(3): 287–93.

Scott, S. and Morgan, D. (1993) 'Bodies in a social landscape', in S. Scott and D. Morgan (eds) *Body Matters: Essays on the Sociology of the Body*. London: Falmer.

Seale, C. (1995) 'Heroic death', *Sociology* 29(4): 597–613.

Sharkin, B. (1993) 'Anger and gender: theory, research and implications', *Journal of Counseling and Development* 71(4): 386–9.

Smith, P. (1992) *The Emotional Labour of Nursing*. London: Macmillan.

Stearns, P. (1992) 'Gender and emotion: a twentieth century transition', in D. Franks and V. Gecas (eds) *Social Perspectives on Emotion*, Vol. 1. Greenwich, CT: JAI Press, pp. 167–89.

Strauss, A., Fagerhaugh, S., Suzcek, B. and Wiener, C. (1982) 'Sentimental work in the technologized hospital', *Sociology of Health and Illness* 4(3): 254–78.

Strong, P. (1979) *The Ceremonial Order of the Clinic: Parents, Doctors and Medical Bureaucracies*. London: Routledge & Kegan Paul.

Sudnow, D. (1967) *Passing On*. Englewood Cliffs, NJ: Prentice-Hall.

Thomas, S. (1990) 'Theoretical and empirical perspectives on anger', *Issues in Mental Health Nursing* 11(3): 203–16.

Turner, B. (1984) *The Body and Society*. Oxford: Blackwell.

United Kingdom Central Council (1994a) *Exercising Accountability*. London: UKCC.

United Kingdom Central Council (1994b) *Code of Professional Conduct*. London: UKCC.

Vincent, R. (1991) 'Medical ethics', oral communication at Resuscitation Council of the United Kingdom annual symposium. London.

Wagg, A., Kinirons, M. and Stewart, K. (1995) 'Cardiopulmonary resuscitation: doctors and nurses expect too much', *Journal of Royal College of Physicians* 29(1): 20–4.

Walsh, M. and Ford, P. (1989) *Nursing Rituals: Research and Rational Actions*. Oxford: Butterworth-Heinemann.

Walter, T. (1991) 'Modern death: taboo or not taboo?', *Sociology* 25(2): 293–310.

Walters, A. (1995) 'Technology and the lifeworld of critical care nursing', *Journal of Advanced Nursing* 22: 338–46.

Watson, J. (1988) *Nursing, Human Science and Human Care: A Theory of Nursing*. New York: National League of Nursing.

Wolf, Z. R. (1988) *Nurse's Work: The Sacred and the Profane*. Philadelphia, PA: University of Pennsylvania Press.

Wolf, Z. R. (1989) 'Uncovering the hidden work of nursing', *Nursing and Health Care* 10(8): 463–7.

Wolf, Z. R. (1991) 'Nurses' experiences giving post-mortem care to patients who have donated organs', *Scholarly Inquiry for Nursing Practice: An International Journal* 5(2): 73–87.

Zijderveld, A. C. (1983) 'The sociology of humor and laughter', *Current Sociology* 31(3): (Winter): 15–33; Menlo Park, CA: Sage.

17 Emotions in rationalizing organizations

Conceptual notes from professional nursing in the USA

Virginia Olesen and Debora Bone

INTRODUCTION

The highly dynamic domain of health and healing contains the great human themes of life and death, separation and reconciliation, greed and generosity, hope and despair accompanied by a gamut of emotions: joy, sorrow, rage, grief, pride, embarrassment, all sociologically constituted. These themes and emotional expressions occur in organizations that are already highly bureaucratized or are becoming bureaucratized in varying degrees, as well as in informal settings. Thus, health care organizations present opportunities to analyse the interplay between structures and emotions. As Lutz and White remind us, 'principles of social organization construct size, stability and status characteristics of the audience for performance of emotions' (1986: 420).

The interplay of emotions and structure is an old question in the sociology of organizations, reaching back at least as far as Weber's observation that conflicts emerge when 'substantive justice oriented to the concrete instance and person collide' with the 'formalism and rule-bound and cool "matter of factness" of bureaucratic administration' (Gerth and Mills 1958: 229–31). However, a new dimension in this question emerges out of pressures induced by the fiscal crisis in American health care for organizations to rationalize and become more efficient. This new dimension, changes in organizational structures, poses the issue of how emotions and emotional behaviours fare in altering contexts, an issue in the sociology of emotions which has received relatively little sustained attention.

Here we try to lodge the analysis and understanding of emotions and emotional behaviour in changing organizational contexts as a beginning move to a more dynamic sociology of emotions. To examine this we review the current situation of professional nursing in the United States. Like many other providers in the American health care system, nurses face increasing rationalization of organizational contexts (hospitals, clinics, health maintenance organizations (HMOs), hospices) as the system struggles to become more cost-efficient. Early dismissal of patients, larger workloads, substitution of other personnel for nurses, all figure in the cost-conscious scenario. Because expression of emotions is thought to be significantly embedded in the work of nursing care and nurses' professional orientation, this trend creates the potential for tension between structural demands for efficiency and the expression of emotion. This is particularly intriguing, if one accepts the view of some nurses that emotional work is central to care and the nurse's professional identity.

Our choice of nursing does not imply that other health care professionals, such as physicians, physical therapists, or social workers, who work in these changing organizations are not affected with regard to the emotional components of their work. Along with other observers, we recognize the possibility that many medical and helping professionals may experience tensions between 'the unrealizability of empathetic, personal concern and rational universal detachment' (Weigert and Franks 1989: 210; see also Fox 1989: 100–1). We have limited our discussion to professional nursing (registered nurses and licensed vocational nurses) in order more effectively to focus on and draw out conceptual problems which bear on issues of emotions in changing organizations. To further narrow the analysis and avoid ill-founded generalizations we restrict our discussion to nursing in the United States, while recognizing that rationalizing trends under way in other western societies – the UK for example – also impinge on nurses (Strong and Robinson 1990).

Although we recognize the highly gendered nature of this profession, an issue developed extensively in other analyses (Garmarnikov 1978; Davies 1995), here we do not centre gender. To do so risks an essentialist stance, i.e. women are inherently emotional and are the only ones who can do such work, which obviates analysis of changing emotions in changing structures if emotional expression *is* inherent in femaleness.[1] It also overlooks the wide variety of emotional experience and expression in women (and men) and necessitates comparative discussions beyond the scope of this chapter. Thus the chapter does not reveal women's or females' emotional labour in changing organizations, though issues of gender and changes in emotional labour would be of interest in a comparative analysis. Rather, it explores how institutional and economic change interacts with emotional labour in a largely female profession oriented to caring as a way to understand the larger problems of emotions in changing organizational contexts.

To set the stage for this discussion we review, first, major themes around emotions in organizations and then material on nursing in changing social and economic contexts.

EMOTIONS IN ORGANIZATIONS

The ideal-typical conceptualization of bureaucracy as completely rationalized and free of subjective or emotional elements has given way to more complex views of the interrelationship of emotions and structures (Gibson 1994). A host of studies from organizational theorists recognize that rationality is bounded, hence space emerges for the exercise of subjectivity and emotion. In contrast to the imagery of a perfectly rational organization where emotion is excluded, rationally designed organizations do not and cannot exclude emotionality (Gibson 1994: 21). Organizational structures and the work contexts within them are seen to contain a mix of rational and emotional elements which are reciprocally influential. Jones's study of a rape crisis organization demonstrates this point by showing that work 'routine may include authentic emotions and strategies that help the worker successfully do the work while being true to their self-expression' and argues that 'simultaneous expression of emotion and distance demonstrates the need to realize the role of emotions in occupational settings and the process of work' (1996: 26).

As Shott has argued, structure and norms 'are the framework of human action, rather than its determinant, shaping behaviour without dictating it' (1979: 1321). Individuals seeking solutions to complex organizational problems draw on emotional resources which are influenced by and in turn influence context and structure (Collins 1981: 994). This contemporary formulation of the interrelationship of structure and emotion still permits, indeed facilitates, examination of the central question in this chapter: how emotions are felt, constructed and enacted within the dynamics of organizational change where structure and emotion intertwine. In particular, this framing leaves open the question of the relationship between expressed and felt emotions, a topic to which we shall return in our discussion of American nursing.

At the heart of these issues is Hochschild's influential concept of 'emotional labour' (1983), which empirically demonstrated and theoretically outlined the impact of culture and economic orientation on emotion and the expression or lack thereof of emotions deemed appropriate to realize entrepreneurial economic interests. For our purposes emotional labour lies at the interstices of individual expression, normative and structural constraints, and the dynamics of change.

With a few exceptions to be discussed shortly, most research on emotional labour has been found in management studies where the question of increasing productivity, profit, etc., is central. These studies nevertheless delineate the important theme of fitting workers' emotions to company goals, hence they bear on our discussion of the increasing rationalization of the American health care system, which clearly raises questions of competition, profit and productivity.

Studies of emotional labour in service occupations can be divided into inquiries into occupations where the recipient of service is a customer and those where he or she is a client or patient. This distinction points to the sociological boundary, not always clear, between occupations and professions. Socialization to emotional behaviour can and does occur in both occupations and professions, but professional mandates which carry moral concern for the person *may* impinge more intensively on emotional behaviour; for example, the admonitions for affective neutrality, universalism, detached concern in physicians' behaviour (Lief and Fox 1963). Moreover, in most cases the relationship between the seller and the customer is more bracketed, less ambiguous and briefer than that between professional and client/patient.[2]

However, as we shall detail shortly, the elements of managed care bring into play themes which shift the definition of 'the patient' and, indeed, of the provider as the search for cost containment impinges on emotional behaviour. It is precisely the blurring of the distinction between patient as patient and patient as customer that becomes significant in the shifting managed-care scenarios. Consequently, the literature on emotions in customer service relations becomes relevant in the health care setting.

The literature on emotions in a wide variety of customer service occupations abundantly documents organizations' formal and informal efforts through recruitment, socialization and rewards or punishments to try to ensure that employees display the desired emotions, whether the emotions be positive, negative or neutral (for informative reviews of this literature see Ashforth and Humphrey 1993; Gibson 1994). Jovial employees at Disneyland (Van Maanen and Kunda 1989), neutral or angry bill collectors (Sutton 1991), fast food servers' routinized responses (Leidner 1993), all reflect a display of organizationally mandated emotions which, one could argue, have become the property of the organization, hence rationalized and commodified (Hochschild 1983; Sugrue 1982).

Whereas the literature on consumer service organizations reveals management efforts to commodify workers' emotions, an important theme, mostly ignored in that literature, is explored in material on patient/client settings, namely, how experience and expression of emotion are juxtaposed (Ashforth and Humphrey 1993). A study of case-workers in a public housing office shows that clients' tears led case-workers not only to feel and express sympathy, but to make decisions favourable to the client (Garot 1995), while angry clients were handled neutrally and did not receive favourable decisions. Detectives faced with victims who would dissolve in emotional outbursts had difficulty in expressing emotional support even if they felt empathetic (Stenross and Kleinman 1989). Nurses working with terminally ill patients, troubled by the bureaucratic necessity to undertake neutral, heroic measures when they preferred to give emotionally supportive care, experienced 'outlaw emotions': shame, guilt, dysphoria (Jaggar 1989; Burfoot 1994). In short, the bureaucratic requirement that emotional labour *not* be performed had emotional consequences for these nurses.

A critical factor in the tension between experience of and expression of emotion in care settings is temporality. Bureaucratic strictures in rationalized settings which demand a certain amount of physical work done within specific time-limits create tensions for care-givers who experience certain emotions for patients, but who are restricted from expressing them. Foner's ethnographic study of nurses and nurses' aides in a nursing home documents how this tension constrains the emotional labour of nurses' aides, sometimes to patients' detriment (1994: 73–4). This study and Diamond's ethnography of a nursing home (1992) detail the problems in emotional expression when bureaucratization occurs. A nurses' aide nostalgically recalled a less rule-bound era, 'Everything was nice in those days' (Foner 1994: 73), to capture the shift in rules and emotional expression.

There are, however, some exceptions, which are found in settings where emotional expression is valued as a means of recruiting or retaining patients – not unlike certain commercial enterprises. Studying a dedicated AIDS ward, Kotarba *et al.* found a free range of emotions and emotional involvement which they attribute to the fact that 'a warm environment is useful for attracting patients and ensuring repeat visits in an increasingly competitive market for middle class (privately insured) HIV/AIDS patients' (1996: 12). Thus, there is a range of relationships in the experience and expression of emotion, running from instances where contexts work against expression of emotions which nurses may wish to express, to settings where they must express emotion whether or not they wish to do so.

To understand emotional dynamics in contemporary nursing practice in institutional settings, it is useful to review briefly the history of nursing in the United States, situating the emotional labour of nurses within the structural conditions that shaped the development of the profession.

NURSING HISTORY AND EMOTIONAL LABOUR

During colonial times, nursing care in America was provided informally by family members and neighbours. Overseeing nutrition, hygiene, first aid and convalescent care were among the household skills women settlers acquired (Donahue 1985). Modern American nursing traces its origins to the Civil War, in the 1860s, when women served as nurses in field hospitals, tending wounded and sick soldiers (Donahue 1985). Nursing expertise in managing the environment of, and care for, sick patients was kept rigorously distinct from the medical skills of diagnosis and cure. Building on gendered *domestic* divisions of labour, the work of providing nurturance and emotional support fell 'naturally' to the nurse.

By the end of the nineteenth century, nursing became an acceptable vocation for young middle-class women. Hospitals and training schools were established in many of the large eastern cities. Student nurses lived a regimented, semi-military lifestyle, received on-the-job training for two or three years, and provided the majority of nursing care in hospitals (Flood 1981). Graduate nurses moved quickly into the community, working as private duty nurses in the homes of better-off families.

Early nursing texts gave instructions in 'hospital etiquette', indicating the proper manners of the professional nurse. Advice on issues such as greeting doctors, handling difficult patients or how to maintain good relations among the staff was offered (Hampton 1949 [1893]). Nurses were expected to control personal feelings and adhere to ideals of devotion and calling. Their work was motivated by a sense of duty and an obligation to care (Reverby 1987).

By the early twentieth century, the modern health professions were dominated by two masculinist ways of organizing work and setting priorities: the bureaucratic rationalization of hospital administration and the scientific rationality of medicine. The mundane and feminine 'details' of nurses' care-giving work, including emotion work, tended to be devalued and under-recognized (Davies 1995). This presented a dilemma for elite nurses, educators and superintendents, who sought to professionalize nursing by aligning themselves with rationality and efficiency without losing the traditionalists, who emphasized 'maternalist' qualities in nurses (Melosh 1982; Brannon 1994).

After the Second World War, an influx of economic resources, medical and technological innovations, and social policies transformed American health care services into a formidable health care industry, with nurses as its largest single group of employees (Melosh 1983). As nursing care became much more complex, conscious interest in 'nurse–patient interactions' and the 'psycho-social status' of patients reflected both the impact of the social sciences in nursing and attempts to articulate non-technical aspects of clinical care. During the postwar decades, efforts to balance 'high tech' with 'high touch' aspects of nursing took place under conditions of rapid expansion and a relative availability of resources.

NURSING IN MANAGED CARE

The 1990s are a time of massive restructuring and change in the American health care system, characterized by cost containment measures and new managerial strategies, which affect the delivery of nursing care services. Key issues include temporality, as labour speed-ups reduce nursing time with the patient; role adjustments, as nurses move into advanced practice and team management; and customer relations, as patients are reconceptualized as clients. The emotional work of providing support to patients and managing feelings of staff, families and clients often falls to the nurse, who is being asked to adapt quickly to fundamental shifts in the organization of work.

These changes are highly complex, occurring within diverse nursing practices differentiated by speciality, geographical region, type of organization and level of skill. Some trends contradict others. Older models overlap and coexist with newer formats, creating a pastiche or bricolage from which it is difficult to draw specific conclusions. Though hospital managers have designed new work systems, outlining and understanding the implications at the level of patient care is an empirical task for the future and well beyond the scope of this chapter. Nevertheless, it is possible to identify a number of characteristics of managed care and integrated health care systems, driven by economic pressures, that are currently shaping nursing practices both in and out of the hospital.

The impetus to redesign the delivery of health care in the USA began during the 1980s as both privatized and federally subsidized hospital and insurance systems grappled with escalating costs of providing care. Previously, reimbursement for health care was designed as a 'cost-based retrospective system' (DeLew *et al.* 1992: 162), in which insurance plans or government programmes paid some or all of the health care costs of qualified participants to the providers.

In the 1980s, new 'fixed-priced prospective payment systems' (DeLew *et al.* 1992), linked to diagnostic related groups (DRGs), were instituted in part as incentives for hospitals to be efficient. Both the streamlining of public spending and the principles of market competition in the private sector gave financial impetus to a new round of rationalization in the delivery of health care services. Management consultants were recruited from other industries to instruct hospital administrators how to reduce labour costs, streamline mid-level management, shorten hospital stays and render operations 'leaner and meaner' (MacLaren 1994; Riley 1994; Sovie 1995).

Health maintenance organizations developed capitated plans by which insurees' health needs would be met for a flat fee, encouraging decreased use of services. Preferred provider organizations negotiated reduced fees with physician groups, promising increased numbers of clients in exchange for lower rates. Hospital mergers reduced duplication of services, thereby cutting costs while making some services less accessible to clients. Each of these changes has made an impact on the organization of nursing work. Shorter hospitalizations, increases in outpatient services and increases in home health care have been effective in reducing expensive hospital stays. However, with outpatient procedures and home care expanding, only the sickest patients are hospitalized. Nurses are attending to the needs of patients with highly complex medical problems and these sicker patients have more acute emotional needs as well (Himali 1995).

Managed-care plans strive for efficiency by rationalizing the organization of work and streamlining the delivery of services (McLaughlin *et al.* 1995). Since nursing labour costs are expensive, hospitals are redesigning the utilization of nursing staff. Where a decade ago there was much talk about nursing shortages, today hospital managers attempt to use fewer nurses more effectively (Zimmerman 1995). Nurses are expected to move flexibly from one speciality unit to another, or take 'call off' time, according to variations in census. Hospitals have fewer permanent staff and save benefits costs by using part-time and per diem nurses. New information systems, standardized care plans and labour-saving hospital equipment are employed to reduce nursing hours. While working conditions for staff nurses deteriorate, better educated and more experienced nurses are moving away from direct patient care into case manager or supervisory roles (Buerhaus 1994).

Hospitals are also changing the 'skill mix', increasing the numbers of less trained licensed vocational or practical nurses (LVN and LPN), and utilizing unlicensed assistive personnel (UAP). Care is organized by team models in which various tasks are performed by specialized ancillary providers (Fritz and Cheeseman 1994). Registered nurses intervene with technical skills and oversee and document the work performed by others (Campbell 1988). They may be responsible for a greater number of patients, but are no longer providing primary care. In this instance, the emotion work becomes that of managing other personnel more than interacting with patients.

The overall impact of managed care has been to decrease the number of nurses involved in direct patient care while increasing the levels of responsibility for patient outcome. In general, this has reduced the amount of time available for all aspects of work, including emotional labour. Here it is useful to distinguish between the nurse's expression of emotion as part of the service work of caring for patients, and the experience of emotion as she responds both to the organizational changes and to their consequences for patient care. During this time of change, the emotional standards for expression, as well as expectations and feelings about new organizational processes, are in flux. Adapting to change is itself emotionally demanding. Nurses' responses to organizational restructuring have included feelings of uncertainty, impotence, anger, grief, frustration, resentment and insecurity (DeMoro 1996; Droppleman and Thomas 1996).

While hospitals and care-providers have not specifically addressed the emotional dynamics of health care workers, most hospitals have introduced multiple educational and organizational incentives to engage staff, including nurses, in the restructuring process. One such strategy, Total Quality Management (TQM), borrowed from industrial management,[3] is a managerial rationalization strategy in which work processes are monitored and evaluated according to specific outcome criteria. The patient is conceptualized as a client and indicators of customer satisfaction are used to determine quality. Data are collected on an ongoing basis and multidisciplinary teams are rewarded for devising and implementing 'action plans' to improve service delivery (Flarey 1995; Kelly 1995; Zonsius and Murphy 1995). The TQM approach to health care management claims to be 'patient focused' and builds on hospitality models of customer relations. However, the criteria developed for organizational efficiency and cost containment may differ from clinical criteria based on nursing standards of care. Nurses find themselves caught between competing models with contradictory demands.

The emphasis on patient relations creates an interesting paradox of emotion work under managed care. On the one hand, organizational restructuring has reduced the amount of time available for nurse–patient interactions, yet on the other hand, efforts to improve customer satisfaction have drawn attention to the clients' subjective needs. The complexity of the 'psychosocial' dimensions of care makes them an important focus of attention in nursing.

This has not gone unnoticed in nursing. A growing body of advice literature, in-services and continuing-education options for nurses indicates renewed interest in gaining emotional skills for handling the complexity of patient care in the redesigned settings of today's health-care system. In wide-ranging articles, attention is focused on clarification of what emotional assessments and interventions might be appropriate in a variety of clinical situations in the managed-care context. Topics include conflict resolution, empathic relationships, caring for the dying, dealing with grief and loss, handling difficult people, reassuring anxious patients and creating a sense of security and trust (Baker 1995; Davidhizar 1992; Davidhizar and Bowen 1993; Ellis 1993; Raudonis 1993; Schaefer and Peterson 1992; Teasdale 1995).

In sum, nurses working in today's rapidly changing health care services face multiple demands in which sophisticated emotional skills and flexibility are needed to handle the increased workloads, high levels of patient acuity and labour speed-ups. Nurses manage their own feelings, those of their patients and those of other workers, each interaction grounded in the shifting contexts of cost containment (see Thoits 1996 for an illuminating discussion of managing others' emotions). Paradoxically, managed care is simultaneously diminishing the structural support for nurses to provide traditional emotional support, and increasing the emphasis on customer relations and patient satisfaction as quality measures of successful outcomes.

EMPIRICAL QUESTIONS ABOUT THE EMOTION WORK OF NURSES

What these observations about emotional dynamics in the changing work of nurses mean for the conceptualization of emotions in changing structures can be glimpsed in a series of questions which contain themes or implicit concepts that lead to our final discussion. These might also guide empirical research to explore the question of emotions in changing institutions.

Regarding emotions, will the newly redesigned organization of work require new or different emotional competencies? Is the labour-intensive work of providing emotional support during illness being replaced with stylized performances of hospitality and routinized niceness? As service workers experience labour speed-ups and are required to do more faster, how might emotions be felt and experienced differently? When individuals confront restructuring of emotional work, do flexible emotionalities emerge, replacing earlier, more uniform emotional standards? What adaptations of expression and communication of feelings transpire during the emotional nano-seconds of the brief and efficient encounter between nurse and patient in the managed-care environment? For some nurses, emotional involvement is considered one of the rewards of care-giving work. Does renewed professional interest in caring and empathy represent efforts of nurses to reclaim this role, holding firm to traditional emotional turf?

On a micro level, what political economy of emotion management might emerge? If nurses are not performing some of the emotion work needed to assist patients through illness, how has this work been redistributed among other practitioners such as psychotherapists, social workers and pastoral care workers? In what ways are families taking on more emotional labour? Are patients assuming greater responsibility for their own emotional needs as providers of this care become scarce or are limited in what they do? What, if any, will be the influence of textually mediated emotional labour, that is, the emotional responses set down in in-service educational writing or ward procedures? Will these alter the 'sentimental order' (Strauss *et al.* 1982)? All of these questions, grounded in health care systems, suggest the utility of a theoretical framework that links emotional dynamics, structural contexts and variations of self within rapidly changing organizations. We now discuss a few conceptual approaches with which to interpret the complexities of performing emotional labour within commodifying service economies.

CONCEPTUAL AND THEORETICAL IMPLICATIONS

Where the organization of work in health care organizations was relatively stable and predictable for many decades, recent mergers, downsizing and restructuring have resulted in levels of worker insecurity in health care settings hitherto more familiar in other industries. Economic uncertainties, rapid redesign of services provided, and role redefinitions all contribute to a highly labile work climate wherein both workers and work are transformed. Thus, the economic realities of flexible accumulation (Harvey 1989; Jameson 1992) have important implications for contemporary subjectivities, as is well documented elsewhere (Giddens 1991; Flax 1993; Martin 1994). These are not only visible, but palpable for those working in health care contexts; for example, the stress on measuring patient satisfaction as a quality measure of successful outcomes (Fuller and Smith 1991). The economic uncertainties and rapid redesign of services and role definitions contribute to a highly fluid work climate wherein workers and work undergo transformation.

This suggests that the conceptual properties of a frame with which to understand emotions in changing structures must include and intertwine self, emotion and structure, a view notably articulated in Lofland's analysis of grief (1985). However, we cannot assume a unified, static self, and particularly not a unified, static professional self in the case of American nurses. What is required is a conceptualization that captures the fluidity of multiple selves.

In organizational contexts – and others as well – individuals bring a multiplicity of selves emergent from and influenced by the multiple realities which characterize their lives (Schutz 1962: 207–29). The work setting is not impermeable; it is but another site on which and in which histories, relationships, trajectories and valences play on and through the interacting individuals. The experiences in that worksite are not merely of the worksite *qua* worksite, but are constructed of these multiple historical moments and dimensions, even as are selves in those contexts (Scott 1991). Thus worksites represent fragmented possibilities that can be shaped and reshaped.

Theoretically, those interacting in shifting, unstable, rationalizing organizations themselves possess shifting, unstable, emergent 'mobile subjectivities' (Ferguson 1993). These move along many trajectories: race, class, gender, age, sexual orientation, familial position, regional origin, to name but a few. In the case of the nurse these are nested within and run through the individual's professional self, which is diversified by type of schooling, specialization, views on issues within nursing, likes or dislikes of certain kinds of patients (Liaschenko 1995). This does not deny that there may be, indeed is, varying agreement among nurses as to what 'good' professional care is. There is a moral core to the profession which is shared in varying degrees. However, those sharing that moral core to whatever degree are not static entities frozen in a timeless mould of 'the nurse' but are constantly emergent and altering as they construct themselves, their work, and their being in the changing care contexts.

This recognizes that those who provide care in shifting, rationalizing organizations both experience and express emotion not only in terms of what the organizations' demands are (and the demands may be fragmentary and diverse), but also because the selves brought to the context and created within it are multiple, hence providing the opportunity for many diverse responses. One has only to read Foner's (1994) or Diamond's (1992) accounts of the care in nursing homes to realize the layered complexities of emotional experience and expression in rationalized contexts.

Further, in understanding the complexities of intersubjectivity, it is helpful to consider that social actors shift adeptly and sometimes concurrently between different experiential modes – physical, cognitive and emotional – as well as between solo and joint levels of interaction (Clark *et al.* 1994). Intensity of feelings and cognitive reflexivity may be high or low (Mills and Kleinman 1988) depending on the situation, making it impossible to suggest any simplistic predictability. However, one consequence of working under conditions of rapid structural change may be 'emotional lag' (Olesen 1990). This refers to one of several possible relationships between a self or selves socialized to experience and express certain emotions and what is demanded or arises in changing structures and contexts. For example, as we have noted earlier, some altering structures pose normative demands for more neutral or even cooler responses than nurses socialized to a more supportive emotional style are comfortable in making (Burfoot 1994; James 1989, 1992).[4] A countering case might be found in the situation where providers, accustomed to relating to clients (formerly patients) in modes which once would have been characterized as 'affectively neutral' (Parsons 1953), now must present much warmer emotional responses. In both cases, the lag occurs between one part of the self, socialized to experience and express certain emotions, and another part emergent from the changed circumstances where expression of emotion differs. In the experience of emotional lag, expression might register along a wide continuum, ranging from authentic to fake, expressed in terms of diverse sets of realities, contexts and work criteria.

Because the self in its many facets continually reflects on multiple emotional encounters, assessing those encounters and the required or created emotional expression, the discrepancy between feeling and expression, past and emergent selves, may well generate another level of emotion. This might take the form of ambivalence, shame, or anger in discrepant situations or perhaps even pride in being able to transcend emotions experienced by an older self and to realize those in a newly emergent self. This second-order emotional reflexivity may lead to resistance to expected norms ranging from outlaw emotions to glazed numbness, alternatively defying local convention, or being unable to assimilate or perform appropriately. What will be of theoretical interest is whether new emotional skills emerge as individuals succeed or fail to develop an agility to adapt to the increased fluidity and ambivalences of emotionality required in contemporary work settings (Martin 1994).

The dynamics of how such new skills, emotional perceptions and expressions emerge are in part grounded in the important context of the workplace. The case of Total Quality Management illustrates this. As the emphasis on interpersonal skills in TQM philosophies suggests, the emotion work of service providers is a priority in managed-care contexts. While there are some efforts to standardize this work, it cannot be totally rationalized. Workers are embedded in workplace cultures which derive from workers' interactions and interpretations of the setting and their own multiple subjectivities (Foner 1994; Kotarba *et al.* 1996). This means they have the potential to select among numerous possible emotional experiences and expressions at the point of service; this type of emotional decision-making cannot be determined ahead of time. The microdynamics of emotional expression in the shifting scenarios of managed care will enter and play through those scenarios, shaping interactions and framing new levels of emotional definition and competencies which may or may not fit structural imperatives.

Using the case of American nursing in the highly rationalizing climate of contemporary managed care, we have attempted to delineate some elements with which to explore emotional experience and expression in shifting social structures. Such exploration requires that the elements of emotion, self, structure be intertwined in a framework which is sensitive to multiple subjectivities, temporality and the dynamics of workplace culture. It should also attend to second-order emotions emergent from the ruminations of the reflexive self or selves assessing emotional lag or congruence. Further conceptual refinement and empirical exploration of these elements are key tasks to advance the sociology of emotions and to grasp the emotional dynamics of care in contexts where, in spite of the redefinition of the patient as consumer, suffering, one of the key attributes of the patient, still occurs (Stacey 1976).

NOTES

1 While it is the case that nursing is predominantly female, the gendered nature of the profession in part can be explained by labour force dynamics which allocate less powerful persons (women, women of colour) to dirty work (physical care) and devalued work such as emotional labour (Navarro 1994; Butter *et al.* 1987).
2 A district general manager quoted in Strong and Robinson's study of the NHS neatly poses this distinction between professional and commercial service work: 'A professional dealing with a patient has a one to one relationship which transcends organizational concerns . . . in the NHS there's a personal and emotional side. We have to deal with patients who are frightened and worried. This puts huge pressure on us, far greater than customers put on Burton's' (1990: 190). Nevertheless, emotion displays in customer service organizations must convey some sensitivity and concern if they are not to appear synthetic and offensive (Ashforth and Humphrey 1993: 96).
3 This approach to business is built on work done by W. Edward Deming and others in continuous quality improvement (CQI) during the 1950s. In 1987, the quality movement was applied to health care in a demonstration project by the Harvard Community Health Plan and was later incorporated into the accreditation policies of the Joint Commission on Accreditation of Healthcare Organizations (JCAHO) (Zonsius and Murphy 1995).
4 There are also instances where emotions change too rapidly for structural expectations; for instance, the persistent fear, reported among some health care providers and students, of persons with AIDS (Gillon 1987; Gerbert *et al.* 1988; Bosk and Frader 1990; American Civil Liberties Union 1990; Cooke *et al.* 1990). Fear has outpaced structural and professional expectations for emotional expression in some health care educational contexts and practice settings. Many places as yet do not well or readily accommodate the presence and consequences of these fears, although there have been some alterations in structures in schools of nursing regarding how faculty should work with students who express fear of or refuse to care for patients with AIDS and in professional nursing associations which offer train-the-trainer sessions to resocialize providers who fear giving such care.

BIBLIOGRAPHY

American Civil Liberties Union (1990) *Epidemic of Fear: A Survey of AIDS Discrimination in the 1980s and Policy Recommendations for the 1990s*. New York: ACLU.
Ashforth, B. E. and Humphrey, R. H. (1993) 'Emotional labour in service roles: the influence of identity', *Academy of Management Review* 1: 88–115.
Baker, K. M. (1995) 'Improving staff nurse conflict resolution skills', *Nursing Economics* 13(5): 295–8.

Bosk, C. L. and Frader, J. E. (1990) 'AIDS and its impact on medical work: the culture and politics of the shopfloor', *Millbank Quarterly Supplement on the Impact of AIDS* 68: 40–60.

Brannon, R. L. (1994) *Intensifying Care, the Hospital Industry, Professionalization, and the Reorganization of the Nursing Labour Process*. Amityville, NY: Baywood Publishing.

Buerhaus, P. I. (1994) 'Economics of managed competition and consequences to nurses, Part I and Part II', *Nursing Economics* 12(1): 10–17 and 12(2): 75–80, 106.

Burfoot, J. H. (1994) 'Outlaw emotions and the sensual dynamics of compassion: the case of emotion as instigator of social change', unpublished paper, Department of Sociology, Middlebury College, Burlington, VT.

Butter, I. H., Carpenter, E. S., Kay, B. J. and Simmons, R. (1987) 'Gender hierarchy in the health labour force', *International Journal of Health Services* 17(1): 133–49.

Campbell, M. (1988) 'Management as "ruling": a class phenomenon in nursing', *Studies in Political Economy* 27 (Fall): 29–51.

Clark, C., Kleinman, S. and Ellis, C. (1994) 'Conflicting reality readings and interactional dilemmas. Part I: The conceptual model', in J. Wentworth (ed.) *Social Perspectives on Emotion*. Greenwich, CT: JAI Press.

Collins, R. (1981) 'On the microfoundations of macrosociology', *American Journal of Sociology* 86: 984–1014.

Cooke, M., Koenig, B., Beery, N. and Folkman, S. (1990) 'Which physicians will provide AIDS care?', unpublished paper presented at the 6th International Conference on AIDS, San Francisco, CA (UCSF Center for AIDS Prevention Studies).

Davidhizar, R. (1992) 'When the nurse encounters crying', *Today's OR Nurse* (March): 28–32.

Davidhizar, R. and Bowen, M. (1993) 'Responding to irritable people in the OR setting', *Today's OR Nurse* (September/October): 43–7.

Davies, C. (1995) *Gender and the Professional Predicament in Nursing*. Milton Keynes, Bucks: Open University Press.

DeLew, N. *et al.* (1992) 'A layman's guide to the US health care system', *Health Care Financing Review* 14(1): 151–69.

DeMoro, R. A. (1996) 'It's the reality that's scary in current health care trends', *California Nurse* 92(1): 3, 10.

Diamond, T. (1992) *Making Grey Gold: Narratives of Nursing Home Care*. Chicago: University of Chicago Press.

Donahue, M. P. (1985) *Nursing, The Finest Art: An Illustrated History*. St Louis, MO: C. V. Mosby.

Droppleman, P. G. and Thomas, S. P. (1996) 'Anger in nurses: don't lose it, use it', *American Journal of Nursing* 96(4): 26–32.

Ellis, C. (1993) 'Incorporating the affective domain into staff development programs', *Journal of Nursing Staff Development* 9(3): 127–30.

Ferguson, K. E. (1993) *The Man Question: Visions of Subjectivity in Feminist Theory*. Berkeley, CA: University of California Press.

Flarey, D. L. (1995) *Redesigning Nursing Care Delivery: Transforming Our Future*. Philadelphia, PA: J. B. Lippincott.

Flax, J. (1993) *Disputed Subjects: Essays on Psychoanalysis, Politics and Philosophy*. New York: Routledge.

Flood, M. E. (1981) 'The troubling expedient: general staff nursing in United States hospitals in the 1930s: a means to institutional, educational, and personal ends', unpublished dissertation, University of California School of Education, Berkeley, CA.

Foner, N. (1994) *The Caregiving Dilemma: Work in an American Nursing Home*. Berkeley, CA: University of California Press.

Fox, R. C. (1989) *The Sociology of Medicine: A Participant Observer's View*. Englewood Cliffs, NJ: Prentice-Hall.

Fritz, D. J. and Cheeseman, S. (1994) 'Blueprint for integrating nurse extenders in critical care', *Nursing Economics* 12(6): 327–31.

Fuller, L. and Smith, V. (1991) 'Consumers' reports: management by customers in a changing economy', *Work, Employment and Society* 5(1): 1–16.

Garmarnikov, E. (1978) 'Sexual divisions of labour: the case of nursing', in A. Kuhn and A. M. Wolpe (eds) *Feminism and Materialism*. London: Routledge & Kegan Paul.

Garot, R. (1995) 'Substantive rationality in a bureaucratic setting', unpublished paper, Department of Sociology, University of California, Los Angeles, CA.

Gerbert, B., Maguire, B., Badner, V., Altman, D. and Stone, G. (1988) 'Why fear persists: health care professionals and AIDS', *Journal of the American Medical Association* 260: 3481–3.

Gerth, H. H. and Mills, C. W. (eds) (1958) *From Max Weber: Essays in Sociology*. New York: Oxford University Press.

Gibson, D. (1994) 'The struggle for reason: the sociology of emotion in organizations', unpublished paper, Anderson Graduate School of Business, University of California, Los Angeles, CA.

Giddens, A. (1991) *Self and Society in the Late Modern Age*. Stanford, CA: Stanford University Press.

Gillon, R. (1987) 'Refusal to treat AIDS and HIV positive patients', *British Medical Journal* 294: 1332–3.

Hampton, I. (ed.) (1949 [1893]) *Nursing of the Sick*. New York: McGraw-Hill.

Harvey, D. (1989) *The Condition of Postmodernity*. Cambridge: MA: Blackwell.

Himali, U. (1995) 'Managed care: does the promise meet the potential?', *The American Nurse* 1: 15–16.

Hochschild, A. R. (1983) *The Managed Heart: The Commercialization of Human Feeling*. Berkeley, CA: University of California Press.

Jaggar, A. M. (1989) 'Love and knowledge: emotion in feminist epistemology', in A. M. Jaggar and S. R. Bordo (eds) *Gender/Body/Knowledge: Feminist Reconstructions of Being and Knowing*. New Brunswick, NJ: Rutgers University Press.

James, N. (1989) 'Emotional labour: skill and work in the social regulation of feelings', *Sociological Review* 37(1): 15–42.

James, N. (1992) 'Care = organisation + physical labour + emotional labour', *Sociology of Health and Illness* 14(4): 488–509.

Jameson, F. (1992) *Postmodernism, or, The Cultural Logic of Late Capitalism*. Durham, NC: Duke University Press.

Jones, L. (1996) 'Rape crisis work and the unpersonal relationship: the delicate balance of intimacy and social distance', unpublished paper, Department of Sociology, University of Arizona, Tucson, AZ.

Kelly, K. (ed.) (1995) *Health Care Work Redesign*. Thousand Oaks, CA: Sage.

Kotarba, J. A., Ragsdale, D. and Morrow, J. R., Jr (1997) 'Everyday culture in a dedicated HIV/AIDS hospital unit', *Sociology of Health and Illness*, forthcoming.

Leidner, R. (1993) *Fast Food, Fast Talk: Service Work and the Routinization of Life*. Berkeley, CA: University of California Press.

Liaschenko, J. (1995) 'Artificial personhood: nursing ethics in a medical world', *Journal of Nursing Ethics* 2(3): 185–96.

Lief, H. I. and Fox, R. C. (1963) 'Training for detached "concern" in medical students', in H. E. Lief *et al.* (eds) *The Psychological Basis of Medical Practice*. New York: Harper & Row.

Lofland, L. H. (1985) 'The social shaping of emotion: the case of grief', *Symbolic Interaction* 8: 171–90.

328   *Virginia Olesen and Debora Bone*

Lutz, C. and White, G. M. (1986) 'The anthropology of emotions', *Annual Review of Anthropology* 15: 405–36.

MacLaren, E. (1994) 'Basics of managed care', *Nurseweek* (June): 10–11.

McLaughlin, F. E., Thomas, S. and Bates, M. (1995) 'Changes related to care delivery patterns', *JONA (Journal of Nursing Administration)*, 25(5): 35–46.

Martin, E. (1994) *Flexible Bodies*. Boston, MA: Beacon Press.

Melosh, B. (1982) *'The Physician's Hand', Work, Culture and Conflict in American Nursing.* Philadelphia, PA: Temple University Press.

Melosh, B. (1983) 'Doctors, patients, and "big nurse": work and gender in the postwar hospital', in E. C. Lagemann (ed.) *Nursing History: New Perspectives, New Possibilities.* New York: Teachers College Press.

Mills, T. and Kleinman, S. (1988) 'Emotions, reflexivity, and action: an interactionist analysis', *Social Forces* 66(4): 1009–27.

Navarro, V. (1994) *The Politics of Health Policy: The US Reforms, 1980–1994.* Cambridge, MA: Blackwell.

Olesen, V. L. (1990) 'The neglected emotions: a challenge to medical sociology', *Medical Sociology News* 16(1): 11–25.

Parsons, T. (1953) 'Illness and the role of the physician', in C. Kluckhohn and H. A. Murray (eds) *Personality in Nature, Society and Culture.* New York: Knopf.

Raudonis, B. M. (1993) 'The meaning and impact of empathic relationships in hospice nursing', *Cancer Nursing* 16(4): 304–9.

Reverby, S. (1987) *Ordered to Care: The Dilemma of American Nursing, 1850–1945.* Cambridge: Cambridge University Press.

Riley, D. W. (1994) 'Integrated health care systems: emerging models', *Nursing Economics* 12(4): 201–6.

Schaefer, K. M. and Peterson, K. (1992) 'Effectiveness of coping strategies among critical care nurses', *Dimensions of Critical Care Nursing* 11(1): 28–34.

Schutz, A. (1962) 'On multiple realities', in his *Collected Papers: The Problem of Social Reality*, ed. M. Natanson. The Hague: Martinus Nijhoff.

Scott, J. (1991) 'The evidence of experience', *Critical Inquiry* 17: 773–9.

Shott, S. (1979) 'Emotion and social life: a symbolic interactionist analysis', *American Journal of Sociology* 84: 1317–34.

Sovie, M. D. (1995) 'Tailoring hospitals for managed care and integrated health systems', *Nursing Economics* 13(2): 72–83.

Stacey, M. (1976) 'The health services consumer, a sociological misconception' *Sociological Review*, Monograph 22.

Stenross, B. and Kleinman, S. (1989) 'Highs and lows of emotional labour, detectives' encounters with criminals and victims', *Urban Life* 17(4): 435–52.

Strauss, A. L., Fagerhaugh, S., Suczek, B. and Wiener, C. L. (1982) 'Sentimental work in the technological hospital', *Sociology of Health and Illness* 12: 254–78.

Strong, P. M. and Robinson, J. (1990) *The NHS: Under New Management.* Milton Keynes, Bucks: Open University Press.

Sugrue, N. M. (1982) 'Emotions as property and context for negotiation', *Urban Life* 11(3): 280–92.

Sutton, R. I. (1991) 'Maintaining norms about expressed emotions', *Administrative Science Quarterly* 36: 245–68.

Teasdale, K. (1995) 'Theoretical and practical considerations on the use of reassurance in the nursing management of anxious patients', *Journal of Advanced Nursing* 22: 79–86.

Thoits, P. A. (1996) 'Managing the emotions of others', *Symbolic Interaction* 19(2): 85–110.

Van Maanen, J. and Kunda, G. (1989) '"Real feelings": emotional expression and organizational culture', in M. M. Staw and L. L. Cummings (eds) *Research in Organizational Behaviour* 11: 43–103; Greenwich, CT: JAI Press.

Weigert, A. and Franks, D. D. (1989) 'Ambivalence: a touchstone of the modern temper', in D. D. Franks and E. D. McCarthy (eds) *The Sociology of the Emotions.* Greenwich, CT: JAI Press.

Zimmerman, P. G. (1995) 'Replacement of nurses with unlicensed assistive person- nel: the erosion of professional nursing and what we can do', *Journal of Emergency Nursing* 21(3): 208–12.

Zonsius, M. K. and Murphy, M. (1995) 'Use of total quality management sparks staff nurse participation in continuous quality improvement', *Nursing Clinics of North America* 30(1): 1–12.

Index

accommodation 242; phases in process 242–4
action, communicative *see* communicative action
adjacency pairs 100, 117–18
Adult Children of Alcoholics (ACOA) 97, 99, 100–2, 113–17 *passim*, 124–5
adulthood, models of 139–40
age 165
age brinkmanship 177
ageing xx–xxi, 173–89; ages and stages model 175–82; creative tensions 182–7
ahistoricism 66–8
AIDS ward 317
alt.recovery.codependency newsgroup (a.r.c.) 97–119, 124–5; history 102–3; threads 104–13
Amis, K. 185
anger 208, 302–3
anti-pornography movement 233–5, 237
anxiety 303
argument 30–2
Aristotle 254
Arnold, J.V. 185
associative functions 52–3
authenticity 216–18, 220–5; 'doing gender' and 'doing emotion work' 217–8; loss of 216–17; trade-off with emotion work 220–4
Averill, J.R. 177

Bachelier, J.J. 181
Balkans War 91
Barbalet, J.M. 170, 272
Baudrillard, J. 121–2
Bauman, Z. 89–90
Bendelow, G. 182, 278
blasé attitude 90–3, 95

blunting of emotional experience 121–3
Bly, R. 202
body 195, 255–6; children and daily life xxi, 135–54; cultural constructionism 48–52; masculinity and 206; mind–body and performances 271–3; and pain 257–62, 265; re–embodiment of social science 52–5; and self 182–3; somatic responses 274–8; 'virtual' 120–32; *see also* embodiment
body consciousness 274
boundaries 186; dramaturgical work 269–71; self–other 269–70, 279–80
Bourdieu, P. 156–7
bourgeoisie 68–70
boys 155–72; doing emotion work xxi, 169–70; emotion, embodiment and school 159–65; and groups 163–5, 166–7; hierarchies and cycles of embodied masculinity 162–3; learning to endure 166–7; physical touch 167–9; size 160–2, 164, 165, 167; use of space 159–60, 165–6
bride 3–12
Brinkgreve, C. 236–7
Bulger, Jamie 93
bureaucratization *see* rationalizing organizations
Buytendijk, F.J. 156

capitalism 10–12
cardiopulmonary resuscitation (CPR) xxv, 295–312; death, drama and indignity 306–8; emotion work 300–6; emotional labour and caring 296–300; procedure 295–6; theory and practice 299–300
caritas romana ('Roman charity') 181–2

for emotion management 9–12; view of a bride 5–8
sociophysical space 280–7
Sokoloff, J. 184
somatic vulnerability 288–9
space: boys' use of 159–60, 165–6; psychosomatic 271–80; sociophysical 280–7
spatial metaphors 268–71
specificity theory 253
speech acts 16; *see also* communicative action
Spence, J. 181
Spender, D. 213
splitting of consciousness 276–7
sport 123
status, social 53–4, 281, 286–7
status passages 176
Stolk, B. van 241
Stoltenberg, J. 200
story-time 141–2
Strauss, A. 176, 298
stress 288; dramaturgical *see* dramaturgical stress
structure 315, 322–5
strut, the 161
subjective emotions 173–5
subordinate status 281, 286–7
symbols 39–40, 44–5; unresolved contradictions in the concept 45–52

teachers *see* school
television 67; responses to horrific images xix, 83–96
theory: and practice 299–300
Thurm, M. 182–3
Tierney, J. 285
time 151–2
Total Quality Management (TQM) 320, 324
touch: boys and 167–9; cyberspace 128; sexuality and 229
traditionalization of television 88
tranquillity: postures of 275–6
transformation 184–5

trend-followers 242
Turner, B. 254

US health care system xxvi, 313–29; impact of change 318–21
Usenet 97–119, 124–5

Vaughan, D. 220
vibrators 239
victimism 239
violence: Hollywood and TV 67; masculinity and emotional life 193–210; sexual 231–2, 283–4; *see also* television
virtual: and real 99–100
'virtual' body 120–32
visual imagery 257
vulnerability 168–9, 209; somatic 288–9

Wall, P. 253
Walsh, M. 307
Walter, T. 122–3, 307
weakness 203
Weber, A. 83–6
Weber, M. xv, 3
Weiner, H. 287, 288–9
Weiss, R. 214, 215
welfare state 243
Wentworth, W.M. 270, 289
Williams, S. 182, 278
Wolf, Z.R. 299
women 228; emotion work 65, 197, 212–14, 217, 222–4; and male violence 196–7, 198
workplace: culture 324; emotion work 65–6, 158; stress 284–5
Wouters, C. 64, 73–4, 241
Wright, A. 181–2
Wyatt-Brown, A. 184, 185–6

Yardley, D. 270, 289
Young, I.M. 165

Zeegers, W. 229, 242
Zijderveld, A.C. 304